Male Genital
Skin Disease

Commissioning Editor: Sue Hodgson
Project Development Manager: Joanne Scott
Project Manager: Rory MacDonald
Illustration Manager: Mick Ruddy
Design Manager: Jayne Jones
Illustrator: Joanna Cameron

Male Genital Skin Disease

Christopher B Bunker MA(Cantab) MD(Cantab) FRCP(London)

Consultant Dermatologist
Chelsea & Westminster Hospital
London, UK

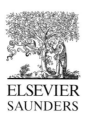

ELSEVIER
SAUNDERS

Edinburgh   London   New York   Oxford   Philadelphia   St Louis   Sydney   Toronto 2004

SAUNDERS
An imprint of Elsevier Limited

First published 2004
  Reprinted 2005 (twice)

ISBN 0 7020 2760 X

British Library Cataloguing in Publication Data
A catalogue record for this book is available from the British Library

Library of Congress Cataloging in Publication Data
A catalog record for this book is available from the Library of Congress

Notice
Medical knowledge is constantly changing. Standard safety precautions must be followed, but as new research and clinical experience broaden our knowledge, changes in treatment and drug therapy may become necessary or appropriate. Readers are advised to check the most current product information provided by the manufacturer of each drug to be administered to verify the recommended dose, the method and duration of administration, and contraindications. It is the responsibility of the practitioner, relying on experience and knowledge of the patient, to determine dosages and the best treatment for each individual patient. Neither the Publisher nor the author assume any liability for any injury and/or damage to persons or property arising from this publication.

The Publisher

ELSEVIER   your source for books,
            journals and multimedia
            in the health sciences
www.elsevierhealth.com

Working together to grow
libraries in developing countries
www.elsevier.com | www.bookaid.org | www.sabre.org
ELSEVIER   BOOK AID   Sabre Foundation
            International

Printed in China

Last digit is the print number: 9 8 7 6 5 4 3

Contents

Dedication

To the many thousands of men from whom I have been privileged to learn; to the women in my life: my wife, daughters, and mother; and to my late father, Sqn Ldr N V D Bunker BA MB BChir MBE RAF, who was not fated to live long enough to develop his own medical career, nor to see his children grow up.

Preface

Over the last few years I have developed an interest in male genital dermatoses and have established a liaison out-patients clinic with a Genitourinary Physician, Dr David Hawkins, and a Urologist, Mr Mike Dinneen. This book has emanated from my experiences.

Patients with non-venereological skin complaints commonly present to genitourinary clinics. There is a widespread belief that skin diseases of the male genitalia are poorly understood, difficult to diagnose and unsatisfactory to treat—especially in the UK, the USA and the antipodes where dermatology and venereology are practiced separately.

I hope that this book will serve gently to disabuse non-dermatology specialists of these misapprehensions but that it will also be useful to general practitioners, primary care physicians and trainee dermatologists.

Emphasis is placed on obtaining a meticulous dermatological history and performing a complete cutaneous examination (both usually neglected outside Dermatology Departments and a common cause of diagnostic confusion and error). Although clinical chapters and contents are arranged according to the nature of the *presenting clinical problem* (itch, pigmentary change, balanoposthitis, patches and plaques, erosions and ulcers etc.) the *natural history* of the common dermatoses (such as psoriasis, seborrhoeic dermatitis, contact dermatitis, lichen planus, lichen sclerosus, vitiligo) that often affect the anogenital area and diseases specific to the penis (such as Zoon's balanitis, erythroplasia of Queyrat) are comprehensively described. Common perianal and rarer penile (and perianal) manifestations of other diseases (Crohn's disease, HIV, diabetes mellitus) are included, although this book does not purport to do full dermatological justice to perianal dermatoses.

Where sexually transmitted diseases such as syphilis and gonorrhoea enter the differential diagnosis, a dermatologist's account of them is given. It is not the aim of this book to be an atlas or textbook of sexually transmitted disease, of which there are already several classics.

An essential theme is the importance of clinically achieved, precise diagnosis in directing suitable treatment. The indications for performing a skin biopsy of the penis are expounded although it is generally not as frequently needed as suggested, requested or performed.

I hope that the chief value of this book to the user will be the clinical illustrations. Most of this material and information is not readily available elsewhere. Skin diseases affecting the genitalia look different compared with other sites, but genital dermatoses are only scantily illustrated in standard dermatologic textbooks and are represented even more sparsely in books about sexually transmitted disease. The literature abounds in pictures of chancroid, granuloma inguinale and lymphomogranuloma venereum diseases, which are rarely diagnosed in the developed world, yet there are few pictures of anogenital psoriasis, lichen planus, lichen sclerosus, Zoon's balanitis etc. which are the commonest diagnoses made in the patients sent to dermatologists for a second opinion.

But the pervading ideology is about accurate diagnosis and effective management. The purpose being to exclude sexually transmitted disease, abolish or minimise sexual (and urinary) dysfunction, both of which can cause a lot of misery in different ways, and to prevent or reduce the risk of penile cancer.

C B Bunker, London, 2004.

How to use this book

No apology is made for repeating important pieces of information at different places (e.g. in the tables) or in presenting the same information in different ways (e.g. in the text and clinical figures); indeed it is hoped that this very attribute of the book will enhance its usefulness in the library, at the bedside or, especially, in the clinic.

The book is arranged according to *clinical presentation* which leads deliberately to overlap of entities as listed in the tables. Unnecessary overlap in the text has been avoided by confining the account of any entity to one chapter only.

Acknowledgements

It has taken nearly ten years to write and to assemble this book. It would not have been possible without the assistance and kindness of many people. My greatest gratitude is to those listed below; if I have omitted anyone it has been unwittingly and I hope that I will be forgiven.

Katie Loughlin (nee Partridge) my private secretary has been a stalwart: the extra work she has cheerfully shouldered because of this folly of her 'boss' cannot be calculated.

Nick Francis has been my Pathologist partner and ally in this and other endeavours. He has taught me a lot more than I thought was known in many spheres of dermatopathology and also provided most of the photomicrographs.

Tamara Basarab helped me with the 'contact' content. Richard Groves lent me an office during my 'penis sabbatical' in 2002.

Bhushan Kumar has been one of many who have generously loaned me photographs from their collections but his contribution has been the most voluminous and I am extremely grateful to him. Peter Copeman my predecessor in the Skin Department of the old Westminster Hospital magnanimously gave me the run of his esoteric collection.

Nick Soter at NYU read and criticised the first draft and provided several slides.

The late Gerald Levene first got me thinking about penis pre-cancer; unfortunately we never completed the paper we started to write in 1986 on this topic (during the time when I was most fortunate to have been his Registrar/Senior Registrar).

Paul Thiruchelvam started to collect references for me in 1996 and Hina Bhutta worked studiously on the Bibliography in 2001 and 2002, both whilst they were Medical Students. Reinhard Wentz, the Head Librarian at the CWH campus (ICSM), has helped me with literature searches and several *ad hoc* German translations.

Mike Nelson and Chris Priest of Medical Illustration at CWH/ICSM and their staff have provided the photographic support to the clinic and the vast majority of illustrations have emanated from that Department.

The following figures were reproduced, with permission, from University College, London: 2.1h; 2.1q; 4.11; 6.9; 6.40; 6.67; 6.77; 6.166; 6.169; 6.211; 6.223; 6.257; 6.255; 7.7; 7.23; 8.3; 8.11; 8.12; 8.38; 8.39; 8.40; 8.45; 8.46; 8.50; 8.78; 8.84; 8.89; 10.1; and 10.12.

Mike Dinneen and David Hawkins have been steadfast in their attendance at the Penis Clinic since inception. I am grateful to them for the clinical wisdom and experience that they have imparted to me over the years.

Janet Ross, Anne Farrell, Eleanor Mallon, Louise Fearfield and Bill Porter have been the Registrars who have helped me the most with the 'penis project' over the last decade.

My colleagues Richard Staughton, Jeff Cream and Nerys Roberts have been supportive and encouraging throughout; Richard Staughton, particularly, when an end seemed unachievable.

Although I had much help from her predecessors if it had not have been for the persuasive enthusiasm of Sue Hodgson at Elsevier, I do not believe I would ever have 'got round' to 'finishing off' in 2002 the manuscript I first drafted in 1995. Joanne Scott and Rory MacDonald are people at Elsevier I have only more recently met but their energy, professionalism and cheerfulness have made the last year much easier (and such fun).

Finally, to the people named in the Dedication I owe everything.

1 Structure, function, normal variation

Although the whole skin organ is concerned with sexual expression and activity the *penis* is the male structure most intimately involved in sexual intercourse; and it is also the conduit for urinary excretion. The *scrotum* is the extracorporeal sack for the containment of the *testes* at the ideal ambient temperature for spermatogenesis. The *anus* may be an orifice of sexual utility (especially in the male homosexual) but its principal purpose is for the evacuation of feces from the gastrointestinal tract (Leiberman 1984). The *natal cleft* and the *inguinal (crural) folds* (and to a limited extent the infragluteal folds) are special sites because they are areas where two layers of skin come into close apposition. Together these sites function as part of the hinge between the lower limbs and the trunk as well as surrounding the mucocutaneous junctions of the anus and genitalia. The *perineum* interposes between the anus and the scrotum and the skin at this site is tightly tethered to the underlying tissues.

The essential structures of the penis, scrotum and testes, and their important landmarks, are illustrated in **Figures 1.1–1.18**. The groin, anus and natal cleft are also illustrated.

As at other sites, topographical and regional anatomical nomenclature is an essential part of the vernacular for a dermatologist. This requirement engenders precise description and the accurate communication of salient clinical features, whether for the clinical record, for a letter about the patient, for teaching or for clinical research. A common source of confusion is the convention that designates the dorsal aspect of the penis as that surface which is in direct contiguity with the abdomen, which is the ventral surface of the body. The *anatomical position* is that of full penile erection.

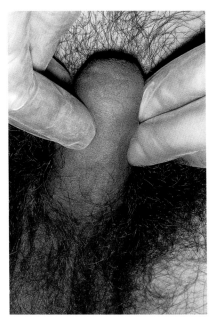

Fig. 1.1 Normal uncircumcised penis. Flaccid, 'short' foreskin, ventral aspect.

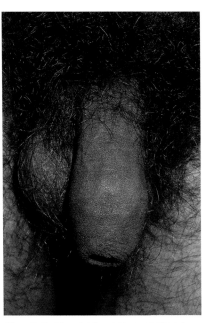

Fig. 1.2 Normal uncircumcised penis. Flaccid, 'short' foreskin, dorsal aspect.

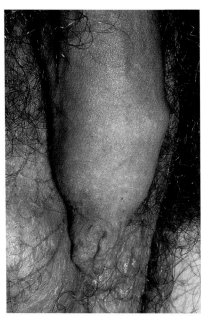

Fig. 1.3 Normal uncircumcised penis. Flaccid, 'long' foreskin, dorsal aspect.

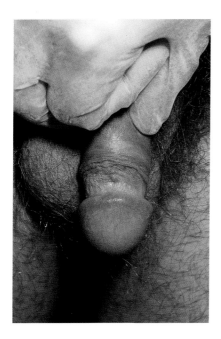

Fig. 1.4 Normal uncircumcised penis. Flaccid, foreskin retracted, dorsal aspect.

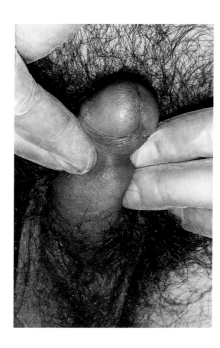

Fig. 1.5 Normal uncircumcised penis. Flaccid, foreskin retracted, ventral aspect.

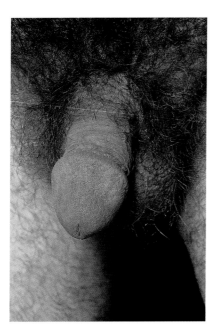

Fig. 1.6 Normal circumcised penis. Flaccid, dorsal aspect.

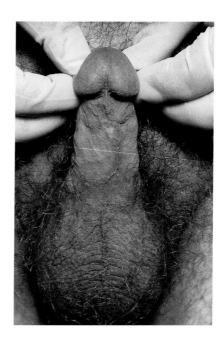

Fig. 1.7 Normal circumcised penis. Flaccid, ventral aspect.

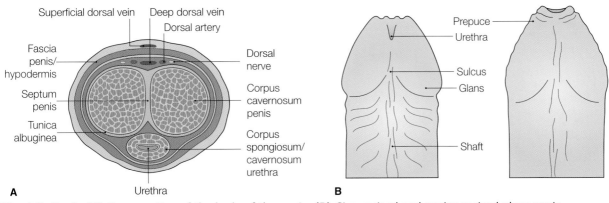

Fig. 1.8 Penis (A) Cross-section of the body of the penis. (B) Circumcised and uncircumcised glans penis.

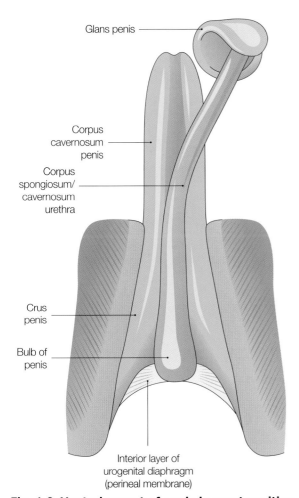

Fig. 1.9 Ventral aspect of penis in erect position.
The glans penis and the distal part of the corpus spongiosum are shown detached from the corpora cavernosa penis and turned to the left.

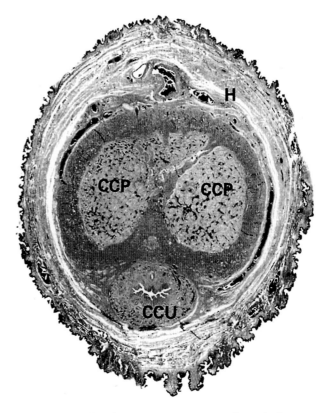

Fig. 1.10 Penis. This transverse section through the penis of an adult human male demonstrates the general arrangement of the penile tissues. The penis consists of three cylindrical masses of erectile tissue: the paired corpora cavernosa penis CCP in the dorsal aspect, and the midline corpus cavernosum urethrae CCU (formerly called the corpus spongiosum) which surrounds and supports the penile urethra and distally forms the glans penis. Condensed fibro-elastic tissue, the tunica albuginea, invests the cavernous bodies, being thickest around the corpora cavernosa penis which are incompletely separated by a midline septum. This dense collagenous tissue is continuous with the very loose hypodermis H which allows the thin penile skin to move freely over the underlying structures. Note the prominent blood vessels of the hypodermis. Reproduced with permission from Young & Heath, Wheater's Functional Histology, 4th Edition. © Churchill Livingstone, 2000.

3

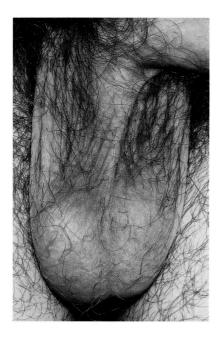

Fig. 1.11 Normal scrotum. This patient complained of scrotal burning and redness.

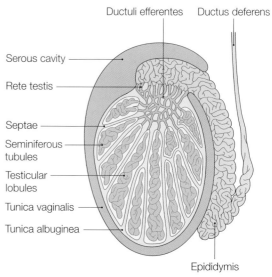

Fig. 1.12 Testis.

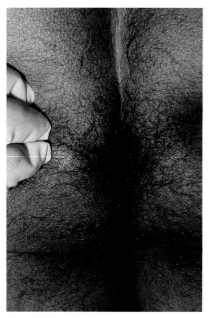

Fig. 1.13 Normal natal cleft.

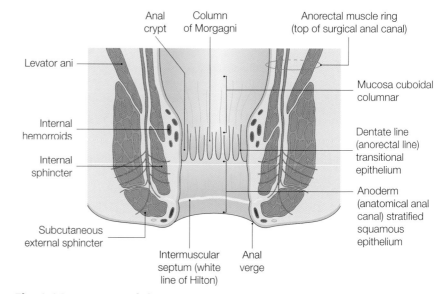

Fig. 1.14 Anatomy of the anus.

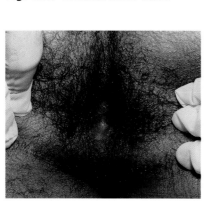

Fig. 1.15 Normal anus.

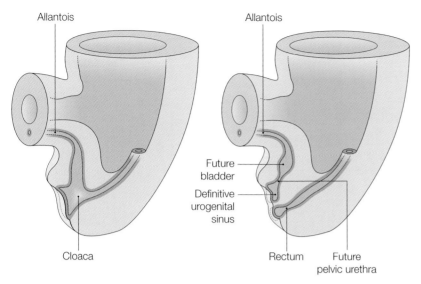

Fig. 1.16 Development of the primitive urogenital sinus. Between 4 and 6 weeks, the urorectal septum splits the cloaca into an anterior primitive urogenital sinus and a posterior rectum. The superior part of the primitive urogenital sinus, continuous with the allantois, forms the bladder. The constricted pelvic urethra at the base of the future bladder forms the membranous urethra in females and the membranous and prostatic urethra in males. The distal expansion of the primitive urogenital sinus, the definitive urogenital sinus, forms the vestibule of the vagina in females and the penile urethra in males.

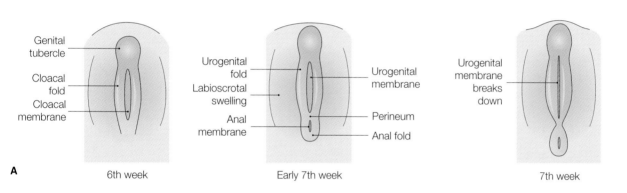

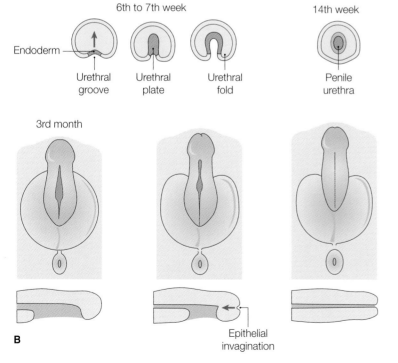

Fig. 1.17 Formation of the external genitalia in males and females (A) the external genitalia form from a pair of labioscrotal folds, a pair of urogenital folds and an anterior genital tubercle. Male and female genitalia are morphologically indistinguishable at this stage. (B) In males, the urogenital folds fuse and the genital tubercle elongates to form the shaft and glans of the penis. Fusion of the urogenital folds encloses the definite urogenital sinus to form most of the penile urethra. A small region of the distal urethra is formed by the invagination of ectoderms covering the glans. The labioscrotal folds give rise to the scrotum.

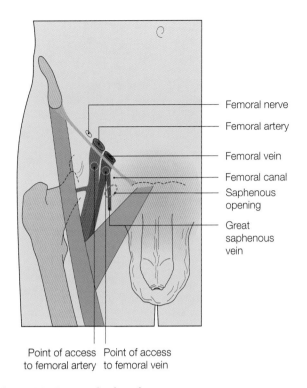

Femoral nerve

Femoral artery

Femoral vein

Femoral canal

Saphenous opening

Great saphenous vein

Point of access to femoral artery   Point of access to femoral vein

Fig. 1.18 Femoral triangle.

The anatomical position and the arrangement of all of the structures in the area are explained by the *embryology* (**Figs 1.16, 1.17**) (Ammini et al 1997). Around the third week of fetal development mesenchymal cells derived from the primitive streak form ridges of tissue around the cloacal membrane. These cloacal folds are joined anteriorly and cranially and form the genital tubercle. Posteriorly and caudally they are partially joined to form an annulus. The underlying cloacal membrane is subdivided into urogenital and anal membranes craniocaudally by about six weeks. During the same period lateral genital swellings are occurring that will form either the scrotum or labia majora.

From this point differentiation of the external genitalia occurs in a sexually specific manner driven in the male by fetal testicular androgens. The genital tubercle lengthens creating an urethral groove. This eventually becomes the urethral canal when the folds fuse at about 12 weeks. This *penile urethra* has an epithelium derived therefore from endoderm. It is incomplete cranially where the glans has developed from the genital tubercle. The glanular urethra and the meatus are derived from an invading cord of ectoderm that eventually becomes canalized. The scrotal swellings fuse posteriorly at about 14 weeks but are not occupied by the testes until about the time of birth.

The *prepuce* (Glenister 1956; Cold & Taylor 1999) is formed by a midline collision of ectoderm, neuro-ectoderm and mesenchyme resulting in a pentilaminar structure consisting of (inner) squamous mucosal epithelium, lamina propria, dartos muscle, dermis and glabrous skin (outer). The preputial fold progressively extends but there is also an ingrowth of a cellular lamella. It then fuses with the mucosa of the glans. The female counterpart of the prepuce is the clitoral hood.

The cloacal membrane is where ectodermal and endodermal tissues are in direct apposition caudally. The separation into urogenital membrane and anal membrane with the formation of the perineum at about seven weeks is due to the separation of the cloacal portion of the hindgut by the urorectal septum growing caudally between the allantois anteriorly and the hindgut and partitioning the cloaca into the urogenital sinus anteriorly and the anorectal canal posteriorly. The anal membrane disintegrates at about 9 weeks to open into an ecto-dermal anal pit formed in the posterior cloacal (anal) folds. **Figure 1.19** conveys the stylized normal structure of skin.

There are several thousand named *skin diseases*. This fact is explained by consideration of the pathological possibilities due to the principal morbid processes (*neoplasia, inflammation, degeneration* and *fibrosis*) impacting on such an heterogeneous organ as skin with its numerous different cell types and organ structures and its wide regional, racial, sexual and physiological variation as well as differences in environmental exposure. Obviously the anogenital area differs between the sexes, but it is a good example of regional human variation; variation in contrast with other mucocutaneous sites and variation within the specialized anogenital area itself.

An important difference from other sites is that the perineal area possesses numerous eccrine and apocrine (some functionless) *sweat glands*. Also in plentiful number are (holocrine) *sebaceous glands* usually in association with *hair follicles* (pilosebaceous units) but also occurring as free glands at some sites, such as the anal rim or around the coronal sulcus (Tyson's glands). These secretions are to lubricate the hinge between limb and torso, to lubricate hair, to lubricate the mucocutaneous junctions to assist in the voiding of excreta and to protect the epithelia from irritation, and to lubricate the penis for sexual activity (the retraction of the foreskin more than the penetration of the vagina).

Pubic hair appears in puberty as vellus hair that is focally replaced by terminal hair. Men have a different pattern of pubic hair compared with women but in practice it is one of degree. The distribution of hair and pubic hair varies widely among men. McGregor (1961) studied approximately 4000 soldiers and defined three patterns (**Fig. 1.20**). Generally, the abdominal wall, pubic mound, groins, scrotum and perineum are hairy but the natal cleft, perianal skin, distal penile shaft, prepuce and glans are hairless. The function of pubic hair is open to interesting but speculative anthropomor-phological debate.

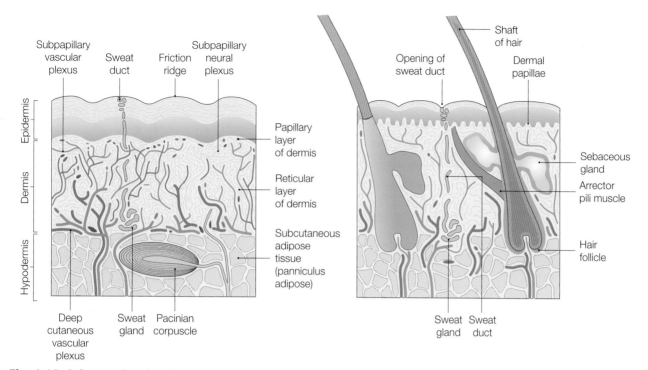

Fig. 1.19 Schema showing the organization of skin. Structures present in thick, hairless (plantar and palmar) skin compared with thin, hirsute skin.

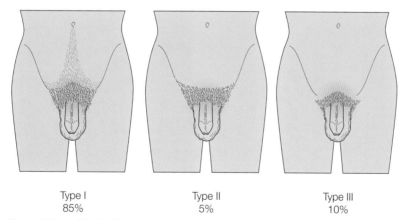

Type I
85%

Type II
5%

Type III
10%

Fig. 1.20 Pubic hair. Normal distribution of pubic hair in men. (After McGregor 1961).

The pattern of keratinization of the epithelium is different throughout the anogenital area, most markedly so at the mucosal junctions, the prepuce and distal penile shaft and especially the glans in the circumcised subject. The wide spectrum of differentiation of the male urogenital tract is accompanied by pronounced changes in the expression of epithelial cytokeratins (Achtstatter et al 1985). Normal regional histology is illustrated in **Figs 1.21–1.25**.

The principal normal variants encountered in and around the male genitalia are listed in **Table 1.1**.

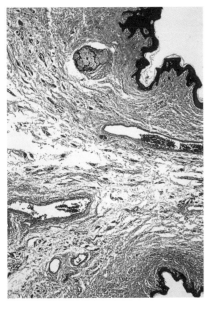

Fig. 1.21 Normal histology. Foreskin. Full thickness of prepuce shows all five layers: keratinized stratified squamous epithelium, dermis with sebaceous glands, dartos, submucosa and squamous mucosa. H&E. (Courtesy of and reproduced with permission from Sternberg, SS, ed. Histology for Pathologists, 2nd edition. Philadelphia: Lippincott, Williams and Wilkins, 1997.)

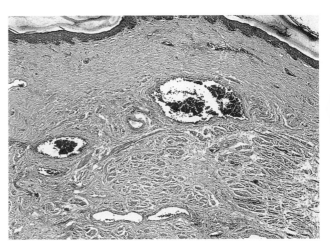

Fig. 1.22 Normal histology. Balanopreputial sulcus. Histologic components of both glans and peneal body are present. This specimen from a circumcised person shows the mucosa at top, lamina proporia below, then dartos, or smooth muscle layer and Buck's fascia. H&E. (Courtesy of and reproduced with permission from Sternberg, SS, ed. Histology for Pathologists, 2nd edition. Philadelphia: Lippincott, Williams and Wilkins, 1997.)

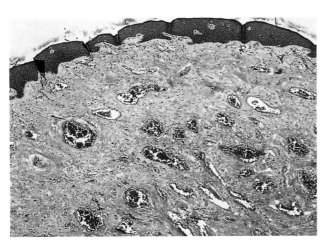

Fig. 1.23 Normal histology. Glans penis. The three layers of glans are noted: nonkeratinized stratified mucosa, lamina propria and corpus spongiosum. H&E. (Reproduced with permission from Sternberg, SS, ed. Histology for Pathologists, 2nd edition. Philadelphia: Lippincott, Williams and Wilkins, 1997.)

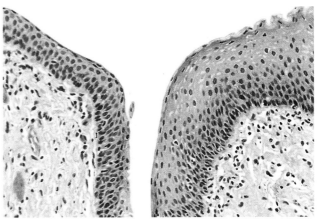

Fig. 1.24 Normal histology. Anal transitional zone (ATZ). Transition from ATZ epithelium (left) to squamous zone (right). H&E. (Reproduced with permission from Sternberg, SS, ed. Histology for Pathologists, 2nd edition. Philadelphia: Lippincott, Williams and Wilkins, 1997.)

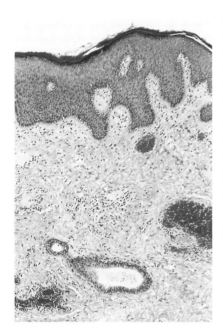

Fig. 1.25 Normal histology. Perianal skin. Keratinized squamous epithelium and an underlying apocrine gland. H&E.(Reproduced with permission from Sternberg, SS, ed. Histology for Pathologists, 2nd edition. Philadelphia: Lippincott, Williams and Wilkins, 1997.)

PIGMENTATION

The most common variation due to race is pigmentation. The amount of pigment in the skin is related to the amount of melanogenesis and not to the number of melanocytes, which is constant in human beings at about 1 in 8–10 of epidermal basal layer cells. Melanin synthesis by melanocytes is not only racially determined (constitutive pigmentation) but also induced by sunlight exposure (facultative pigmentation) and circulating and local melanotropic factors (for example, as part of the cellular response to inflammation). Most races keep the genital skin covered so the former factor is rarely relevant. Physical signs, particularly of inflammation, are harder to detect in pigmented skin. Race may also account for differences in hair type and distribution.

It is not uncommon to find linear hyperpigmentation of the ventral penile shaft, along the median raphe (Fig. 1.26).

Table 1.1 Normal variants

Pigmentation

Skin tags (acrochordons)

Pearly penile papules (angiofibromas)

Sebaceous prominence

Melanocytic nevi

Prominent veins

Bier's vascular spots

Angiomas

Angiokeratomas

Congenital abnormalities

Circumcision

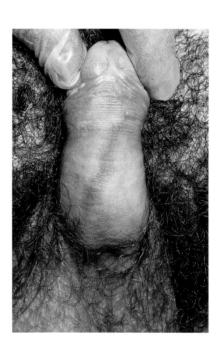

Fig. 1.26 Hyper-pigmentation of the median raphe. Ventral penis shaft. Normal variant.

SKIN TAGS (ACROCHORDONS)

Skin tags are common in the groins especially in those of obese men. They may catch on clothing, bleed and get infected (**Figs 1.27, 1.28**). The histology is of squamous papilloma. Treatment is by electrocautery or scissor amputation and cautery.

Fibrosed hemorrhoids result in perianal skin tags.

Larger, fleshier more oedematosus skin tags should arouse the suspicion of Crohn's disease. They can predate gastrointestinal disease by several years. Sigmoidoscopy and biopsy are essential (Alexander-Williams & Buchmann 1980).

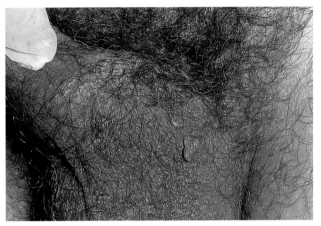

Fig. 1.27 Skin tag. Scrotum.

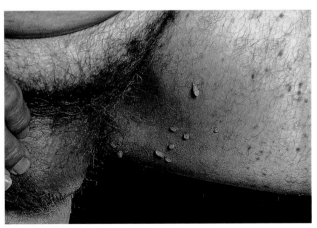

Fig. 1.28 Skin tags. Groin and thigh.

PEARLY PENILE PAPULES (ANGIOFIBROMAS)

Pearly/pink penile papules/hirsutes papillaris (Johnson et al 1964; Tanenbaum & Becker 1965; Oates 1997) are common: they may be found in up to 15–48% of men (Glicksman & Freeman 1966; Neinstein & Goldenring 1984; Sonnex & Dockerty 1999) depending upon how officiously they are sought.

They manifest as flesh-colored, smooth, rounded papules (1–3 mm) occurring predominantly around the coronal margin of the glans, rarely on the glans. Often there are rows or rings of the papules (**Figs 1.29–1.32**). Ectopic lesions, for example on the penile shaft, have been reported (O'Neil & Hansen 1995) including in children (Neri et al 1997) (**Fig. 1.33**). They are frequently mistaken for warts by both patients and physicians and can be mislabeled Tyson's glands or ectopic sebaceous glands by physicians. As Oates (1997) has put it, pearly penile papules 'commonly present to clinics for sexually transmitted diseases as one of the minor "rarities" and the source of much anxiety for worried adolescents'.

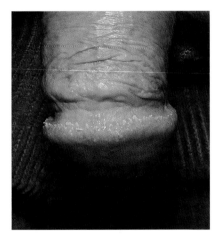

Fig. 1.29 Pearly penile papules. Glans penis and coronal rim.

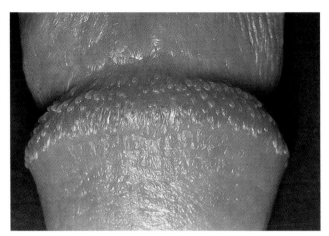

Fig. 1.30 Pearly penile papules. Glans penis, coronal rim.

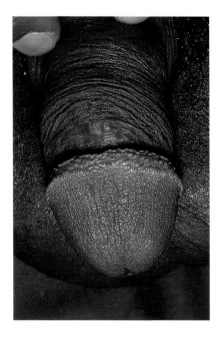

Fig. 1.31 Pearly penile papules. Glans penis and coronal rim.

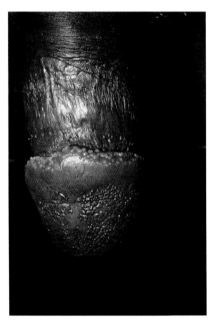

Fig. 1.32 Pearly penile papules. Glans and distal shaft, penis. (Courtesy of Dr Peter Copeman, London, UK).

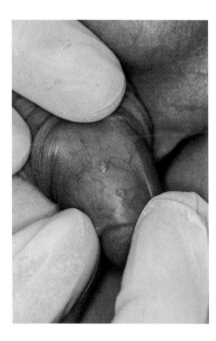

Fig. 1.33 Pearly penile papules. Shaft of penis. Ectopic lesions. Child. (Courtesy of Dr Iria Neri, Bologna, and reproduced from Neri I et al. Genitourin Med 1997; 73: 136, with permission from BMJ Publishing Group).

The histology is that of angiofibroma and the lesion is analogous to other acral angiofibromas such as adenoma sebaceum (a misnomer due to James Pringle), subungual and periungual fibromas, fibrous papule of the nose, acquired acral angiofibroma and oral fibroma (Ackerman & Kornberg 1973). HPV DNA is absent (Ferenczy et al 1991). Confident reassurance is the conventional line of management. Cryotherapy can be effective (Porter & Bunker 2000). Laser treatment has been advocated (McKinlay et al 1999).

SEBACEOUS GLAND PROMINENCE

Sebaceous gland prominence, Tyson's glands, sebaceous hyperplasia, ectopic sebaceous glands (Fordyce's condition) are all virtually synonymous, common, normal variants of the skin of the scrotal sac and penile shaft but may cause concern to patients (**Figs 1.34–1.38**). Fordyce's condition commonly affects the vermilion border of the lips (**Fig. 1.37**) and the genitalia.

I have seen a nevoid linear lesion on the penile shaft (**Fig. 1.39**), and something similar has been reported by Kumar & Kossard (1999). For the lesions to occur on the glans (**Figs 1.39, 1.40**) is unusual, but documented nonetheless (Massmanian et al 1995). Reassurance is usually adequate but the patient illustrated in **Figure 1.36** developed somatopsychic symptoms amounting to dysmorphophobia. The patient discontinued a course of isotretinoin, which can help with sebaceous hyperplasia on the face, after three months because of side effects and lack of therapeutic response and he then defaulted from follow-up.

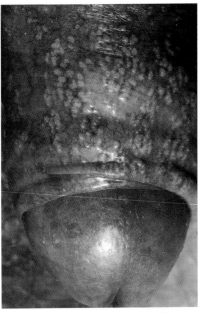

Fig. 1.34 Sebaceous hyperplasia (Fordyce's condition). Penis, prepuce.

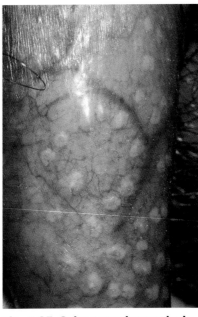

Fig. 1.35 Sebaceous hyperplasia (Fordyce's condition). Penis, shaft.

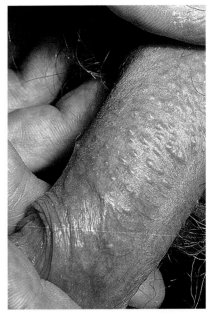

Fig. 1.36 Sebaceous hyperplasia (Fordyce's condition). Penis shaft. Patient with dysmorphophobia.

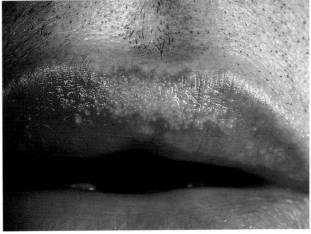

Fig. 1.37 Ectopic sebaceous glands (Fordyce's condition). Vermilion upper lip.

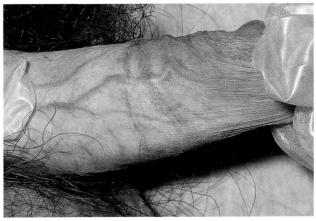

Fig. 1.38 Sebaceous hyperplasia. Penis. Nevoid linear distribution.

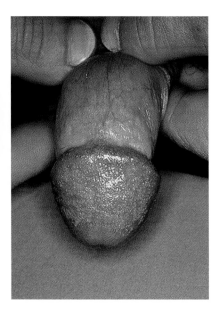

Fig. 1.39 Ectopic sebaceous glands. Glans penis. (Courtesy of Dr Antranick Massmanian, Valencia, Spain, and reproduced by permission of Blackwell Science Ltd from Massmanian A et al. Fordyce spots on the glans penis. Br J Dermatol 1995; 133: 498–500.)

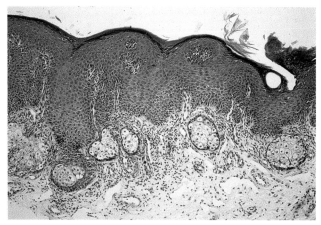

Fig. 1.40 Ectopic sebaceous glands. Histology. Glans penis. H&E × 500. (Courtesy of Dr Antranick Massmanian, Valencia, Spain, and reproduced by permission of Blackwell Science Ltd from Massmanian A et al. Fordyce spots on the glans penis. Br J Dermatol 1995; 133: 498–500.)

MELANOCYTIC NEVI

Melanocytic nevi may be congenital or acquired. Congenital nevi (**Fig. 1.41**) have a risk of malignant transformation of between 0–15% depending on size. Large 'bathing-trunk' nevi may involve the anogenital area and pose significant management problems (**Fig. 1.42**): they carry a very high risk of multifocal malignant transformation.

Acquired melanocytic nevi are extremely common in white-skinned people. Cullen (1962) reported an incidence of approximately 15% of males having at least one acquired melanocytic nevus (**Figs 1.43–1.47**) of their genitalia (9.5% whites; 21.5% Latins; 3.5% blacks).

It is possible that nevi on the penis occur more frequently in patients with the atypical nevus syndrome (**Figs 1.48, 1.49**) but this has not been formally documented. Individuals with the atypical/dysplasic nevus syndrome classically have a family or personal history of melanoma and numerous acquired nevi. They also have many nevi that are atypical: larger, more irregular of

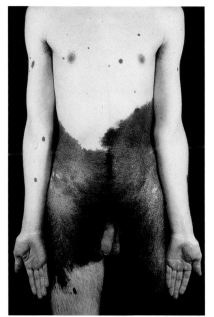

Fig. 1.42 Congenital 'bathing-trunk' melanocytic nevus. Pelvic girdle and thighs. Very high risk of multifocal malignant change. (Courtesy of Medical Illustration UK, Chelsea and Westminster Hospital, London, UK).

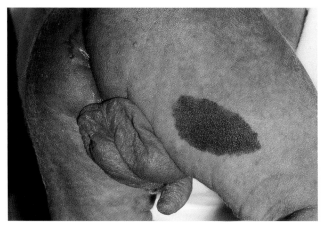

Fig. 1.41 Congenital melanocytic nevus. Right thigh.

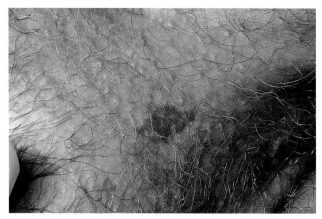

Fig. 1.43 Junctional melanocytic nevus. Left scroto-inguinal fold.

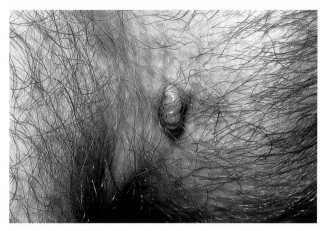

Fig. 1.44 Cellular intradermal melanocytic nevus. Right scroto-inguinal fold.

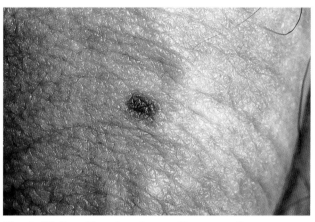

Fig. 1.46 Junctional melanocytic nevus. Prepuce. Same case as Fig. 1.45.

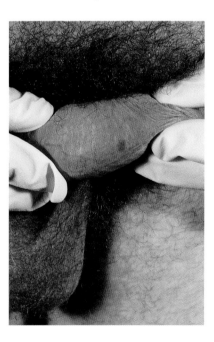

Fig. 1.48 Atypical/ dysplastic nevus. Penis, shaft. This patient and his brother have had a melanoma.

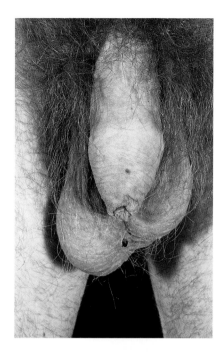

Fig. 1.45 Junctional melanocytic nevus. Prepuce.

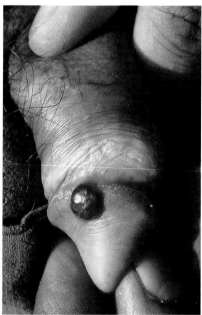

Fig. 1.47 Intradermal melanocytic nevus. Coronal rim, glans penis. (Courtesy of Prof. Bhushan Kumar, Chandigarh, India).

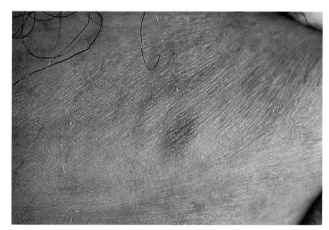

Fig. 1.49 Atypical/dysplastic nevus. Penis, shaft. This patient presented with a melanoma elsewhere.

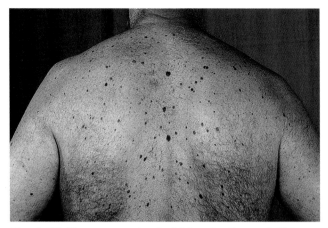

Fig. 1.50 Numerous atypical/dysplastic nevi. This patient and his brother have had a melanoma.

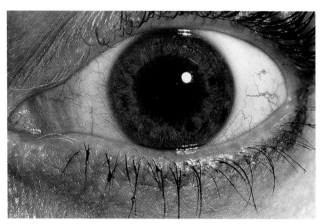

Fig. 1.51 Iris lentigines. Atypical nevus syndrome.

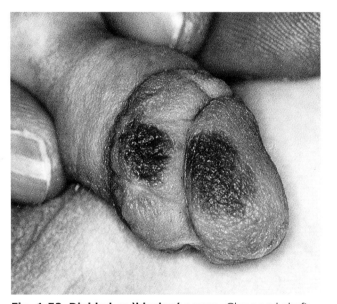

Fig. 1.52 Divided or 'kissing' nevus. Glans and shaft, penis. (Courtesy of Dr François Desruelles, Nice, France, and reproduced from Desruelles F et al. Arch Dermatol 1998; 134: 879–80. Copyright 1998 American Medical Association.)

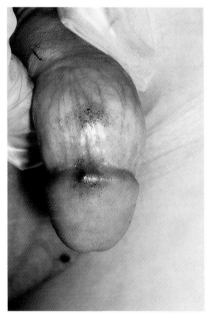

Fig. 1.53 Divided or 'kissing' nevus. Glans and shaft, penis.

edge, of pigment, and surface (**Fig. 1.50**) and atypically distributed on the scalp, buttocks, feet and have iris lentigines (**Fig. 1.51**). The syndrome in its complete and incomplete forms is important because of the increased risk of melanoma that the phenotype represents.

Any one acquired melanocytic nevus has been estimated to have a 1/1 000 000 risk of becoming melanoma. Approximately 50% of melanoma arises from pre-existing normal skin and not from a pre-existing nevus.

Cases of divided or 'kissing' nevus (**Figs 1.52, 1.53**) have been reported with one half located on the glans and the other on the distal penile shaft separated by uninvolved skin across the coronal divide (Desruelles et al 1998; Choi et al 2000). An analogous condition is recognized on the eyelids. Epithelioid blue nevus of the genitals is very rare (Izquierdo et al 2001).

PROMINENT VEINS

Prominent veins are common (**Figs 1.54, 1.55**) and very occasionally give rise to concern but very rarely cause complications.

BIER'S SPOTS

Vascular white spots are sometimes seen on the glans. I propose that they are analogous to Bier's spots seen on the palms and forearms where there are macular foci of relative cutaneous vasoconstriction against a background of more confluent erythema representing relative vasodilatation. The cutaneous microvasculature is under multifactorial control but endogenous tone is modulated

15

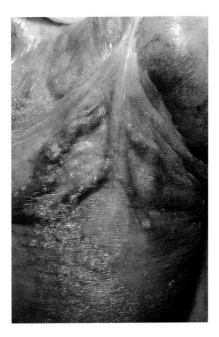

Fig. 1.54 Prominent veins. Subcoronal, perifrenulum, ventral penis.

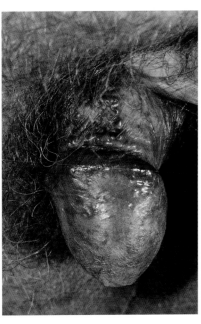

Fig. 1.55 Prominent veins. Dorsal, distal shaft, penis.

who described them. They are idiopathic age-related lesions (Dowd & Champion 1998) of vascular ectasia and tightly coiled tortuosity that may vary with the season or temperature and may be more common in diabetics for obscure reasons. They have the histological features of angiokeratomas and under the electron micrscope show reduplication of the basement membrane and endothelial fenestration (Stehbens & Ludatscher 1968).

The differential diagnosis includes angiokeratoma, acquired capillary and cavernous hemangiomas (Dehner & Smith 1970), Masson's tumour (see page 199), glomus tumour (see page 201), epithelioid hemangioma (see page 202), bacillary angiomatosis (page 182), Kaposi's sarcoma (page 119) and epithelioid hemangio-endothelioma (see page 232).

Clinical diagnosis of cherry angioma is usually reliable. To most physicians the history and physical signs are pathognomic. Odder, angiomatous lesions may require biopsy.

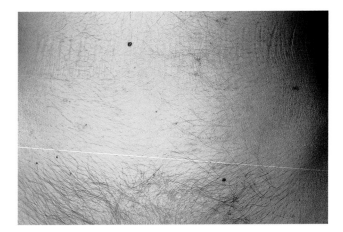

Fig. 1.56 Angiomas. Campbell de Morgan spot. Suprapubic skin.

by powerful endothelial-derived mediators such as nitric oxide (vasodilator) and endothelin (vasoconstrictor). Bier's spots may be due to predominant focal endogenous endothelin influence (Bunker et al 1996). The glans of the penis is as vascular as the palm of the hand.

ANGIOMA

Cherry angiomas are found as centripetal, pinhead to small berry-sized, cherry red to port-colored, dome-shaped papules, usually not blanchable. Unusually they may be confined to the genitalia but frequently they are sparsely, sometimes abundantly distributed over the rest of the torso (**Figs 1.56, 1.57**).

In the British literature these are called Campbell de Morgan spots after the Middlesex Hospital surgeon

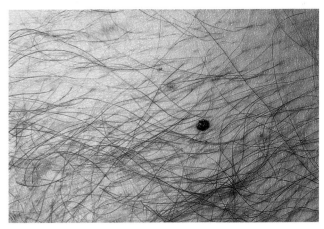

Fig. 1.57 Angioma. Campbell de Morgan spot. Suprapubic skin.

For cherry angiomas, usually no treatment is desired or indicated. The response to cryotherapy with liquid nitrogen is indifferent. Electrocautery probably gives better results, as does possibly the tunable dye laser.

CONGENITAL ABNORMALITIES

The complicated embryogenesis of the anogenital region involving sexual differentiation and pubertal determination of secondary sexual characteristics mean that congenital and developmental anomalies are common. The dermatologist will rarely be involved in making a primary diagnosis but needs to recognize anatomical and functional abnormality because this will increase the vulnerability of the area to dermatoses and infections.

Congenital (and acquired) melanocytic nevi are discussed on page 196. Other common abnormalities include meatal pit (**Fig. 1.58**), sacral pit (**Fig. 1.59**), hypospadias (Ammini et al 1997; Ellsworth et al 1999), median raphe cysts, canals and sinuses (see page 171) and ambiguous genitalia (**Fig 1.60**). These entities may be features of other syndromes: for example, hypospadias occurs frequently in the Smith-Lemli-Opitz syndrome (autosomal recessive: mental retardation and multiple congenital anomalies). Some congenital anomalies are discussed in Chapter 9.

Even rarer anomalies include hypospadias variants (Duckett & Keating 1989; Attalla 1991), epispadias (Mollard et al 1998), segmental urethral hypospadias (see page 221), meatal stricture (**Fig. 1.59**), penile hypoplasia (Austoni et al 1999), mucoid or urethral cysts (**Fig. 1.61**, see also page 175), dermoid cysts (see

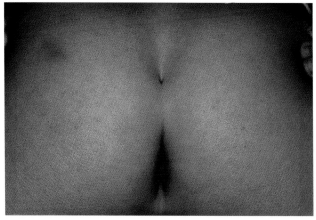

Fig. 1.59 Congenital pit. Sacrum. Not a precursor of pilonidal sinus. (Courtesy of Prof. Tim Allen-Mersh, London, UK).

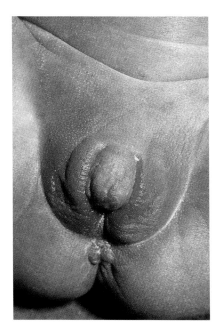

Fig. 1.60 Ambiguous genitalia.

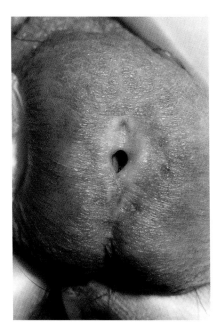

Fig. 1.58 Meatal pit and stricture. Glans penis.

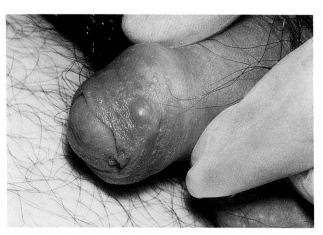

Fig. 1.61 Urethral/mucoid cyst. Ventral distal penile shaft.

page 194), divided or kissing nevus (Desruelles et al 1998; Choi et al 2000; see above **Figs 1.53, 1.54**), buried penis (**Fig. 1.62, Table 1.2**), either congenital due to maldevelopment of the elasticity of the Dartos fascia that prevents the skin from sliding freely over the deeper layers of the penile shaft (Shenoy et al 2000; Brisson et al 2001; Chuang et al 2001) or acquired, urethral atresia: for example with Fraser syndrome where serious renal and pulmonary damage occurs during fetal life (Andiran et al 1999), penoscrotal transposition (Kolligan et al 2000), congenital lymphoedema (Bolt et al 1998), giant prepucial sac (Philip & Nicholas 1999), megaprepuce (Shenoy & Rance 1999; Summerton et al 2000), accessory scrotum (Syzlit et al 1986), hemangiomas (Eastridge et al 1979; Gotoh et al 1983; Tsujii et al 1998), strawberry nevus (more common in girls) (Achauer & Vander Kam 1991), os penis (Champion & Wegrzyn 1964), true aposthia (Cold & Taylor 1999), faun tail (**Fig. 1.64**; see also page 57).

Table 1.2 Causes of acquired buried or concealed penis

Congenital

Radical circumcision

Abdominoplasty

Penile lengthening

Obesity with descent of the escutcheon

(after Casale et al 1999, Alter & Ehrlich 1999).

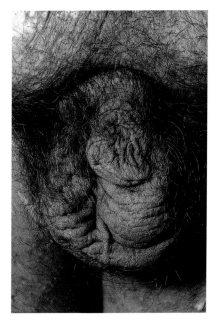

Fig. 1.62 Buried penis. Obesity. (Courtesy: Dr Peter Copeman, London, UK).

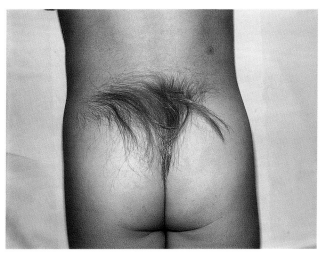

Fig. 1.63 Faun tail. Central lumbosacral area. Underlying spinal dysraphism.

THE FORESKIN

The prepuce has been present in primates for at least 65 million years and may be up to 100 million years old.

The embryology is described on page 8. At birth the prepuce is still developing histologically and it is usually incompletely separated from the glans. Only 4% of boys have a retractable foreskin at birth, 15% at six months, 50% at one year and 80–90% at three years (Gairdner 1949). The separation of the mucosa of the prepuce and glans is usually complete by 17 years (Øster 1968; Hsu 1983; Cold & Taylor 1999).

The prepuce is a specialized protective and erogenous structure. The protection it affords is both physical and immunological (Cold & Taylor 1999). Its structures (e.g. the penile dartos muscle and the corpuscular receptor-rich ridged band) and secretions are held to be important for 'normal copulatory behavior'.

The foreskin is of variable length and retractability in uncircumcised men: individuals with 'short' and 'long' foreskins are encountered (see **Figs 1.1, 1.2, 1.3**).

The foreskin is also a useful resource for tissue culture research and skin grafting (Emory & Chester 2000).

CIRCUMCISION

Harold Ellis (2000) says that 'circumcision might well be claimed to be the most ancient "elective" operation' (other surgical procedures performed in prehistoric times include trephination of the skull and cutting for the bladder stone). He records that 'it was practiced in Ancient Egypt by assistants to the priests on the priests and on members of royal families' and cites 'remarkable evidence for this carved on the tomb of a high-ranking royal official that was discovered in the Sakkara cemetery in Memphis and is dated between 2400 and 3000 BC' (**Fig. 1.64**). It 'represents two young boys or

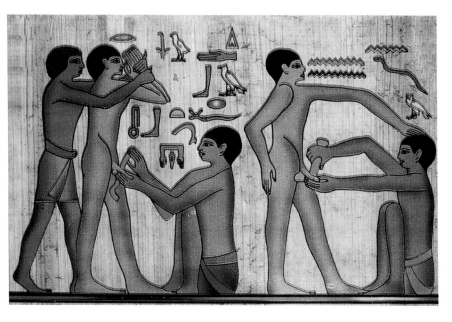

Fig. 1.64 Circumcision. Tomb carving, circa 3000 BC, Memphis, Egypt.

young men being circumcised. The operators are employing a crude stone instrument. While the patient on the left of the relief is having both arms held by an assistant, the other merely braces his left arm on the head of his surgeon. The inscription has the operator saying, "hold him so that he may not faint" and "it is for your benefit" (Ellis, 2000). The ancient Jews may have learned the art of circumcision during their bondage in Egypt'.

The operation has been performed for religious, cultural or medical reasons throughout history (Dunsmuir & Gordon 1999). There are approximately 100 references to the foreskin or circumcision in the Bible; indeed it is the only surgical procedure alluded to in the Old Testament (Ellis 2000). Ethnologists have shown that circumcision was practiced widely among

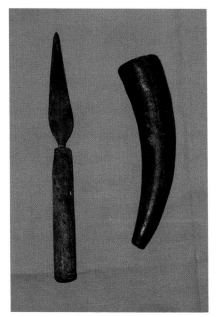

Fig. 1.65 Circumcision tools. Central Africa. (Courtesy of Mr Joseph Schlesinger, London, UK.)

the primitive communities of Africa (**Fig. 1.65**), Australasia and South America and became 'traditional amongst Jews, Moslems and Copts' (Ellis 2000). Although practiced from earliest times by Moslems it is not mentioned at all in the Koran (Mansfield 1992). Its origins were probably as 'a fertility or initiation rite or possibly for cleanliness and hygiene' (Ellis 2000). I suspect that the operation was developed as prophylaxis against cancer.

Contemporaneously, circumcision is a contentious issue. It has been estimated that globally 25% of men have been circumcised (Moses et al 1998). The prevalence of circumcision in any population reflects racial, religious, cultural and medical differences.

The risks and benefits of neonatal circumcision have been the focus of much debate. Opinions are strongly held. The arguments have been well covered in a supplement of the urology journal *BJU International* (Whitfield 1999). The UK General Medical Council (GMC) undertook a consultative review of the circumcision of infants in 1997, which 'demonstrated widely conflicting views in society that neither doctors nor the GMC can resolve' (Anon 1997). Yet the legal basis of circumcision is not beyond question (Dalton 1997, van Howe et al 1999).

During infancy circumcised boys have a higher incidence of penile problems than the uncircumcised but after infancy the situation is significantly reversed (Fergusson et al 1988; van Howe 1997). Many recent reviews have concluded that there is considerable evidence to support the long-held opinion (see, for example, the American Academy of Pediatrics 1989 'Report of the Task Force on Circumcision' by Schoen et al) that circumcision protects men from cancer of the penis and urinary tract and sexually transmitted infections including HIV (Parker et al 1983; Roberts 1986; Wiswell et al 1987; Fussell et al 1988; Wiswell &

Geschke 1989; Schoen 1990; Moses et al 1998; Wijesinha et al 1998; Halperin & Bailey 1999; O'Farrell & Egger 2000; Schoen et al 2000). However, the incidence of penis cancer is low in Japan and Denmark where circumcision is rare (Williams & Kapila 1993; Frisch et al 1995) so other factors are important in the carcinogenesis (see page 208). Recently data has emerged to suggest that female partners of circumcised men have a lower risk of cervical cancer (Castellsague et al 2002). But some have argued that the effects of circumcision on the other outcomes may be small (Poland 1990; Laumann et al 1997): for example urethritis may be more common in the circumcised and ulcerative genital disease more common in the uncircumcised (van Howe 1999).

Data from my clinic suggest that circumcision protects against inflammatory genital dermatoses including psoriasis, seborrheic dermatitis, lichen planus and lichen sclerosus. About 50% of men attending general clinics were uncircumcised, whereas uncircumcised men were in the majority in the penis clinic (Mallon et al 2000; Laumann 2001; Newson 2001). Balanitis is much less common in the circumcised male (Fakjian et al 1990).

Uncontroversially, circumcision is indispensable in the management of disease of the penis and foreskin, including dermatological conditions. However, there may be confusion and disagreement about what are the medical and surgical indications in different age groups: overall, in the UK it is estimated that 1–2% of boys need circumcision for clinical reasons (Gordon & Collin 1993).

The indications for circumcision in childhood and adulthood (Escala & Rickwood 1989; Rickwood 1999) include true phimosis, recurrent balanoposthitis, lichen sclerosus, penile lymphoedema, intraepithelial neoplasia and carcinoma. The idea that circumcision might be a useful strategy in the epidemiological management of HIV is under investigation (Bailey et al 2002).

Rickwood & Walker (1989) estimated that 30 000 circumcisions were being done annually in England (21 000 on boys under 15 years old) and that too many circumcisions were being done because true phimosis was being over diagnosed.

Although the long-held consensus is that there is little evidence of significant adverse effects on health, including psychosexual function (Harnes 1971), circumcision undoubtedly has side effects and complications.

Possible risks or complications of circumcision are bleeding (Williams & Kapila 1993), postoperative infection including overwhelming fatal Group B β-hemolytic sepsis (Cleary 1979; Wiswell et al 1991; Williams & Kapila 1993) salmonella scrotal abscess (Uwyyed et al 1990) and syphilis (Rosenbaum 1899) adhesions (**Fig. 1.66**, Ponsky et al 2000), including skin bridge (Kaplan 1983; Sathaye et al 1990), fistula (Williams & Kapila 1993), hair coil strangulation (Bashir & El-Barbary 1979; **Fig. 1.67**), keloid (Warwick & Dickson 1993; Gurunluoglu et al, 1999; **Fig. 1.68**, see also page 179), concealed or buried penis (Alici et al 1998; Yildirim et al 2000; Esen et al 2001), amputation (Coskunfirat et al 1999), excision of excessive penile skin (Quintela et al 2000), meatal stenosis (meatal irritation and damage to the frenular artery supplying the anterior urethra), meatitis and meatal ulcer, cysts, chordee, hypospadias

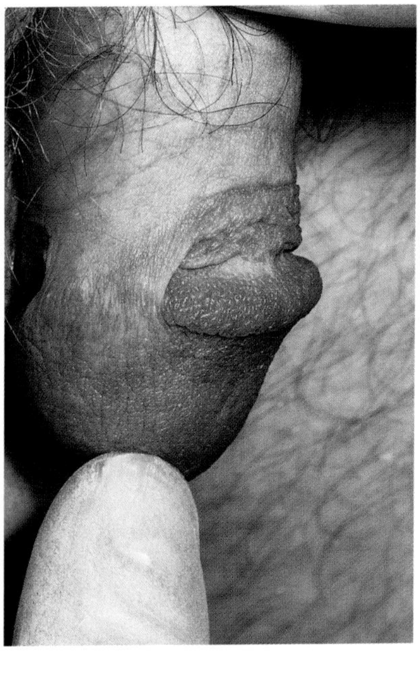

Fig. 1.66 Adhesions. Glans and shaft, penis. Transcoronal bridging adhesions since neonatal circumcision.

Table 1.3 Complications of circumcision

Bleeding

Post-operative sepsis

Adhesions including skin bridge

Fistula

Hair coil strangulation

Keloid

Concealed or buried penis

Amputation

Excision of excessive penile skin

Meatal stenosis

Meatitis and meatal ulcer

Cysts

Chordee

Hypospadias and epispadias

Amputation neuroma

Abnormal sexual behavior

Psychological distress and dysmorphophobia

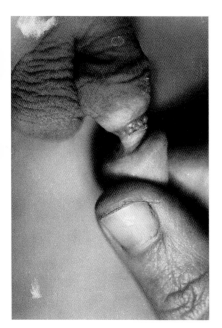

Fig. 1.67 Hair coil strangulation. Penis shaft. Boy aged four years, 10 days post-circumcision. (Courtesy of Dr Abdullah Al-Bashir, Amman, Jordan and reproduced by kind permission of Blackwell Science Ltd from Bashir AY, El-Barbary M. Hair coil strangulation of the penis. JR Coll Surg Edinb 1980; 25: 47–51.)

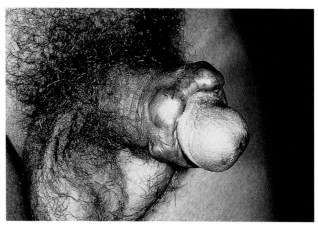

Fig. 1.68 Keloid. Penis shaft. Black 10-year-old boy. Post-circumcision. (Courtesy of Mr W. A. Dickson, Swansea, Wales, UK, and reproduced with permission from Warwick DJ, Dickson WA. Keloid of the penis after circumcision. Postgrad Med J. 1993; 69: 236–7.)

and epispadias (Kaplan 1983), amputation neuromas in the scar, loss of the penile dartos muscle and the corpuscular receptor-rich ridged band of the male prepuce, leading to abnormal sexual behavior (Cold & Taylor 1999), psychological distress (Goldman 1999) and dysmorphophobia (Williams & Kapila 1993). Some of the risks or complications of circumcision can be reduced by different techniques, such as the Gomco circumcision (Peleg & Steiner 1998). See **Table 1.3.**

'*Uncircumcision*' refers to the practice of preputial restoration, desired and performed throughout history for a variety of reasons (Schultheiss et al 1998; Brandes & McAninch 1999).

2 Dermatological diagnosis

Achieving a dermatological diagnosis depends upon the conventional clinical process of *history* taking, physical *examination*, elaboration of a *differential diagnosis* (and problem list), and by special *investigations* if needed.

It has been observed that clinical diagnosis of penile dermatoses is frequently inadequate (Hillman et al 1992). There is a widespread misconception about dermatological practice that supposes that skin physicians diagnose all their patients by near-instant pattern recognition or 'spot diagnosis'. Nothing could be further from the truth. Although it is possible in some instances and with considerable experience, it is an approach fraught with dangerous pitfalls. The practical reality is that a recognizable pattern emerges, as reliably in the skilled elicitation of the history, as in the examination. Most dermatologists will agree that if they do not have a good idea what the patient's problem is after thorough enquiry then they stand a good chance of being hard-pressed when the patient has his clothes off and the rash or lump is displayed. A full history is mandatory (**Table 2.1**).

The symptomatic presentation of skin disease is limited. Essentially, patients complain of *itch* (soreness or pain), a *rash*, a *lump*, *bump* or *breach* of the skin, or of a problem with *hair* or *nails*. In obtaining the history the nature of the symptoms is explored, especially the time and space relationships.

Additional symptoms generated by anogenital skin disease include those due to sexual dysfunction particularly *preputial dysfunction* e.g. soreness, pain, bleeding or tearing on intercourse i.e. male dyspareunia, or difficulty with the mobility of the prepuce – phimosis or paraphimosis, *urinary dysfunction* e.g. frequency, discharge, dysuria or *colorectal dysfunction* e.g. pain, bleeding, discharge. It is often forgotten that male sexual function amounts to much more than just the ability to achieve an erection (Gasser & Lehmann 1995): libido, erection, ejaculation and orgasm are the principal components.

The responsibility for the diagnosis of anogenital symptoms may need to be shared with the genitourinary physician, pediatrician or the urologist or colorectal surgeon.

Patients with anogenital skin complaints are often worried about sexual transmission so a *sexual history* is vital. Knowing a patient's job provides a double function: there could be an occupational component to the skin problem and a physician obtains early on in the consultation a good idea at what intellectual level to communicate with his patient.

Table 2.1 Key facets of the history

Age

Job

Symptom
  Itch, soreness, pain
  Rash
  Lump, bump
  Ulcer, blister

History of presenting complaint
  Time and space relationships (especially to sexual activity and urinary function)

Personal and family history
  Circumcision
  Atopy
  Psoriasis

Drugs and allergies
  Systemic medication
  Topicals
  Over the counter

Sexual history
  Single/married
  Hetero/homo/bisexual
  Regular partner
  Last sexual activity
    When
    How (vaginal, oral, anal)
    Contraception
  Partner symptomatology

Urological history and symptomatology

Smoking

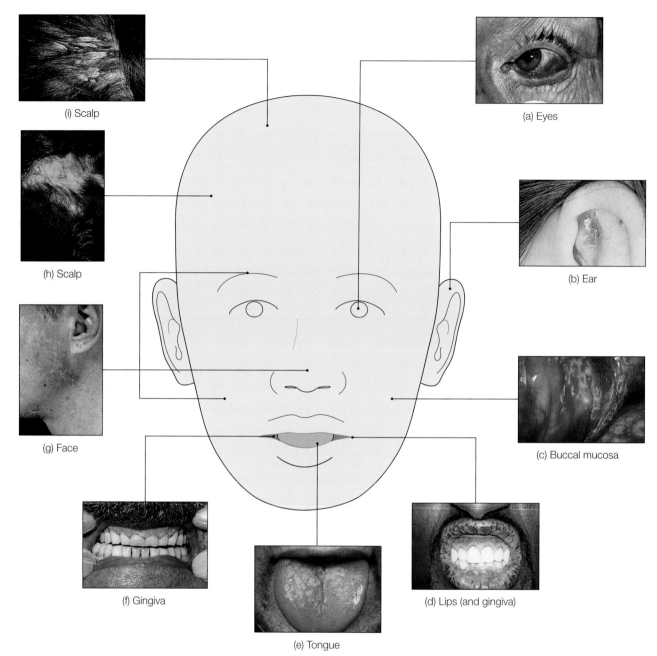

(i) Scalp

(a) Eyes

(h) Scalp

(b) Ear

(g) Face

(c) Buccal mucosa

(f) Gingiva

(d) Lips (and gingiva)

(e) Tongue

Fig. 2.1a–i
a **Eyes.** Cicatricial pemphigoid. (Courtesy of Dr Jane Setterfield, London, UK).
b **Ear.** Psoriasis. External auditory meatus.
c **Buccal mucosa.** Lichen planus.
d **Lips (and gingiva).** Lichen planus.
e **Tongue.** Lichen planus.
f **Gingiva.** Lichen planus.
g **Face.** Epidermodysplasia verruciformis. White papules, cheek and jaw. HIV.
h **Scalp.** Lichen planus. Scarring alopecia.
i **Scalp.** Pityriasis amiantacea (psoriasis). Tenacious asbestos-like scale.

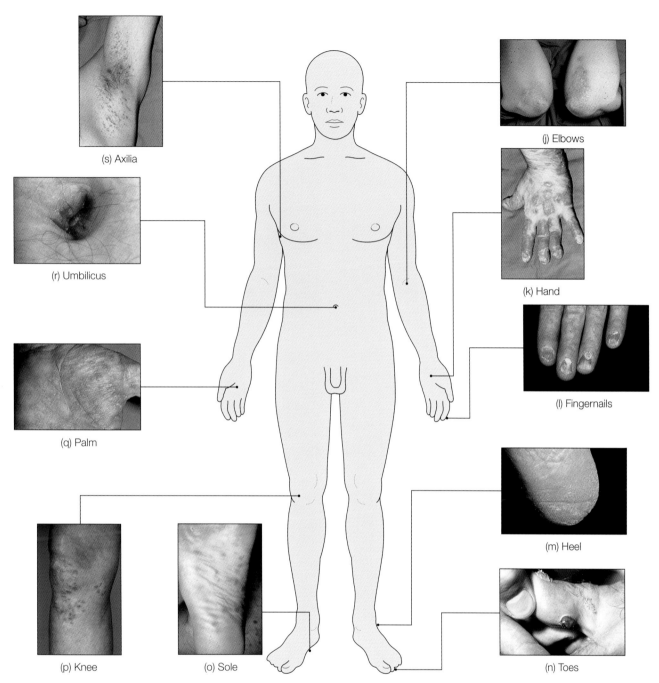

(s) Axilia

(r) Umbilicus

(q) Palm

(j) Elbows

(k) Hand

(l) Fingernails

(m) Heel

(p) Knee

(o) Sole

(n) Toes

Fig. 2.1j–s
j   **Elbows.** Psoriasis.
k   **Hand.** Psoriasis. Severe involvement including arthritis mutilans and gross nail dystrophy.
l   **Fingernails.** Psoriasis. Dystrophy.
m   **Heel.** Psoriasis.
n   **Toe.** Kaposi's sarcoma. Single digital lesion masquerading as pyogenic granuloma in HIV.
o   **Sole.** Secondary syphilis. Coppery-hued papulosquamous eruption.
p   **Knee.** Psoriasis.
q   **Palm.** Multiple papules of lichen planus.
r   **Umbilicus.** Psoriasis.
s   **Axilia.** Lichen planus.

The past *medical history* (especially of skin disease) is crucial as is the family history: asthma, hay fever or eczema in a patient or first-degree relative defines atopy; people may not know what psoriasis is, so explain; ask about dandruff, cradle cap, warts, skin cancer, etc.

The crude dermatological maxim 'any drug, any rash' explains why a rigorous, even obsessive *drug history* is encouraged. Culprits are sometimes not even regarded by patients as drugs – cough medicines, laxatives, pain killers, vitamins, etc. And, does the patient have any allergies to drugs or other substances? Also, when people develop a skin problem and are particularly troubled with the fear of a sexually transmitted disease they frequently resort to highly unsuitable topical preparations (disinfectants, antihistamine creams, a variety of over-the-counter agents, etc.), and they may have been misdiagnosed and given an inappropriate prescription by another physician (potent topical corticosteroids, creams containing common allergens, etc.).

Knowing whether a patient *drinks* or *smokes* is not always peripheral to diagnosing and managing anogenital skin problems; smoking is a risk factor for penis cancer. Enquiring about sporting and washing habits is very rewarding; the pernicious effects of over washing with soap are not widely appreciated.

The patient should then be examined all over, in a good light, preferably natural sunlight (**Table 2.2**). It is totally inadequate to examine just the genitalia because the common diagnoses will be reached with the assistance of important clues at other sites. Conversely, it is interesting how frequently in general medical practice a patient will not have his genitalia examined, although the chest will be conscientiously auscultated and the fundi diligently illuminated. More than once, in my experience, has the dermatologist been the *first* physician to examine the genitalia of a hospitalized male patient (despite that patient being the subject of otherwise meticulous clinical interrogation and examination and cutting-edge laboratory and radiological investigation). An old urological adage states that the physical examination of the male at any age is incomplete without examination of the scrotum and urologists teach that there are three primary reasons for careful examination of the scrotum: pain, swelling and absence of contents.

A checklist for complete examination takes us from head to toe: scalp, brows, eyes, ears, elbows, hands,

Table 2.2 Key facets of the examination

Prepuce	Present/absent
	Phimosis/paraphimosis
Rash	Distribution
	Morphology
Lump	Site
(or other focal lesion)	Morphology

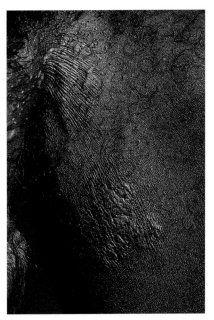

Fig. 2.2 Hyperpigmentation. Left groin. Hyperpigmented psoriasiform plaque. HIV-positive patient. Dermatological signs are harder to interpret in pigmented skin. (Reproduced from Bunker CB. Skin conditions on the male genitalia. Medicine 2001; 29:7. By kind permission of the Medicine Publishing Company.)

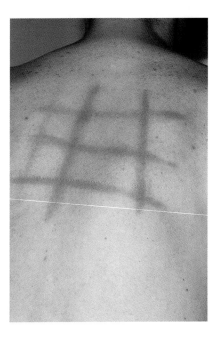

Fig. 2.3 Dermatographism Back.

nails, umbilicus, anus, groins, genitals, knees, feet, toes (**Fig. 2.1a–s**). Wear gloves, establish the presence or absence of the *prepuce*, *phimosis* or *paraphimosis*, and retract the foreskin gently if present, part the gluteal and crural folds, part the meatal lips, do a rectal examination, use a magnifying lens.

Note the *distribution* of the rash and describe the *morphology* of its constituent lesions; observe the *site* of any lump, bump, erosion or ulcer and define its *morphology* (**Table 2.3**). Be aware that the interpretation of morphology is altered by several factors. In black skin erythema is hard to discern and the pigmentary response may be prominent (**Fig. 2.2**). In HIV infection cutaneous and systemic immunodysfunction attenuate or enhance the host response and hence modulate the classical morphological features of disease. Elicit *dermatographism* (**Fig. 2.3**). Do *urinalysis*.

Table 2.3 Glossary of dermatological vocabulary

Macule	Small flat lesion	Fig. 2.4
Patch	Larger flattish lesions	Fig. 2.5
Papule	Small raised palpable lesion	Fig. 2.6
Micropapule	Tiny palpable lesions	Fig. 2.7
Nodule	Large raised palpable lesion	Figs 2.8, 2.9
Plaque	Raised thick flattish bulky lesion	Fig. 2.10
Vesicle	Small fluid-filled lesion	Fig. 2.11
Pustule	Small pus-filled lesion	Fig. 2.11
Erosion	Shallow breach of surface: denuded epithelium only	Fig. 2.11
Bulla	Large fluid-filled lesion	Fig. 2.12
Ulcer	Full thickness breach of surface: epithelial loss and dermal involvement	Fig. 2.13
Cyst	Papule or nodule with a lining and contents	Fig. 2.14
Scar	Replacement of skin with fibrous tissue	Figs 2.15, 2.24
Atrophy	Loss of skin substance	Fig. 2.16
Purpura	Small (macular or papular) cutaneous hemorrhage	Fig. 2.16
Ecchymosis	Larger area of cutaneous hemorrhage	Fig. 2.16
Erythema	Redness	Figs 2.17, 2.29
Erythroplakia/ erythroplasia	Red patches or plaques with connotations of dysplasia or neoplasia	Fig. 2.18
Leucoderma	White patch or plaque	Fig. 2.28
Leukoplakia	White patches or plaques with connotations of dysplasia or neoplasia	Fig. 2.18
Telangiectasia	Visible cutaneous microvessels because of dilatation	Fig. 2.19
Lichenification	Thickening – exaggerated skin markings (like tree bark)	Figs 2.20, 2.21
Phimosis	Foreskin unretractable	Figs 2.22, 2.23, 2.24
Paraphimosis	Foreskin fixed in retraction	Fig. 2.25
Waisting	Preputial sclerosis	Figs 2.26, 2.27

For the non-dermatologist a simple glossary of dermatological vocabulary is given in Table 2.3 (**Figs 2.4–2.28**).

Phimosis (**Figs 2.22, 2.23, 2.24**) refers to a non-retractable foreskin (phimosis = 'muzzling'). Rickwood et al (1980) has defined it as scarring of the tip of the foreskin. There are several possible causes of phimosis (**Table 2.4**). In adults acquired phimosis is probably usually the consequence of disease processes such as lichen sclerosus (see page 79), lichen planus (Itin et al 1992; Aste et al 1997), cicatricial pemphigoid (Ridley & Neill 1993) and hidradenitis (Chaikin et al 1994). I have seen a case where an aute complete phimosis was due to Kaposi's sarcoma in previously undiagnosed AIDS: the patient also had stridor from laryngeal involvement and needed emergency tracheostomy as well as circumcision (Morris-Jones et al 2000). It has been ascribed to titanium formulated in proprietary skin topicals (Dundas & Laing 1988).

Phimosis may complicate scarring following sexually transmitted infections if there has been a significant

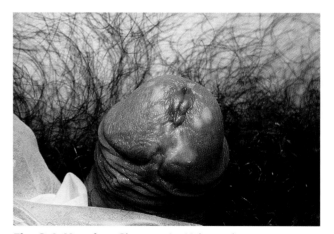

Fig. 2.4 Macules. Glans penis. Lichen sclerosus.

posthitis e.g. due to *Trichomonas* (Michalowski 1981) and herpes.

Chopra et al (1982) reported that diabetes was diagnosed in 36% of men between 17 and 59 years of

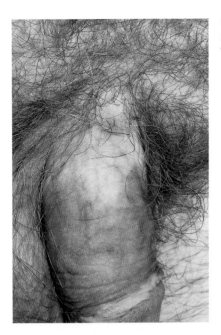

Fig. 2.5 Patch. Shaft penis. Vitiligo.

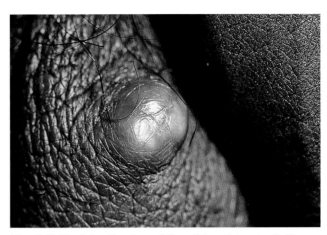

Fig. 2.8 Nodule. Scrotum. Idiopathic calcinosis. Solitary rock-hard lesion.

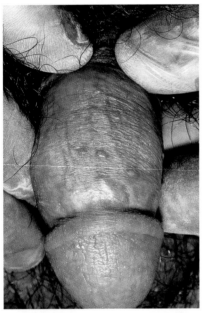

Fig. 2.6 Papules. Dorsal shaft penis. Viral warts.

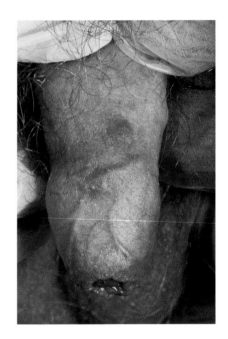

Fig. 2.9 Nodules. Shaft penis. Scabies.

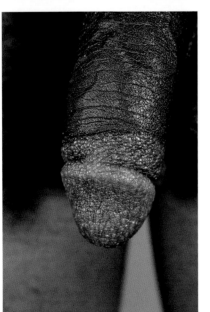

Fig. 2.7 Micro-papule. Tiny raised palpable lesions.

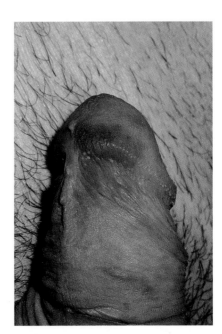

Fig. 2.10 Plaque. Penis, ventral coronal rim. Kaposi's sarcoma. (Courtesy of and reproduced from Bunker CB. Skin conditions on the male genitalia. Medicine 2001; 29: 7. By kind permission of the Medicine Publishing Company.)

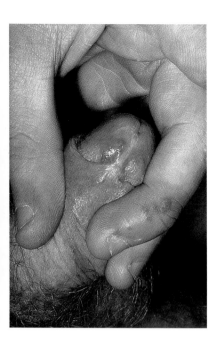

**Fig. 2.11
Erosion and
vesicopustules.**
Glans penis and
digits. Herpes
simplex (erosion
on glans and
vesicopustules on
fingers).
(Courtesy of
Dr Richard
Staughton,
London, UK).

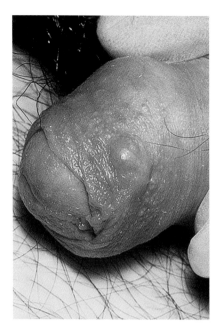

Fig. 2.14 Cyst.
The ventral penis.
Urethral/mucoid
cyst.

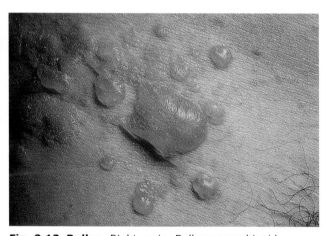

Fig. 2.12 Bullae. Right groin. Bullous pemphigoid.

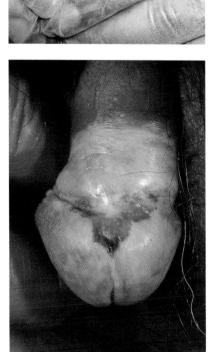

**Fig. 2.15
Scarring.** Ventral
glans penis and
coronal sulcus.
Lichen sclerosus.

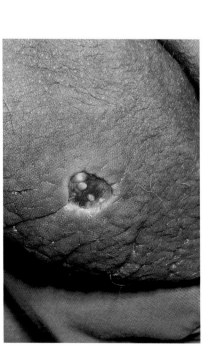

Fig. 2.13 Ulcer.
Scrotum.
Idiopathic or
trophic. Patient
with spina bifida
confined to a
wheelchair.

**Fig. 2.16
Atrophy
ecchymosis and
purpura.** Glans
penis. Lichen
sclerosus.
(Courtesy of
Dr Nick Soter,
New York, NY,
USA).

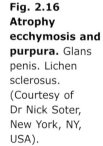

29

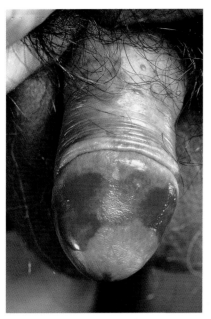

Fig. 2.17 Erythema. Glans penis. Zoon's balanitis.

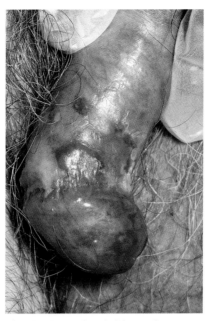

Fig. 2.18 Leukoplakia and erythroplasia (of Queyrat). Penile intraepithelial neoplasia. Glans and distal prepuce, penis. Widespread carcinoma in situ.

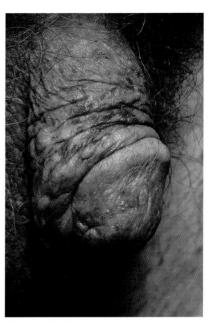

Fig. 2.19 Telangiectasia (also atrophy and hyperpigmentation – poikiloderma) and lymphedema. Glans and shaft, penis. Radiodermatitis.

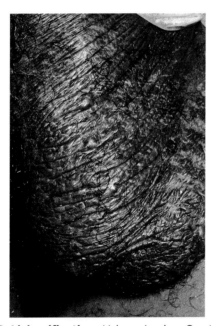

Fig. 2.20 Lichenification. Lichen simplex. Scrotum.

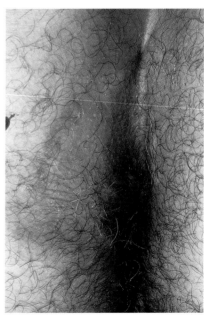

Fig. 2.21 Lichenification. Lichen simplex. Perianal skin.

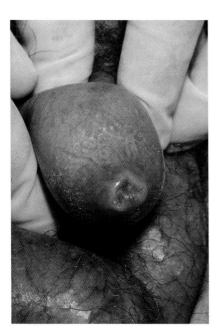

Fig. 2.22 Phimosis. Penis. Probable lichen sclerosus.

Table 2.4 Causes of phimosis

Congenital

Non-specific balanoposthitis (e.g. in diabetes)

Lichen sclerosus

Lichen planus

Hidradenitis suppurativa

Crohn's disease

Cicatricial pemphigoid

Chronic penile lymphedema

Sexually transmitted diseases

Kaposi's sarcoma

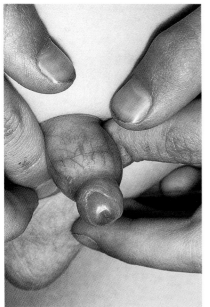

Fig. 2.23 Phimosis. Penis, infant. Circumcision was performed but histology was not obtained.

age presenting with phimosis of less than 2 years duration. On histology no specific preputial pathology was identified. In boys the histological findings may be normal in nearly half those circumcised (Clemmensen et al 1988).

Paraphimosis (**Fig. 2.25**) refers to a foreskin fixed in retraction. Although some authors have used the term to describe a foreskin that is tight in retraction around the flaccid penile shaft (**Figs. 2.26–2.27**), I call this '*waisting*'. Rickwood (1999) has said that paraphimosis results from abuse not disease of the foreskin but I believe that some medical causes can be identified (**Table 2.5**).

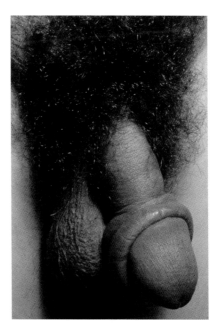

Fig. 2.25 Paraphimosis. Idiopathic.

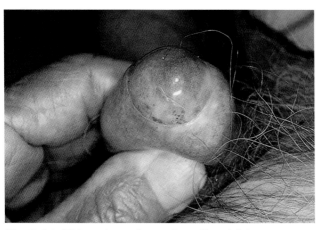

Fig. 2.24 Phimosis and scarring. Cicatricial pemphigoid. Three years after therapy. (Courtesy of Dr Brian Adams, Cincinnati, OH, USA and reproduced with permission from Fueston JC et al. Cicatricial pemphigoid-induced phimosis. J Am Acad Dermatol. 2002; 46(5 Suppl): S128–9 with kind permission of Mosby Inc.)

Table 2.5 Causes of paraphimosis

Acute contact urticaria

Acute allergic contact dermatitis

Lichen sclerosus

Idiopathic

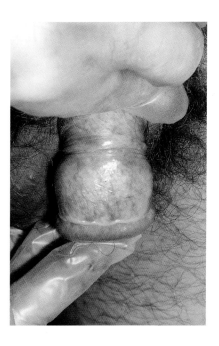

Fig. 2.26 Waisting. Penis, prepuce retracted. Paraphimosis incipient. Lichen sclerosus.

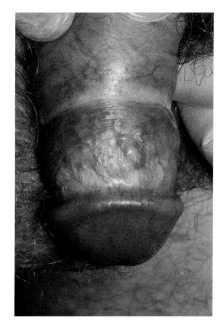

Fig. 2.27 Waisting. Prepuce. Posthitis with sclerotic band. Lichen sclerosus.

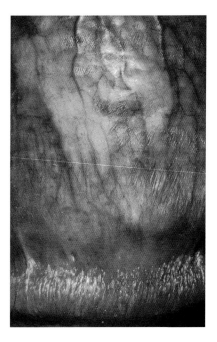

Fig. 2.28 Leukoderma. Distal penis shaft. Lichen sclerosus.

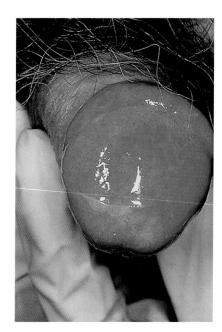

Fig. 2.29 Photography. Cicatricial pemphigoid. At presentation. (Courtesy of Dr Brian Adams, Cincinnati, OH, USA and reproduced with permission from Fueston JC et al. Cicatricial pemphigoid-induced phimosis. J Am Acad Dermatol. 2002; 46(5 Suppl): S128–9 with kind permission of Mosby Inc.)

Photography is an invaluable adjunct to the clinical process enabling *clinicopathological* correlation and follow-up and dialogue between physicians (**Fig. 2.29**).

The most commonly required special investigations are a *swab* or *smear* for microbiology or virology, *scrapings* for fungal microscopy and culture, scrapings for mite identification, and *skin biopsy*. Dermatologists enjoy exhibiting *Wood's light* (a source of ultraviolet light at 360nm) because it is very helpful in the clinical diagnosis of vitiligo (**Fig. 2.30**; see also page 51), erythrasma (**Fig. 2.31**; see also Fig. 7.75) and fungal infections and rarely porphyria. Occasionally, blood tests or imaging are indicated.

Deliberately, those investigations pertinent to the evaluation of sexually transmitted diseases are not discussed further but it is worth emphasizing that if a diagnosis of a potentially sexually transmitted disease is reached (warts, mollusca, herpes simplex, scabies, pediculosis, etc.) then the patient should be referred for a genitourinary opinion and advised to inform his partner(s) so that they may be screened.

It is widely and erroneously supposed that a *skin swab* for microbiology is useless unless the skin is wet, broken or pustular. Dipping the swab in the transport medium before wiping it over the surface of the skin is recommended, for example where *cellulitis* (**Fig. 2.32**) is suspected. Make sure that you understand your local

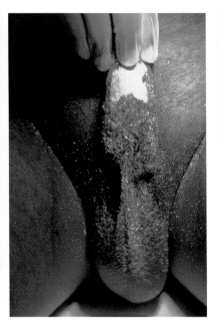

Fig. 2.30 Wood's Light. Vitiligo. Ventral penis shaft. Note also coral-pink fluorescence of concomitant erythrasma. See also Fig. 4.14, page 51.

laboratories' requirements for samples for *virological* diagnosis and then be forearmed with the necessary swabs, media and slides.

Scrapings from the skin for *mycological* purposes should be obtained with a flat linear pre-blunted blade. With practice they can be examined directly. Whilst a portion is sent to the laboratory (preferably between black paper and thin transparent plastic) some scale can be smeared on a slide under a coverslip and a few drops of warm potassium hydroxide solution (10–30%) used for several minutes to clear the keratin from the specimen allowing the microscopic identification of fungal elements (**Figs 2.33, 2.34**). Most microbiology laboratories also provide this service as well as putting the specimen down to culture for four weeks.

A more important skill for the dermatologist to acquire is the clinical (Latin: at the bedside) *demonstration of the scabies mite*. In a good bright artificial light (wearing gloves and with a hand lens) identify a suitable lesion, preferably a burrow rather than a papule and certainly

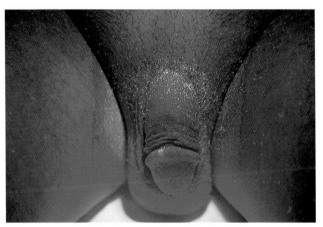

Fig. 2.31 Wood's Light. Erythrasma. Groins.

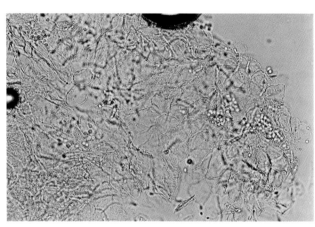

Fig. 2.33 Potassium hydroxide preparations. Superficial skin scrapings from pityriasis versicolor demonstrating yeast and short mycelial forms. (Reproduced with permission from Sobera JO, Elewski BE, Fungal Diseases. In: Bolognia JL, Jorizzo JL, Rapini RP, eds. Dermatology. London: Mosby; 2003: 1171–98.)

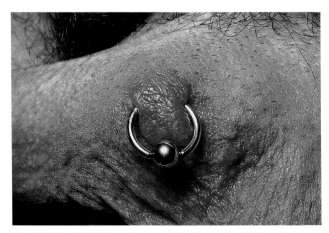

Fig. 2.32 Cellulitis. Proximal shaft, penis. Infected piercing site.

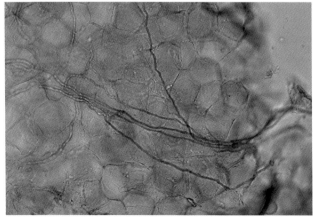

Fig. 2.34 Potassium hydroxide preparations. A dermatophyte, in this case *T. tonsurans,* demonstrating branching hyphae.

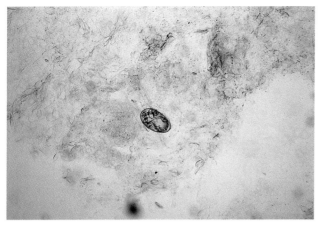

Fig. 2.35 Scabies. Egg ready to hatch. Low power.

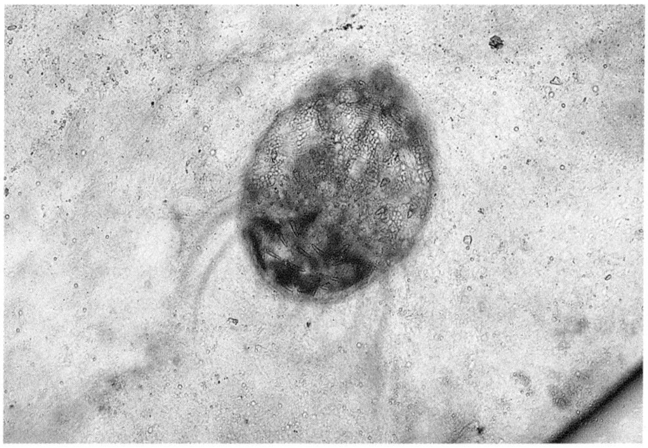

Fig. 2.36 Scabies. Mature mite. High power.

not a nodule. Align the skin plane parallel to the floor. Apply a drop of potassium hydroxide solution (5%) and wait one minute. Hold a pre-blunted scalpel blade perpendicular to the lesion and with one purposeful, but not incisive, scrape, deroof the whole lesion and smear the entire specimen onto a slide to view for mites, eggs and mite parts (**Figs 2.35, 2.36**). Screen the field first at low power.

In genitourinary clinics, application of 3–5% *acetic acid* to the penis is used as an aid to the clinical diagnosis of viral warts and is held to reveal subclinical infection (Steinberg et al 1993). It is not in routine use in dermatological practice, nor my clinic. HPV PCR screening suggests that the acetowhite test is not very specific (Wikström et al 1992; Mazzatenta et al 1993; Voog et al 1997).

A *skin biopsy* is highly informative under selected, advantageous, clinical conditions. Every endeavor should be made to obtain the right specimen from the right site at the right time and to provide the pathologist with the right information and to ask of him the right question(s) (Mallon et al 1997). A regular meeting with your pathologist constitutes 'best practice'.

Some advice follows. It is safe to use small amounts (1:200,000) of adrenaline and then at least you can see what you are doing: the region, especially the penis, is highly vascular. A punch biopsy is not always acceptable even though very convenient. Know your anatomy: neither go too deep or too shallow. Beware the ventral midline structures or where the urethra is perilously close to the surface. It is often not necessary to suture a punch biopsy site. My preference is for fine silk sutures left in for just a few days although increasingly I am using the fine synthetic monofilament, Novafil ®; urologists prefer absorbable sutures. The penis, including the glans, heals very well. **Figures 2.37–2.44** illustrate the punch biopsy procedure performed on the glans penis.

Fill in the request form and label the specimen *yourself*. Give as much information about site and diagnostic considerations as is demanded and as you can. If you want

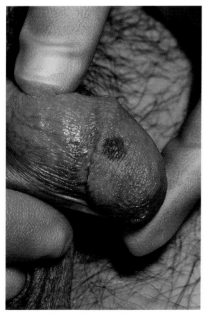

Fig. 2.37 Lesion for biopsy. Glans penis.

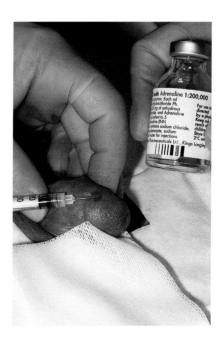

Fig. 2.38 Punch biopsy. A tiny bleb of local anesthetic (2% Xylocaine with adrenaline 1:200 000) is introduced under the skin with an insulin syringe.

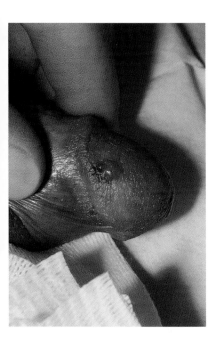

Fig. 2.39 Punch biopsy. Bleb of anesthetic visible.

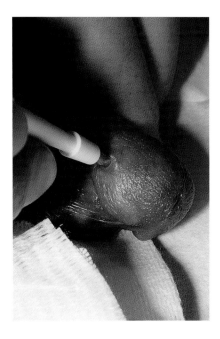

Fig. 2.40 Punch biopsy. A 4mm disposable punch tool is used to incise the skin. A gentle firm rotational technique is used.

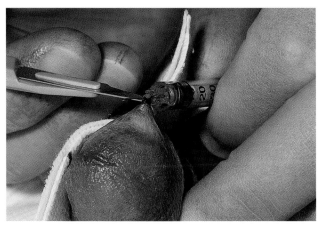

Fig. 2.41 Punch biopsy. The specimen is elevated above the biopsy site by inserting the anesthetic needle through it, horizontal to the skin. The base of the specimen is then cut free from the skin with a scalpel.

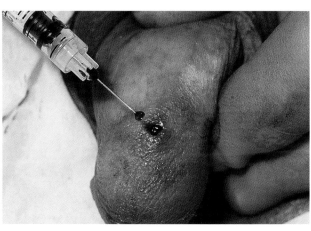

Fig. 2.42 Punch biopsy. Specimen on needle, above the wound.

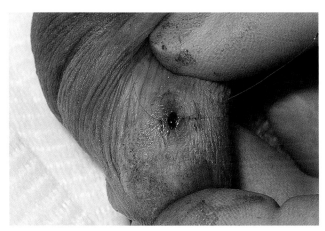

Fig. 2.43 Punch biopsy. Suturing with a 6.0 synthetic suture Novafil ®. The shaft and prepuce do not usually require suturing after a 4mm punch biopsy procedure.

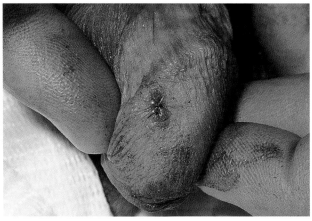

Fig. 2.44 Punch biopsy. Suture in situ. It can be removed after five to six days.

special stains or studies, make sure that you have taken the right size of sample so that it can be divided (or take several samples) and be sure (check with the laboratory) that you have used the correct transport medium (especially if you want *direct immunofluorescence*). Biopsy should *not* be regarded as a substitute for *clinical* diagnosis. **Figure** 2.45 shows the psoriasiform histology of circinate balanitis.

Diagnostic imaging of the penis, scrotum and perineum by ultrasonography or MR can be very helpful under some circumstances (Pretorius et al 2001).

Finally, ask the question: 'does my patient require the additional, complementary or exclusive expertise of another colleague, whether genitourinary physician, urologist, colorectal surgeon, pediatrician, psychiatrist or plastic surgeon?'

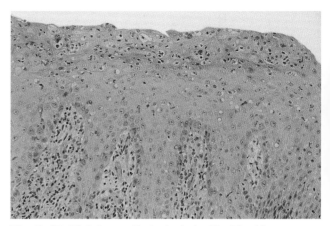

Fig. 2.45 Histology. Circinate balanitis. The biopsy shows epidermal hyperplasia with a psoriasiform pattern of broad and focally clubbed rete ridges with underlying chronic inflammation. Acute inflammatory cells are within the superficial keratin and epidermal layers with the papillary parts of the rete pegs showing chronic inflammation and vascular ectasia. Neutrophils are present within the surface. H&E. (Courtesy of Dr Nick Francis, London, UK).

3 Pruritus

Pruritus (itch) is a cardinal feature of skin disease. Its causes, mediation and central perception are complex. There is a cutaneous nocifensor system of cells, nerves, vessels and mediators that serves basic reflex defense mechanisms against injury (**Fig. 3.1**). Itch is a sensory modality that is centrally perceived when there is activity in this system whereas some of the classical physical signs of inflammation are visible expressions. The wheal-and-flare triple response of Lewis is the simplest and best-known example of the function of part of the nocifensor system.

The response to the sensation of itch is to scratch or to rub (grattage) and both these actions cause skin morbidity in the form of excoriations (often with secondary infection – *impetiginization*) and/or *lichenification* (thickening, with exaggeration of the markings of the skin appearing like the bark of a tree). Lichenification may be a manifestation of an eczematous process, as in atopic dermatitis and is in itself pruritic, so as a response to scratching it contributes to a vicious cycle of symptomatology.

Epidermal neuronal sprig
Langerhans' cell
Basal keratinocyte
Endothelial cell
Papillary capillary loop
Beaded neuro peptide containing neurones
Mast cell
Dermal venule
Dermal arteriole

Fig. 3.1 Cutaneous nocifensor system. (After Bunker et al, 1990).

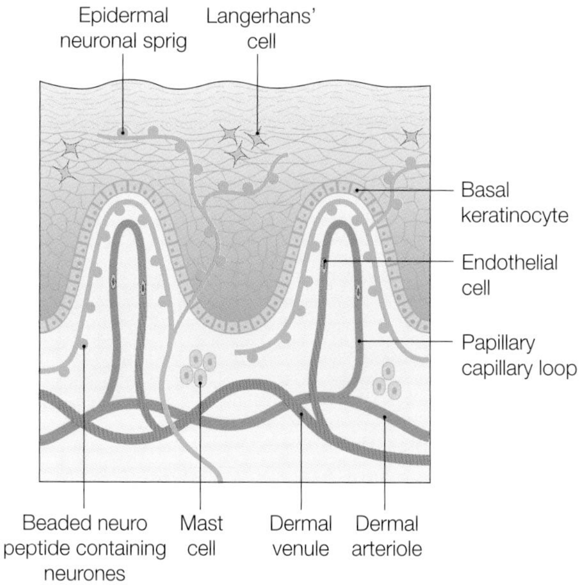

The important pruritic skin diseases that may affect the anogenital region are listed in **Table 3.1**. Itch occurring in the absence of specific diagnostic skin lesions is not usually confined to the area but if so it should not be labeled as psychogenic until all possible causes have been excluded. Generalized pruritus (without an apparent primary cutaneous diagnosis) evokes a catechism of general medical diagnoses and screening investigations beyond the scope of this book (**Table 3.2**).

The intensity with which itch is sometimes perceived in the anogenital area may be a reflection of the development of disproportionate cortical representation of sensory input from the region (see the homunculus in **Fig. 3.2**) but may also be part of more generalized

Hip
Leg
Trunk
Neck
Head
Shoulder
Arm
Elbow
Forearm
Wrist
Hand
Little
Ring
Middle
Index
Thumb
Eye
Nose
Face
Upper lip
Lips
Lower lip
Teeth, gums and jaw
Tongue
Pharynx
Intra-abdominal
Foot
Toes
Genitals

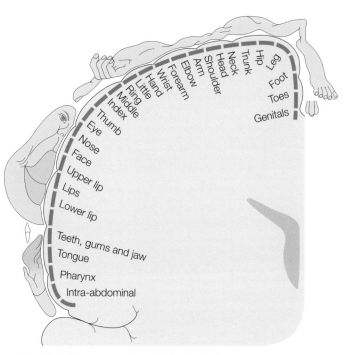

Fig. 3.2 Representation of the body in primary sensory and primary motor fields of the human cerebral cortex. (From: Penfield W, Rasmussen T. The cerebral cortex of man. Macmillan, New York: 1950).

Table 3.1 Causes of anogenital pruritus

Common causes	Rare causes
Pruritus ani	Insect bites/papular urticaria
Eczema/dermatitis	Radiodermatitis
Exogenous	Hirsutes
Contact	Hyperhidrosis
Irritant	Fox-Fordyce disease
Allergic	Urticaria and dermographism
Endogenous	Dermatitis herpetiformis
Atopic	Chlamydia
Seborrheic	Gonorrhea
Lichen simplex	Syphilis
Psoriasis	Other STDs
Lichen sclerosus	Trichosporosis
Lichen planus	Larva currens
Perianal streptococcal	Cutaneous larva migrans
dermatitis	Onchocerciasis (in Western
Erythrasma	practice)
Herpes simplex	Bowen's disease
Candidosis	Extramammary Paget's
Tinea	disease
Onchocerciasis (in the	Langerhans cell histiocytosis
Third World)	Drugs
Pediculosis	Foods
Scabies	Milk products (e.g. yoghurt)
	Coffee
	Tea
	Chocolate
	Tomatoes
	Senile pruritus
	Dysesthesia

Table 3.2 Causes of genital itching in the absence of clinical findings

Symptomatic dermatographism

Contact urticaria
  non-immunological (e.g. mechanical friction of pubic hair, topical substances)
  immunological (latex, body fluids)

Contact dermatitis

Incognito disease
  Psoriasis
  Candidosis
  Scabies

Drugs and foods

Senile pruritus

Delusions of parasitosis

Dermatological non-disease

Dysesthesia

Psychosexual

(after Sherertz 1994)

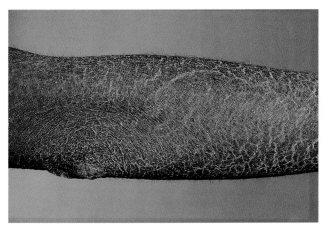

Fig. 3.3 Congenital ichthyosis. Arm.

somatization where there is anxiety about sexual exposure to venereal disease and anogenital cleanliness.

Itching and lichenification particularly around the scrotum and anus are common presenting problems. Twenty percent of the population are atopic by some definitions (e.g. personal or first-degree relative with history of asthma, eczema or hay fever) and this predisposition goes hand in hand with a tendency to itchy, dry, scaly skin called *xerosis* when mild and *ichthyosis* (usually congenital: **Fig. 3.3**) when severe. Two percent of people have psoriasis with a tendency to develop lesions at sites of mild trauma (Koebnerization). These and other diatheses may overlap. The phenotypic possibilities thus created constitute a spectrum of susceptibility to dermatological morbidity.

The chief exogenous mechanism is irritation and it may cause problems at vulnerable sites regardless of the phenotype. Irritation may be due to sweat, sebum, friction from adjacent skin, toilet paper and towels, desquamated corneocytes, dirt, excreta, a partner's sexual secretions, clothing, detergents, toiletries, cosmetics, contraceptives and some therapeutic topical treatments, compounded by friction and maceration and other common human afflictions such as piles, constipation and straining at stool, diarrhea and fecal soiling, urinary dribbling and so on. The present state of male human evolution does not help. We can blame an upright posture, having legs too close together, a dependent scrotum and genitalia, sedentary occupations, motorcar and airplane travel, tight underclothing and trousers.

Of all of these, the most frequently under-rated are over-washing and the over-use of soap and toiletries. Many people wash several times a day and use large quantities of soap on the skin particularly the anogenital areas, particularly if they have a skin disease or urinary or bowel problem and especially if they feel that they might have been exposed to a sexually transmitted disease. People wash their hair in the bath or shower and effectively immerse their skin in concentrated detergent or let it run down and pool in the natal cleft, around the anus, in the groins and under the foreskin. They do not rinse the skin properly and then use abrasive towels over-vigorously.

Patients will bathe themselves or douche themselves or treat themselves with the most extraordinary range of bath additives, shower gels, skin moisturizers, disinfectants, antipruritics, toners, conditioners, vitamins, powders, etc., reserving an especial double dose for the most sensitive skin of all, in and around the perineum and genitalia. It is surprising that the whole Western world does not have xerosis and eczema and it is not difficult to see why they are so common.

PRURITUS ANI

Pruritus ani (Smith et al 1982; Alexander-Williams 1983; Jones 1992; Rohde 2000) is more common in males than in females. It is important to remember that it is a *symptom* not a diagnosis unless qualified as constitutional (Verbov 1984) or idiopathic. Roughly one half of patients with pruritus ani will have a cause after dermatological evaluation (Verbov 1984).

Idiopathic pruritus ani is said to be related to stress and anxiety, high pressure and sedentary jobs. The itch may be triggered by a bowel movement or wiping with toilet paper but often occurs at night, waking the patient from sleep. Feces are themselves irritant and may generate perianal itch (Kocsard 1981). Lichenification, excoriation and secondary bacterial and candidal infection can supervene (**Fig. 3.4**).

It may be related to anal leakage due to coexisting anal disease or an exaggerated rectoanal inhibitory reflex (Allan et al 1987) and anal sphincter dysfunction (Eyers & Thomson 1979) or be precipitated by broad-spectrum antibiotics and diarrhea. Hypertrophy of anal

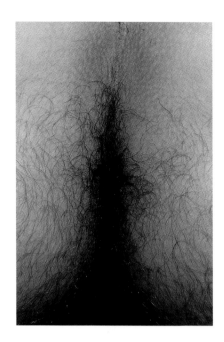

Fig. 3.5 Psoriasis. Natal cleft. Patient with pruritus ani.

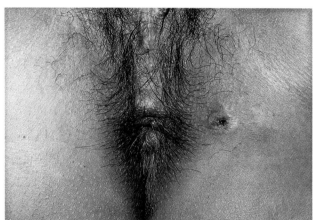

Fig. 3.6 Anal fistula. (Courtesy of Prof. Tim Allen-Mersh, London, UK)

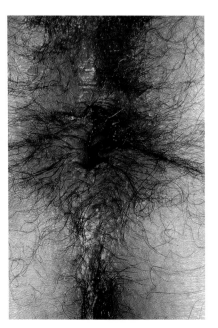

Fig. 3.4 Lichen simplex. Perianal skin.

papillae is probably not relevant (Jensen et al 1988). Whatever, many patients have a dermatosis and some will have irritant contact dermatitis (see page 60) and some patients will have an allergic contact hypersensitivity (see page 62) demonstrated by patch testing (Dasan et al 1999; Bauer et al 2000).

It is important to exclude staphylococcal infection, folliculitis, erythrasma (Bowyer & McColl 1971), candida, tinea, warts and thread/pinworms (*Enterobius vermicularis*) and establish whether there are other underlying skin diseases such as psoriasis (Farber & Nall 1992, **Fig. 3.5**), atopic dermatitis, lichen planus, lichen sclerosus or extramammary Paget's disease (Jensen et al 1988). Patch testing may be important to exclude sensitivity to lanolin, medicaments, rubber, perfumed paper, etc. (see page 62).

Longstanding pruritus ani should raise the suspicion of anorectal and proximal colonic disease so proctoscopy and sigmoidoscopy are mandatory. Anal fistulae (**Fig. 3.6**) are particularly prevalent in chronic pruritus ani (Petros et al 1993). But Verbov (1984) emphasizes that the majority of patients with piles, skin tags, fissures, warts, diarrhea or fecal soiling do *not* itch. Systemic diseases that may predispose to pruritus ani include lymphoma, pellagra, hypovitaminosis A and D and diabetes mellitus.

The patient's washing habits should be explored minutely. Soap is replaced with a suitable substitute and a moisturizer prescribed. Washing in a bidet is preferable to wiping with toilet paper if possible, after defecation. Pre-moistened toilet papers should be avoided because of the potential irritancy of the moisturizing agent, which may be alcohol, and the risk of developing allergic sensitivity to fragrance or preservative components. Some authorities recommend talcum powder after each wash but a moisturizer may suffice. The use of a topical corticosteroid/antibiotic/antifungal preparation is useful for acute episodes. Coffee consumption might be curtailed (Veien et al 1987). Other foodstuffs could be eliminated (Smith et al, 1982), such as yoghurt (Aki, 1992).

Patients are best advised not to use topical anesthetics (Allenby et al 1993 describe a spray of 0.2% hydrocortisone and 1% lignocaine) because they may become sensitized to their constituents (Handfield-Jones & Cronin 1993).

Therapeutic attention to concomitant proctological disorders (hemorrhoids, fissures, anal spasm and occult mucosal prolapse) is important, if found (Pirone et al 1992).

Other treatments that appear in the literature (Verbov 1984) include St. Mark's lotion, half-strength Castellani's paint, weak (0.05–0.25% silver nitrate solution [if wet]), cryotherapy, oral antihistamines, a 10-day tapering course of prednisolone, intralesional triamcinolone and intralesional methylene blue +/– marcaine/epinephrine/Xylocaine (Eusebio 1991).

Some authorities see a psychosexual significance in pruritus ani in men as has been debated in pruritus vulvae in women (Whitlock 1976). Patients need to be reassured that they do not have cancer (Smith et al 1982).

INSECT BITES

Itchy, papular, sometimes vesicular, lesions (with a punctum at the apex of each papule) are found in grouped or linear clusters. Perigenital lesions may occur (**Fig. 3.7**) often if the causative insect has been trapped in clothing or after sunbathing partly clad on grass or sand. The bites of blood-sucking insects are a common cause of morbidity (a pattern of widespread skin involvement is sometimes called papular urticaria) and may present a difficult diagnostic problem. Sometimes there may be secondary infection and post-inflammatory hyperpigmentation, especially severe in black skins. The differential diagnosis includes lice and scabies (see page

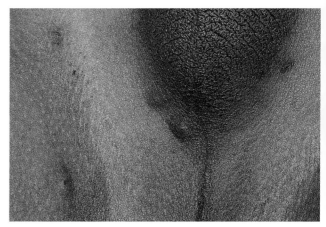

Fig. 3.7 Insect bites. Inguinoscrotal fold and thigh.

34), but it may not be the patient or his or her clothes that are infested, but rather furniture (e.g. bed bugs: *Cimex lectularius*), the house and pets (e.g. fleas: *Ctenocephalides felis*), or pets alone (e.g. sarcoptic mange: *Chyletiella* spp.).

The insecticide lindane, applied topically, may help the patient, but a priority is to establish the source of the bites. Examine the pet or the house, but leave their treatment to the veterinary surgeon or the Environmental Health Officer.

RADIODERMATITIS

This is not usually a diagnostic challenge or a therapeutic problem for the dermatologist in the acute stage after radiotherapy to the skin for skin disease or internal cancer. In the chronic state there may be pruritus; the signs amount to poikiloderma – atrophy, telangiectasia and hyperpigmentation (**Fig. 3.8**). Prior radiotherapy confers a long-term increased risk of skin cancer, especially basal cell carcinoma.

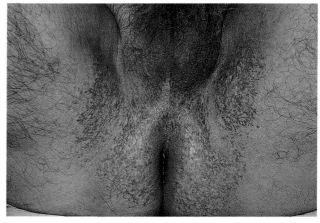

Fig. 3.8 Radiodermatitis. Thighs and perineum. This patient was treated with radiotherapy 50 years previously whilst in the army during World War II (reason unknown).

URTICARIA AND DERMATOGRAPHISM

These are usually generalized eruptions but the topic merits some discussion in this monograph because some focalized forms may occur and because an appreciation of the pathomechanisms and therapeutic approaches has resonance in anogenital dermatology.

Urticaria (hives) describes itchy, erythematous wheals (Fig. 3.9) lasting for a few hours. Urticaria is very common but several clinical types are recognized: common urticaria (acute: a few days, chronic: persisting for several months), angioedema, contact urticaria (immediate response to allergens such as foods: see pages 62 and Table 3.2), physical urticaria (lesions last several minutes, but less than one hour) e.g. dermatographism (in response to a scratch or trauma), cholinergic (in response to heat or exercise), cold urticaria, aquagenic urticaria, solar urticaria and finally urticarial vasculitis and hereditary angioneurotic angioedema.

Urticaria results from mast cell degranulation with the release of histamine and other vasoactive mediators that lead to erythema and edema. This process can affect subcutaneous tissues to cause angioedema. Usually the trigger mechanisms are unknown, but type I immunological mechanisms are thought to be involved. Urticarial vasculitis (5% of all urticarias) is conceived as a type III (serum sickness) immune complex condition: it is associated with systemics lupus erythematosus (SLE) and hepatitis B.

Most cases of chronic common urticaria are idiopathic. Other causes include: drugs: aspirin, codeine, morphine, nonsteroidal anti-inflammatory drugs; foods: fish and shellfish, eggs, nuts, tomatoes; additives: tartrazine, benzoates; inhalants: pollen, spores, house dust; infections: focal sepsis (e.g. urinary tract infection, upper respiratory tract infection, hepatitis, *Candida* spp., protozoa, helminths); systemic disease: systemic lupus erythematosus, reticuloses, carcinoma.

Diagnosis of the type of urticaria can be difficult and is largely based on careful history taking. About 70% of patients with urticaria have common urticaria. The differential diagnosis of urticaria includes insect bites (papular urticaria), the prodrome of pemphigoid, toxic erythema, erythema multiforme and allergic purpura.

If urticaria other than common urticaria is suspected, other investigations may be indicated, e.g. full blood count (FBC), eosinophil count and erythrocyte sedimentation rate (ESR), ANA, complement levels, hepatitis serology, histopathology if urticarial vasculitis is suspected (a leukocytoclastic vasculitis is seen), stool sample (for ova, cysts and parasites).

Counseling and reassurance are the mainstays of treatment. Primary or secondary psychological factors may be present. High doses of non-sedating anti-H1 histamines by day are supplemented by sedating antihistamines at night. The patient should be warned about drowsiness, alcohol and driving. Sometimes the addition of high doses of an anti-H2 agent such as cimetidine is helpful. Systemic steroids are avoided if possible. Angioneurotic edema requires specific treatment beyond the scope of this book. The treatment of urticarial vasculitis depends on the cause, but sometimes oral corticosteroids or other non-specific immunosuppressants are needed.

Dermographism (see above) is a form of physical urticaria where digital contact and pressure causes an itchy, urticarial wheal. It has been proposed that this may be the diagnosis in some patients with pruritus ani and unexplained genital itching (see below). Indeed, stroking could cause itching without any discernible redness or whealing. The importance of accepting these concepts comes in appreciating the need to inhibit the scratch reflex even when overt signs of scratching are absent (Sherertz 1994; Bernhard et al 1995).

THREAD/PINWORMS

Thread/pinworms that parasitize the lower gastrointestinal tract (*Enterobius vermicularis*) can cause pruritus ani. As Watt et al (1991) have pointed out, this is the most common parasite of humans worldwide (yet they have zero prevalence in an urban Australian population). It is prevalent in children in the developed world living in temperate climates as well as in tropical Third World areas. The life cycle of the nematode is such that eggs are released all at once by the female worm at the end of her life so that persistent infestation relies on autoinoculation by ingestion of eggs, which implies poor hygiene.

There may be few physical signs. Excoriations, eczematization and impetiginization may be seen, sometimes away from the site of infestation on the buttocks and upper thighs particularly in the younger child. Perianal abscess may occur very rarely (Mortensen & Thomson 1984).

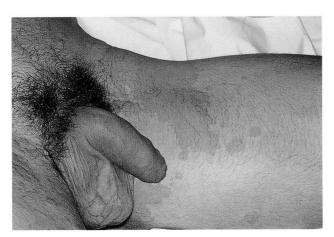

Fig. 3.9 Urticaria. Pelvic girdle and genitalia. Erythematous wheals.

LARVA CURRENS

Larva currens is the term given to the urticarial wheal and flare reaction due to the subcutaneous migration of larvae of the roundworm *Srongyloides stercoralis*, manifesting as linear or serpiginous tracks or papules anywhere on the skin (it is said between the nipples and the knees) but usually around the anus and on the buttocks. The larvae move at several centimeters an hour and the tracks or papules can disappear within a day, helping differentiate the eruption from cutaneous larva migrans. Acute infection is signaled by ground itch, usually of the feet. Gastrointestinal symptomatology is the pointer to chronic infection. Two-thirds of ex-prisoners of war with chronic strongyloidiasis had chronic urticaria and one-third had larva currens. There is an eosinophilia. Diagnosis is by demonstrating the larvae in the stool. Thiabendazole and albendazole are the drugs of choice.

CUTANEOUS LARVA MIGRANS

Cutaneous larva migrans is the name given to the 'creeping eruption' due to the migration in the skin of hookworm parasites of other animals, for which man is a dead-end host. The most common cause is the dog hookworm *Ancylostoma brasiliense* which is usually acquired from walking barefoot or sunbathing on bare sand above the tide-line on exotic holidays (although it is not rare in more temperate climates during warm summers). Ova from infected dogs are deposited with their feces. The larvae hatch and penetrate human skin often of the foot but also commonly around the pelvic girdle and perineum in the sunbathing scenario (**Fig. 3.10**).

An initial rash may be apparent but the larvae can remain quiescent for weeks or months before migrating

(a few millimeters per day) through the skin leaving *behind* them an extremely itchy, raised, linear, serpiginous and figurate, erythematous, sometimes vesicular (and excoriated and sometimes infected), raised papular eruption. Although self-limiting (several weeks or months), treatment with topical thiabendazole 10%, or oral albendazole 400mg/day for three days, or a single dose of ivermectin 12mg, is usually given because of the inordinate pruritus (Bryceson & Hay 1998).

PEDICULOSIS

Pediculosis pubis, phthiriasis or lice (crabs) can cause severe genital itching with little in the way of physical signs unless the hairs are examined very carefully for nits and the base of individual hairs scrutinized (**Figs 3.11, 3.12**) with a hand lens for the lice (*Phthirus pubis*) – 'crabs' (1–2mm in size) which will be tightly adherent to the skin because their mouth parts are embedded in perifollicular blood vessels. Sometimes gray-blue macules (tache bleu; maculae caerulea) are seen on the affected sites. There may be an itchy, non-specific, eczematous

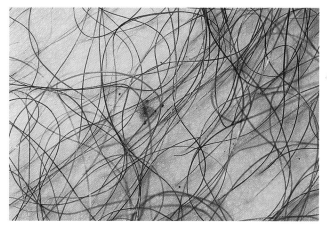

Fig. 3.11 Pediculosis. Pubic hairs. Crab louse (centre).

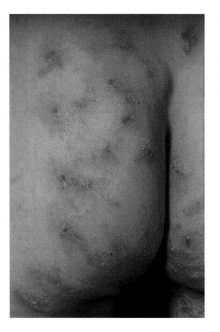

Fig. 3.10 Cutaneous larva migrans. Buttock. Serpiginous and linear raised and excoriated lesions.

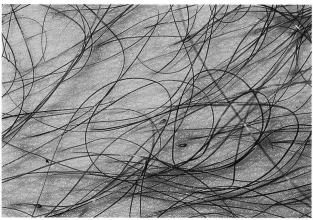

Fig. 3.12 Pediculosis. Pubic hairs. Nits.

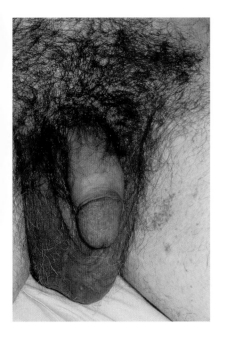

Fig. 3.13
Pediculosis.
Groin. Non-specific eczematous patches (same case as Figs 3.11 and 3.12).

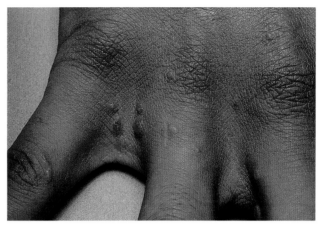

Fig. 3.15 Scabies. Hand. Interdigital linear papules and burrows.

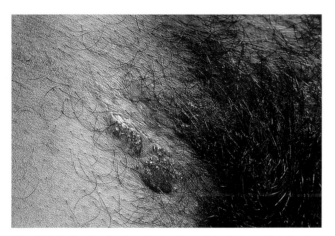

Fig. 3.14 Pediculosis. Groin. Excoriated, impetiginized plaques.

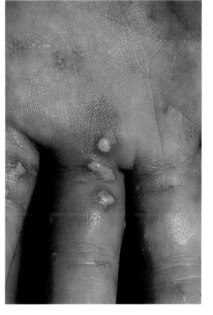

Fig. 3.16 Scabies. Hand. Infected vesicular lesions.

eruption (**Fig. 3.13**) with lichenification, excoriations and secondary impetiginization (**Fig. 3.14**). The pubic area is the site of infestation but in hairy men the abdomen, chest, axillae and thighs are also involved.

Treatment (Roos et al 2001) is with a topical pediculicide and often a topical corticosteroid/antibiotic combination. Screening for other sexually transmitted diseases should be offered to the patient and partner(s).

SCABIES

Scabies is common (Downs et al 1999). Itch is a predominant facet of infestation with the mite *Sarcoptes scabei*. It can be intense and characteristically keeps patients awake at night. Usually there is a rash of diagnostic distribution and morphology (**Figs 3.15–3.20**). Some patients with scabies who may have had it for a

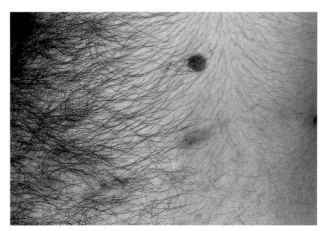

Fig. 3.17 Scabies. Upper groin, lower abdomen. Excoriated nodules.

43

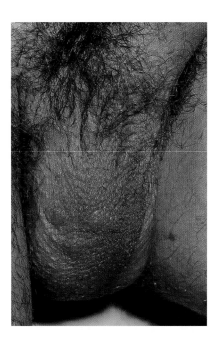

Fig. 3.18 Scabies. Scrotum. Nodules.

long time, or had it before, or been inadequately treated, or been treated adequately but become secondarily eczematized, or develop nodules (Ayres & Anderson 1932), may have itch in the anogenital region only. Such patients require careful and thoughtful assessment because primary or recurrent scabies is easily missed and because unnecessary anti-scabetic treatment can compound the problem due to the essential irritancy of the insecticides. Crusted or Norwegian scabies (Burns 1987) can also be missed (and is highly contagious). Lesions are psoriasiform or eczematous and the scale is teeming with mites (**Figs 3.21–3.24**; see also **Figs 2.14, 2.15** in Chapter 2).

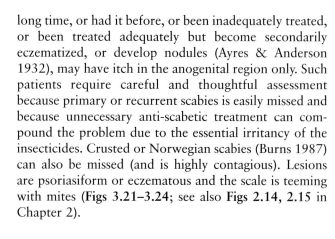

Fig. 3.21 Crusted/ Norwegian scabies. Glans penis hyperkeratotic psoriasiform eruption.

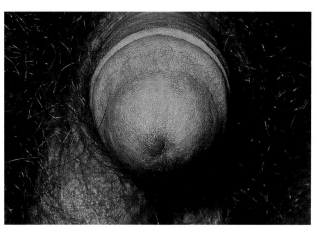

Fig. 3.19 Scabies. Penis. Perimeatal nodule.

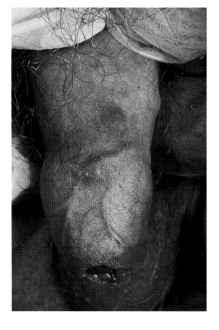

Fig. 3.20 Scabies. Shaft penis. Nodules.

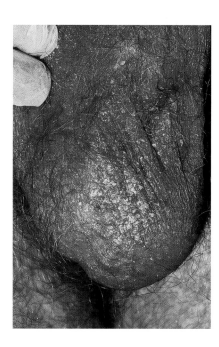

Fig. 3.22 Crusted/ Norwegian scabies. Scrotum. Psoriasiform eruption in HIV.

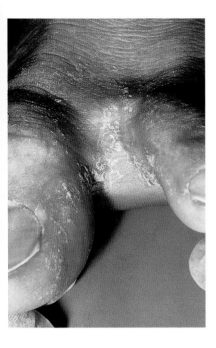

Fig. 3.23 Crusted/ Norwegian scabies. First toe web space. Tinea pedis-like eruption in HIV (same patient as Fig. 3.22).

Scabies is treated (Orkin & Maibach 1993; Roos et al 2001; Scott 2001; Walker & Johnstone 2002) with topical insecticides such as malathion (Hanna et al 1978; Wester et al 1983; Thianprasit & Schuetzenberger 1984), permethrin (Haustein & Hlawa 1989; Taplin et al 1990; Cox 2000; Usha & Gopalakrishnan Nair 2001), gamma benzene hexachloride (Haustein & Hlawa 1989), benzyl benzoate (Haustein & Hlawa 1989; Glaziou et al 1993), crotamiton (Konstantinov et al 1979; Taplin et al 1990) or carbaryl or systemic ivermectin (Glaziou et al 1993; Alberici et al 2000; Nnoruka & Agu 2001). Secondary eczematization and staphylococcal infection should be treated as necessary (Adjei & Brenya 1997). The patient must be told to advise partners and cohabitees to be treated contemporaneously. Screening for other sexually transmitted diseases is mandatory.

DERMATOLOGICAL NON-DISEASE AND DYSASTHESIA SYNDROMES

'Dermatological non-disease' (Cotteril 1980, 1981) may be the diagnosis where florid symptomatology is not commensurate with the absence or paucity of any primary dermatological signs. Genital symptoms include itching, excessive redness, burning and discomfort, in some cases so severe as to prevent the patient from sitting down. Dysmorphophobia, depression and psychosis may be present and attempted or completed suicide is a real risk in such patients.

Itching of the urethra can lead to insertion of a foreign body into the urethra in an attempt to relieve the sensation (Franzblau 1973; Al-Durazi et al 1992). Otherwise this might be done by patients or for sexual gratification (see page 175).

Penile sensitivity is reduced in diabetics and this may correlate with erectile dysfunction in some of these men (Morrissette et al 1999).

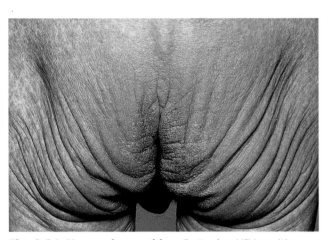

Fig. 3.24 Norwegian scabies. Buttocks. HIV-positive patient.

RED/BURNING SCROTUM SYNDROME

Patients with symptoms of itching, burning and pain focalized to the penis or scrotum are not uncommonly encountered (Markos 2002). The skin may be completely normal. The situation is analogous to vulvodynia in women and terms such as penodynia and scotodynia have emerged to describe the syndrome in men. Doxepin, amitriptyline and paroxetine can afford some relief.

Fisher (1997) has defined this syndrome as 'persistent redness of the anterior half of the scrotum that may involve the base of the penis ... usually accompanied by a persistent itching or burning sensation and hyperalgesia (**Figs 3.25, 3.26**). It is a chronic condition that is resistant to treatment and its cause is unknown' (Fisher 1997; Markos 2002). Accompanying the erythema there may be telangiectasia. It is related to idiopathic penile and scrotal pain syndromes (Wesselmann et al 1997, also see page 222). Prednisolone and antidepressants have given some relief to some patients.

Localized dermatographism (see above) should be sought by stroking the inside of the thigh (**Fig. 3.27**) because such patients may be helped by oral antihistamine treatment.

The possibilities of zinc deficiency (see page 105) and migratory necrolytic erythema (see page 143) should be considered.

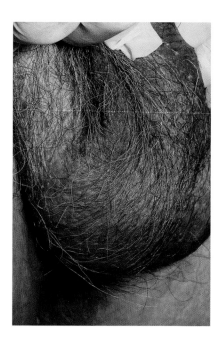

Fig. 3.26 Scrotal rosacea/burning scrotum syndrome. Scrotum. Normal appearance.

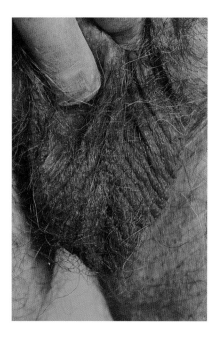

Fig. 3.25 Scrotal rosacea/burning scrotum syndrome. Scrotum. Erythema.

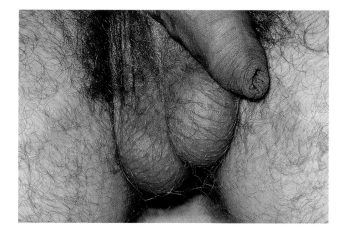

Fig. 3.27 Dermatographism. Thigh. Burning scrotum syndrome. Elicited by a firm downward stroke of the examiners thumbnail plate (not the free edge). Subtle streak (right greater than left thigh). Compare with Fig. 2.3.

4 Pigmentary change

The skin may become *hyperpigmented* because of the deposition of melanin, hemosiderin, amyloid, homogentisic acid (ochronosis in alkaptonuria or following topical hydroquinone usage) or drugs (antimalarials including quinidine, phenothiazine, cytotoxics, amiodarone, tetracycline especially minocycline, rifampacin, phenytoin, clofazimine and AZT), metals (silver, gold, arsenic, bismuth, mercury), other pigments (carotene, hemofuscin, in hemochromatosis alongside hemosiderin) or contact with dyes or bleaching agents containing hydroquinone.

Depigmentation of the skin (leukoderma) may be due to loss of melanin, vasoconstriction or loss of vasculature, sclerosis or scarring.

Causes of anogenital hypo- and hyperpigmentation are given in **Tables 4.1–4.3**.

Causes of post-inflammatory pigmentary change (hypo- and hyperpigmentation) are given in **Tables 4.4** and **4.5**. Causes of *purpura* are listed in **Table 4.6**.

Table 4.2 Causes of anogenital hyperpigmentation

Common causes	Rare causes
Tattoos	Addison's disease
Purpura	Nelson's syndrome
Hyperpigmentation of median raphe	Genital melanosis
	Laugier-Hunziger syndrome
Post-inflammatory hyperpigmentation	Peutz-Jeghers syndrome
	LAMB syndrome
Lentigines/melanosis	LEOPARD syndrome
Pseudo-acanthosis nigricans	Ruvalcaba-Myhre-Smith syndrome
	Acanthosis nigricans
	Acral lentiginous melanoma
	Drugs and metals

Table 4.1 Causes of anogenital hypopigmentation/leukoderma

Common causes	Rare causes
Bier's spots	Squamous hyperplasia
Striae	Paget's disease
Vitiligo	Mycosis fungoides
Post-inflammatory	Melanoma
Lichen sclerosus	
Viral warts	

Table 4.3 Causes of white patches and plaques

Post-traumatic or surgical scar

Lichen sclerosus

Vitiligo

Cicatricial pemphigoid

Peyronie's disease

Syphilis
  leucoderma — post-secondary syphilide
  gumma
  post-gummatous atrophic scar

Viral warts

Pityriasis versicolor

Pseudo-epitheliomatous micaceous and keratotic balanitis (PEMKB)

Table 4.4 Causes of anogenital post-inflammatory hypopigmentation

Post- cryotherapy
electrotherapy
chemocautery
laser surgery

Contact dermatitis
condom leukoderma

Lichen sclerosus

Systemic sclerosis

Lichen planus

Cicatricial pemphigoid

Gonococcal dermatitis

Leprosy

Syphilis
leucoderma – post-secondary syphilide
gumma
post-gummatous atrophic scar

Herpes simplex

Pityriasis versicolor

Onchocerciasis 'leopard skin'

Peyronie's disease

Pseudo-epitheliomatous micaceous and keratotic balanitis (PEMKB)

Table 4.5 Causes of anogenital post-inflammatory hyperpigmentation

Post-traumatic

Lichen planus

Herpes simplex

Fixed drug eruption

Table 4.6 Causes of purpura

Physical, e.g. suction

Zoon's balanitis

Lichen sclerosus

Henoch Schonlein purpura

TATTOOS

Tattoos are occasionally encountered in the anogenital regions (Goldstein 1979).

POST-INFLAMMATORY HYPO- AND HYPERPIGMENTATION

Both patterns of pigmentary change are possible after acute inflammation from diverse causes and both can contribute to the constellation of physical signs observed in chronic inflammatory pathological processes in the skin. These changes usually appear more pronounced in genetically darker skin.

Lichen planus (**Figs 4.1–4.3**, also see page 100), fixed drug eruptions (see page 123) and recurrent herpes simplex (see page 164) are particularly potent at leaving post-inflammatory *hyper*pigmentation (**Fig. 4.4**) which does occasionally complicate lichen sclerosus (**Fig. 4.5**, see page 100). Genital trauma as from a zipper injury can lead to macular pseudo-lentiginous lesions on the glans and shaft of the penis.

Lichen sclerosus and recurrent herpes simplex are the most common causes of post-inflammatory *hypo*-pigmentation. I have seen it with lichen planus (**Fig. 4.6**). Fisher (1989b) describes a man who developed leukoderma of the tip of the penis due to monobenzyl ether hydroquinone (a well-known depigmenting agent) in the condoms he had been using. A post-gonococcal irritant dermatitis of the glans with consequent occurrence of multiple macules of hypopigmentation has been described (Abdul Gaffoor 1983). Pityriasis versicolor (see page 107) due to an aberrant reaction to *Pityrosporum*

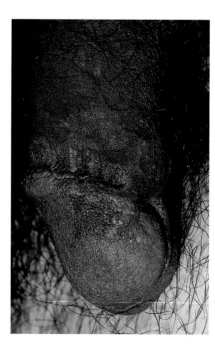

Fig. 4.1 Post-inflammatory hyperpigmentation Glans and distal shaft, penis.

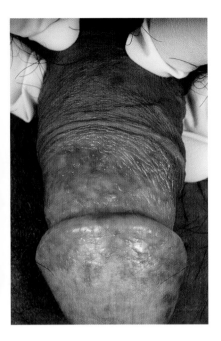

Fig. 4.2 Lichen planus. Glans penis. Post-inflammatory hyperpigmentation.

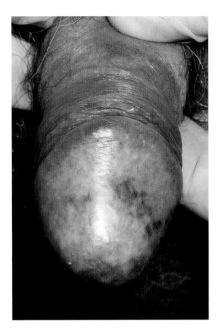

Fig. 4.5 Lichen sclerosus. Glans and distal shaft, penis. Balanitis xerotica, macular post-inflammatory hyperpigmentation, florid lichenoid posthitis.

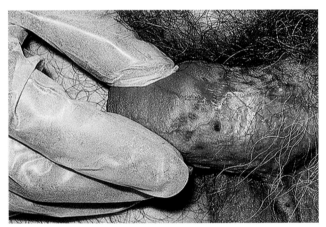

Fig. 4.3 Lichen planus. Lateral penis shaft. Eroded patch and post-inflammatory hyperpigmentation.

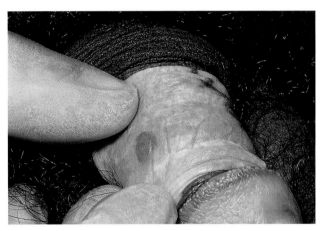

Fig. 4.6 Lichen planus. Post-inflammatory hypopigmentation. Distal prepuce, penis. Lichenoid inflammation with an island of sparing.

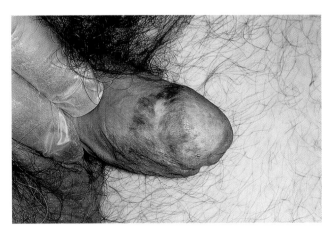

Fig. 4.4 Lichen sclerosus. Post-inflammatory hyperpigmentation. Glans and distal shaft, penis.

ovale can cause hypopigmented scaly macules on the shaft of the penis (**Fig. 4.7**) but, if ever, more often as part of the more widespread corporeal eruption (Aljabre & Sheikh 1994) or a localized anterior pelvic girdle presentation (**Fig. 4.8**). Onchocerciasis (see page 184) can cause hypopigmented spots (leopard skin) usually of the shins but sometimes the scrotum (Akogun et al 1992).

Proposed mechanisms for post-inflammatory pigmentary change include melanocyte damage or loss, pigment spillage and melanocyte stimulation by cells, cytokines or hormones: melanocyte-stimulating hormone (MSH) can be elaborated by cutaneous cells. In lichen sclerosus (see page 81) it has been argued that the leucoderma is due to loss of vasculature rather than hypopigmentation but there is also dermal sclerosis, melanocyte loss and decreased keratinocyte melanization

49

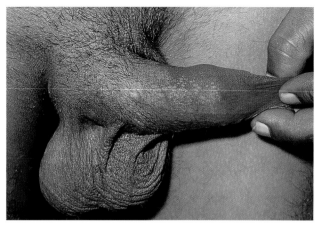

Fig. 4.7 Pityriasis versicolor. Lateral shaft penis. (Courtesy of Prof. Bhushan Kumar, Chandigarh, India).

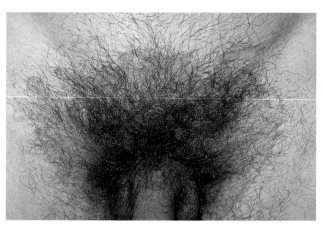

Fig. 4.8 Pityriasis versicolor. Pubis and groins. (Courtesy of Dr Nick Soter, New York, NY, USA).

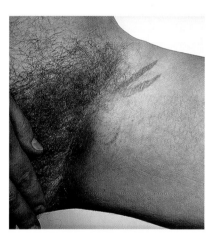

Fig. 4.9 Striae (post-steroidal). Groin. Livid, purple pre-atrophic phase.

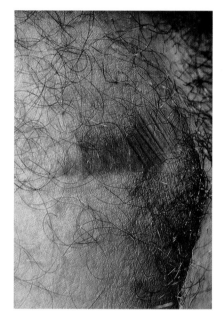

Fig. 4.10 Striae (post-steroidal). Groin. Livid, purple pre-atrophic phase.

(Carlson et al 2002). In onchocerciasis (see page 184) the hypopigmentation is associated with epidermal atrophy and loss of dermal collagen and may be directly related to the bites of the *Simulium* flies and scratching (McMahon & Simonsen 1996).

STRIAE

Striae in the skin are usually due to growth or weight surges or represent an adverse effect of topical corticosteroid application. Initially they are often a purple erythematous hue (**Figs 4.9, 4.10**) before permanent off-white atrophy ensues: such white atrophic striae have been reported on the penis following topical corticosteroid usage (Stankler 1982).

VITILIGO

Vitiligo is consequent upon loss of melanocytes probably due to autoimmune destruction. The genitalia are very commonly affected in men (**Figs 4.11–4.14**), although clinicians might not always notice. It is quite usual for the genitalia to be the only site to be involved (Moss & Stevenson 1981). Perianal involvement is also common (**Fig. 4.15**). Examination with Wood's light (see **Fig. 2.30** in Chapter 2) vividly demonstrates the contrast between the normal and pigmented skin and in the Caucasian allows precise determination of the extent of the disease because the pigment loss may not be obvious at some lightly pigmented sites.

Vitiligo may be one aspect of a tendency to other organ-specific autoimmune diseases such as alopecia areata, halo nevus, lichen sclerosus, pernicious anemia, diabetes mellitus, Addison's disease and thyroid disease.

There are no effective treatments for vitiligo. Topical corticosteroids may arrest the progression of the disease in an active phase. Although PUVA (photosensitization of the skin with psoralens followed by ultraviolet A phototherapy) may help some patients with widespread

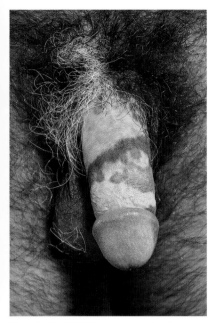

Fig. 4.11 Vitiligo. Penis shaft.

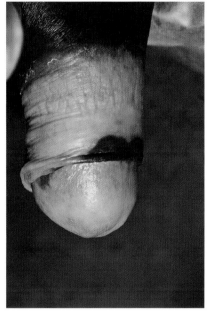

Fig. 4.12 Vitiligo. Penis prepuce and shaft. Black skin.

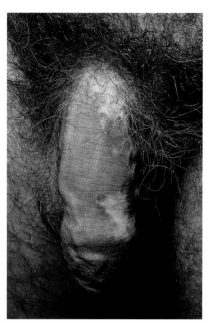

Fig. 4.13 Vitiligo. Penis shaft.

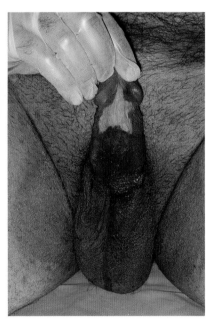

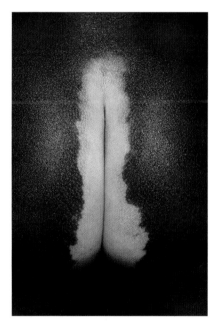

Fig. 4.14 Vitiligo. Ventral penis shaft. Patient also has erythrasma of groins. Same case as Fig. 2.30.

Fig. 4.15 Vitiligo. Buttocks.

disease this cannot really be contemplated for genital vitiligo because some patients treated with PUVA for psoriasis have developed genital skin cancer (Stern et al 1979, 1984, 1990) and one patient treated for vitiligo has developed penile squamous carcinoma. Now, PUVA patients have their genitalia shielded during treatment.

LEUKOPLAKIA

A white patch or plaque (see **Table 4.3**) is sometimes called leukoplakia. It is not, therefore, in itself, a diagnostic term.

Additionally, it is unhelpful in evoking connotations from oral medicine of pre-malignancy or even frank neoplasia.

ADDISON'S DISEASE AND NELSON'S SYNDROME

In Addison's disease and Nelson's syndrome (post-adrenalectomy for Cushing's disease) hyperpigmentation (due to high adrenocorticotrophic hormone levels) is seen on the mucosae, in skin creases and in scars.

PENILE MELANOSIS

Pigmented macules can appear on the glans (**Figs 4.16**, **4.17**) and shaft (**Fig. 4.18**) of the penis (Kaporis & Lynfeld 1998). They are benign but occasionally, because they may be large or enlarging with irregular edges and multifocal and variegated pigmentary patterns, there is concern about atypical melanocytic proliferation and acral lentiginous melanoma under which circumstances they should be biopsied (Kopf & Bart 1982). Some cases have been associated with previous treatment with anthralin or PUVA (Rhodes et al 1983) therapy for psoriasis or diabetes (Barnhill et al 1990). Post-inflammatory changes from prior lichen planus or lichen sclerosus (see **Fig. 4.5** above) may be misdiagnosed as penile melanosis. On histology there may be increased basal epidermal pigmentation with or without benign lentiginous melanocytic hyperplasia and an increase in basal melanocyte number. Breathnach et al (1992) have stated that *depigmentation* is an essential element of the condition and shown that ultra-structurally there may be melanocytic hyperplasia.

Three striking cases (**Figs 4.19–4.21**) have been published where the clinical appearances were extreme with tan to black, retiform macular lesions clinically

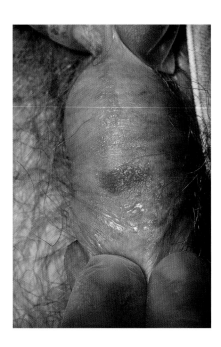

Fig. 4.18 Penile melanosis. Shaft penis.

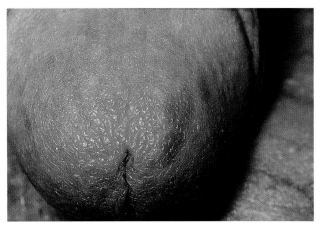

Fig. 4.16 Penile melanosis. Glans penis. Tan macules.

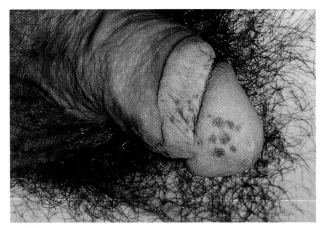

Fig. 4.17 Penile melanosis. Glans penis.

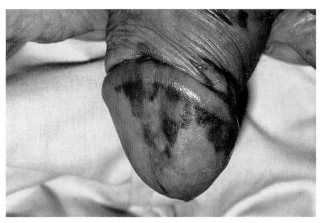

Fig. 4.19 Atypical pigmented penile macules. Glans and distal shaft, penis. Present and unchanging for 50 years, preceded by 'traumatic event'. (Courtesy of Dr. Stuart Leicht, Johnson City, TN, USA).

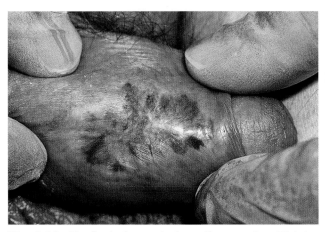

Fig. 4.20 Atypical pigmented penile macules. Distal lateral shaft, penis. Present five years and enlarging. (Courtesy of Dr. Stuart Leicht, Johnson City, TN, USA).

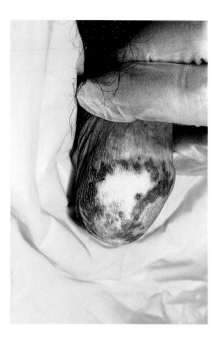

Fig. 4.21 Atypical pigmented penile macules. Glans penis. Present five years and enlarging. (Courtesy of Dr. Stuart Leicht, Johnson City, TN, USA).

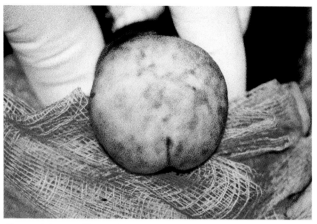

Fig. 4.23 Penile melanosis. Post-treatment with Q-switched ruby laser. Same patient as Fig. 4.22 (Courtesy of Dr. Neil Walker, London, UK).

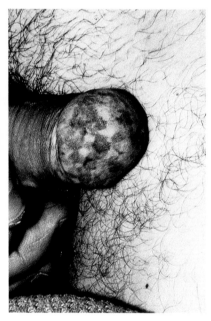

Fig. 4.22 Penile melanosis. Glans penis. Caucasian 28 years old. Shares clinical and histological features with Laugier-Hunziker syndrome. (Courtesy of Drs Neil Walker and Richard Staughton, London, UK, and reproduced by kind permission of Blackwell Science Ltd from Delaney TA, Walker NP. Penile melanosis successfully treated with the Q-switched ruby laser. Br J Dermatol. 1994; 130: 663–4.)

tial melanotic hyperpigmentation of the mucosa. Lenane et al (2000) used the term genital melanotic macules.

Despite being benign, penile melanosis (**Fig. 4.22**) can be unsightly and embarrassing. The Q-switched ruby laser (**Fig. 4.23**) has been advocated as a useful therapeutic modality (Delaney & Walker 1994).

Melanoma has been reported to complicate a congenital macular lentiginous lesion although on histological analysis of the completely resected section the precursor lesion was shown to be a dysplastic nevus similar to those associated with familial and sporadic nevi (Weiss et al 1982).

LENTIGINES

Such lesions may occur idiopathically on the genitals (**Fig. 4.24**) but a lentiginosis syndrome (below) should be considered.

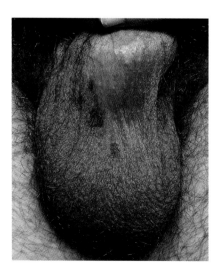

Fig. 4.24 Lentigines. Scrotum.

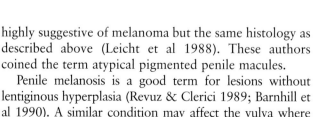

highly suggestive of melanoma but the same histology as described above (Leicht et al 1988). These authors coined the term atypical pigmented penile macules.

Penile melanosis is a good term for lesions without lentiginous hyperplasia (Revuz & Clerici 1989; Barnhill et al 1990). A similar condition may affect the vulva where vitiligo and diabetes are reported associations (Barnhill et al 1990). Revuz & Clerici (1989) proposed the grouping of penile melanosis, vulvovaginal melanosis and the predominantly oral mucosal hyperpigmentation of the Laugier-Hunziker syndrome under the umbrella of essen-

Laugier-Hunziker syndrome

In the Laugier-Hunziker syndrome there is benign non-lentiginous hyperpigmentation of the lips and oral mucosa, but lesions may be found elsewhere including the palms and soles, the penis and vulva and the perineum (Began & Mirowski 2000). The histology is of increased melanin in the basal keratinocytes, melanophages in the upper dermis, and normal melanocyte numbers and appearances.

Peutz-Jeghers syndrome

The most common site for Peutz-Jeghers multiple blue-brown macules is the oral mucosa but anogenital lesions do occur. Other affected sites include face, hand, eyelids and conjunctiva. It is an autosomal dominant disorder and the usual association is with benign gastrointestinal polyps. Malignant change in the jejunal or ileal polyps occurs in 2–3% of cases. A sporadic case with genital involvement and severe ocular disease due to unique uveal melanocytic proliferation has been reported: the patient had rectosigmoid adenocarcinoma (Gass & Glatzer 1991).

Peutz-Jeghers-like melanotic macules (unusual in that they contained proliferating atypical melanocytes histologically) have been reported on the anal mucosa in a patient who also developed the lesions on the face, chin and buccal mucosa. He had metastatic adeno-carcinoma of the oesophagus (Eng et al 1991).

LAMB syndrome

Genital lentiginosis occurs in the LAMB (lentigines, atrial myxoma, blue nevi) and multiple lentigines and hypertrophic cardiomyopathy syndrome (Voron et al 1976; Rhodes et al 1984). The face and lips are also affected.

LEOPARD syndrome

The LEOPARD (lentigines, ECG abnormalities, ocular hypertelorism, pulmonary stenosis, abnormalities of the genitalia, retardation of growth, deafness) syndrome is characterized by widespread lentiginosis of the skin (scalp, face, trunk, limbs, palms, soles) including the genitalia.

Ruvalcaba-Myhre-Smith syndrome

In the Ruvalcaba-Myhre-Smith syndrome pigmented macules on the glans and shaft of the penis are associated with macrocephaly, hamartomatous intestinal polyps, angiolipomas, motor or psychomotor developmental difficulties, ocular abnormalities and an unique lipid storage myopathy (Gretzula et al 1988; Perriard et al 2000).

ACRAL LENTIGINOUS MELANOMA

This has been reported on the penis. Irregularly delineated, irregularly pigmented, coalescent macular hyperpigmentation should arouse the suspicion of this rare event (Jaeger et al 1982).

PURPURA

Purpura may masquerade as a primary pigmentary anomaly. Purpura may unusually be the predominant sign of lichen sclerosus (**Figs 4.25, 4.26**) and be mis-

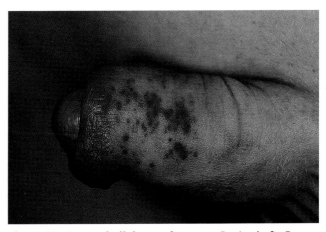

Fig. 4.25 Purpuric lichen sclerosus. Penis shaft. Boy, twelve years old. (Courtesy of Dr Betsy Beers, Gainesville, FL, USA).

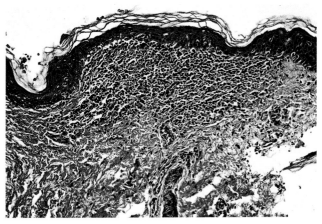

Fig. 4.26 Purpuric lichen sclerosus. Histology. H&E. Penis shaft. Boy, 12 years old. (Courtesy of Dr Betsy Beers, Gainesville, FL, USA).

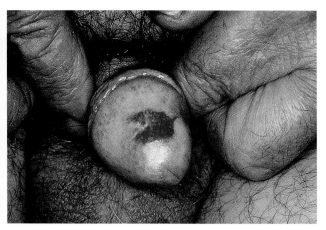 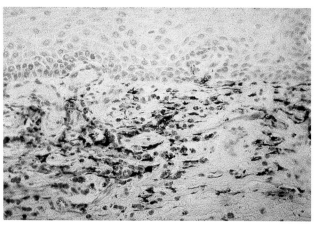

Fig. 4.27 Purpuric Zoon's balanitis. Histology. H&E. 'Lichen aureus' of glans penis. Subsequently this patient developed classical lichen sclerosus of the glans. (Courtesy of Dr Steven Kossard, Darlinghurst, Australia, and reproduced by permission from Kossard S, Shumack S. Lichen aureus of the glans penis as an expression of Zoon's balanitis. J Am Acad Dermatol. 1989; 21: 804–6.)

Fig. 4.28 Purpuric Zoon's balanitis. Same case as Fig. 4.27. Histology, Perl's iron stain × 250. Glans penis. Subsequently this patient developed classical lichen sclerosus of the glans. (Courtesy of Dr Steven Kossard, Darlinghurst, Australia, and reproduced by permission from Kossard S, Shumack S. Lichen aureus of the glans penis as an expression of Zoon's balanitis. J Am Acad Dermatol. 1989; 21: 804–6.)

diagnosed as due to child sex abuse (Barton et al 1993). Purpuric elements of Zoon's balanitis are not unusual (Jonquieres 1971; Jonquieres & de Lutzky 1980) and a lichen aureus presentation (**Figs 4.27, 4.28**) has been reported (Kossard & Shumack 1989), although this patient subsequently developed lichen sclerosus of the glans (Kossard 1997, personal communication). Purpura and ecchymoses may develop after oral sex ('love bites') or the use of vacuum erection devices (Ganem et al 1998) (see **Table 4.6**).

5 Hair

Hirsutes describes hair growth at sites that are normally hairy. *Hypertrichosis* is hair growth at sites that are not normally hairy.

Congenital hypertrichosis over the midline in the lumbosacral area (faun tail) is a sign of underlying spinal dysraphism, e.g. spina bifida occulta (see page 000).

Anogenital hair problems are relatively rare in men who are not generally troubled by hirsutes or pili incarnati (**Figs 5.1, 5.2**) as women may be. Pilonidal sinus is discussed on page 000.

Alopecia areata can affect the pubic hair but usually as part of more widespread involvement as in alopecia universalis (**Fig. 5.3**). It is associated with other organ-specific autoimmune diseases such as vitiligo, pernicious anemia and hypothyroidism. Loss of pubic hair occurs in secondary syphilis and has been reported in primary systemic amyloid (Brownstein & Helwig 1970). Trichotillomania (hair pulling) of the pubic hair has been reported in an adult man (Mazuecos et al, 2001).

Trichomycosis pubis (Rosen et al 1991) is characterized by the appearance of asymptomatic yellow, red or black micro nodules encapsulating affected hair

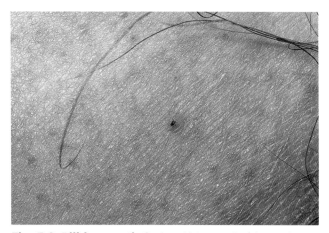

Fig. 5.2 Pili incarnati. Groins. Note: central ingrowing hair and alopecia from progressive follicular destruction. Same patient as Figure 5.1, whose clinical appearance is reminiscent overall of hidradenitis suppurativa.

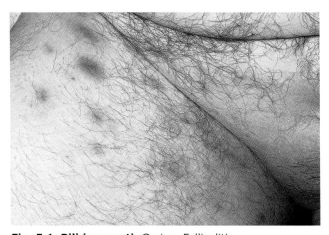

Fig. 5.1 Pili incarnati. Groins. Folliculitis.

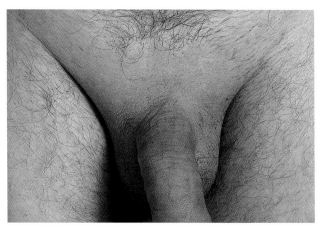

Fig. 5.3 Alopecia areata. Mons pubis and proximal penis shaft.

shafts. Axillary hair may be affected. The skin is normal but the sweat may be discolored. Trichomycosis pubis is probably rather uncommon in everyday Western dermatological practice but is reputedly common in the Middle East (Lestringant et al 1991). It is seen in the groins in India perhaps alongside trichosporosis (Kamalam et al 1988). Trichomycosis is due to *Corynebacterium* sp. and not fungus, despite its name. The differential diagnosis includes true mycoses such as white piedra or black piedra. Treatment is with topical benzoic acid, salicylic acid, clindamycin and naftifine (Rosen et al 1991).

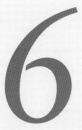

6 Red patches and plaques

RED (SCALY) PATCHES

Patches are thin flat lesions: *plaques* are thicker and raised. White and brown/black (pigmented) patches are discussed in an earlier chapter.

Red patches are usually red because they are *inflamed*. They may or may not be scaly. Scaling may be site dependent, as scale does not readily form on the mucosa. *Erythroplakia* is an alternative term for a red patch on the mucosa and is in common use in oral medicine. More extensive, confluent non-scaly red patches constitute *intertrigo* or *balanoposthitis* and these presentations are discussed in the next chapter. See Tables 6.1–6.3.

ECZEMA AND DERMATITIS

Eczema is not a diagnosis but refers to similar clinical consequences of several different patho-mechanisms in

skin. The symptoms and signs depend on whether the process is acute or chronic (**Table 6.4**) and the clinical subtype (**Table 6.5**). Generally, for practical purposes, the terms eczema and dermatitis may be used synonymously. Eczema is conventionally subdivided into

Table 6.1 Causes of anogenital red patches (non scaly)

Common causes	Rare causes
Eczema	Acrodermatitis
Exogenous	enteropathica
Allergic contact	Hailey-Hailey disease
Irritant contact	Darier's disease
Endogenous	Streptococcal dermatitis
Seborrheic	Gonorrhea
Psoriasis	Leprosy
Reiter's syndrome	Secondary syphilis
Zoon's balanitis	Part of a syphilide
Lichen sclerosus	Mucous patch
Lichen planus	Anal intraepithelial
Candidosis	neoplasia
Tinea	Extramammary Paget's
Erythrasma	disease
Erythroplasia of Queyrat	Kaposi's sarcoma
	Carcinoma erysipeloides
	Fixed drug eruption

Table 6.2 Causes of anogenital red scaly patches

Common causes	Rare causes
Eczema	Eczema
Exogenous	Exogenous
Irritant contact	Allergic contact
Endogenous	Endogenous
Atopic	Asteatotic
Lichen simplex	Inflammatory linear
Seborrheic	verrucous epidermal
Psoriasis	nevus (ILVEN)
Reiter's syndrome	Pityriasis rosea
Lichen sclerosus	Acrodermatitis
Lichen planus	enteropathica
Erythrasma	Hailey-Hailey disease
Tinea	Darier's disease
Scabies	Kawasaki syndrome
Pediculosis	Syphilis
	Primary syphilis
	Balanitis of Follmann
	Secondary syphilis
	Mucous patch
	Part of a syphilide
	Pityriasis versicolor
	Pseudo-epitheliomatous
	micaceous and keratotic
	balanitis (PEMKB)
	Porokeratosis
	Bowen's disease of the
	penis
	Anal intraepithelial
	neoplasia
	Mycosis fungoides
	Extramammary Paget's
	disease
	Fixed drug eruption

Table 6.3 Causes of anogenital red plaques

Giant lichen simplex (of Pautrier)
Inflammatory linear verrucous epidermal nevus (ILVEN)
Psoriasis
Extramammary Paget's disease
Lichen planus
Leishmaniasis
Bowen's disease and Bowenoid papulosis
Anal intraepithelial neoplasia
Kaposi's sarcoma
Carcinoma erysipeloides
Fixed drug eruption

Table 6.4 Physical signs of acute and chronic eczema

Acute	Chronic
Erythema	Lichenification
Edema	Scaling
Vesicles	Pseudoverrucous papules
Serum exudation/crusts	

(After Bunker C 2004 In: Medicine 2nd Edition. J Axford ed. Blackwell Scientific, Oxford)

Table 6.5 Classification of eczema

Endogenous eczema	Exogenous eczema
Atopic	Irritant contact
Pityriasis alba	Allergic contact
Seborrheic	Photodermatitis
Stasis	Photoallergic
Asteatotic	(phytophotodermatitis)
Pompholyx	
Discoid	
Lichen simplex	
Neurodermatitis	
Nodular prurigo	
Eczematous drug reaction	
Perianal dermatitis	
Autosensitization	
Eczema-like eruptions with systemic disease (children)	
Wiskott-Aldrich syndrome	
X-linked agammaglobinemia	
Hyper IgE syndrome	
Chronic granulomatous disease	
Phenylketonuria	
Histiocytosis X (Letterer-Siwe disease)	
Acrodermatitis enteropathica (zinc deficiency)	

(After Bunker C 2004 In: Medicine 2nd Edition. J Axford ed. Blackwell Scientific, Oxford)

endogenous (e.g. atopic, varicose, seborrheic, etc.) or exogenous (contact eczema) types.

Irritant contact dermatitis

It is worth repeating earlier remarks (see Chapter 1) to stress that the response to the sensation of itch is to scratch or to rub (grattage) and both these actions elicit skin morbidity in the form of excoriations, often with secondary infection-impetiginization (**Fig. 6.1**), and/or lichenification (**Fig. 6.2**). Lichenification may be a

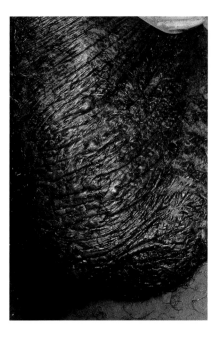

Fig. 6.2 Lichenification. Scrotum.

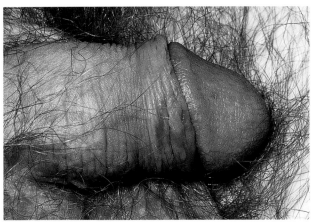

Fig. 6.1 Irritant contact dermatitis. Distal lateral prepuce, penis. Lightly impetiginized dermatitis. Specific irritant not identified. Patient responded to soap substitution and a short course of Trimovate ®.

manifestation of an eczematous process, as in atopic dermatitis and is in itself pruritic so as a response to scratching it contributes to a vicious cycle of symptomatology.

But irritation may cause problems at vulnerable sites regardless of the phenotype. Irritation may be due to friction (Ramam et al 1998) from adjacent skin and clothing, toilet paper and towels, sweat, sebum, desquamated corneocytes, dirt, excreta, partners' sexual secretions, clothing, detergents, toiletries, cosmetics, contraceptives and some therapeutic topical treatments including those used at other nearby sites (e.g. 5-fluorouracil used for keratoses at other sites, Shelley & Shelley 1988), compounded by friction (e.g. cellist's scrotum, Shapiro 1991) and maceration and by common human afflictions such as piles, constipation and straining at stool, diarrhea and fecal soiling, urinary dribbling and so on. Often overlooked is over-washing (**Figs 6.3** and **6.4**), for example the over-usage of soap and toiletries (this topic is expanded below and **Table 6.6** lists potential anogenital irritants) and there may be an association with atopy: Birley et al (1993) diagnosed irritant dermatitis in 72% of patients presenting to a

Table 6.6 Anogenital irritants
Sweat
Sebum
Desquamated corneocytes
Dirt
Excreta
Sexual secretions
Clothing
Soap and detergents
Toiletries
Toilet paper
Cosmetics
Contraceptives
Therapeutic
Friction
Maceration

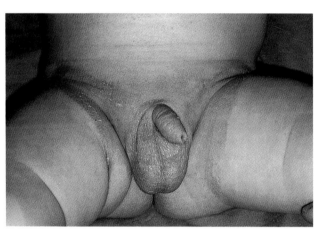

Fig. 6.5 Primary irritant contact napkin (nappy)/diaper dermatitis. Groins, pubis, genitals. If the thighs are spread the inguinal furrows classically are spared: confluent erythema suggests psoriasis.

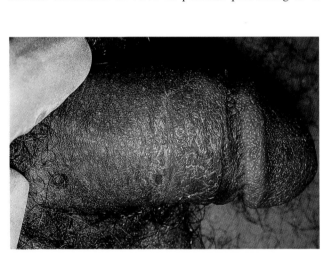

Fig. 6.3 Irritant contact dermatitis. Penis shaft, lateral. Over-washing.

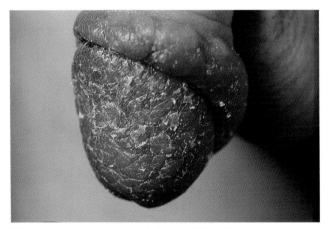

Fig. 6.4 Irritant contact dermatitis. Glans and prepuce. Eczema (glans) and edema (prepuce).

genitourinary clinic with 'balanitis' (they probably meant balanoposthitis) of whom a possible 67% had a history of atopy (but none of these patients was patch tested).

The signs may be acute or chronic, sterile or super-infected with staphylococci or candida or both, eroded or hyperkeratotic depending on the different scenarios. A good example is nappy/diaper rash where urinary moisture; occlusion, friction and candida contribute to the clinical presentation (**Fig. 6.5**). Classically the convex surfaces are affected and the flexures are spared, distinguishing it from psoriasis (Hogan 1999). Nappy rash has become much less common with the availability of absorbent disposable paper napkins. A severe erosive

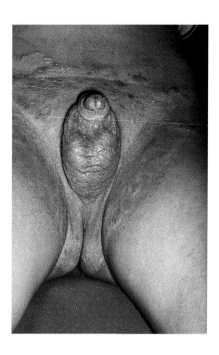

Fig. 6.6 Primary irritant contact napkin (nappy)/diaper dermatitis. Groins, pubis, genitals. Note: erosions (Jacquet's dermatitis). (Courtesy of Dr Peter Copeman, London, UK).

form (Jacquet's dermatitis, **Fig. 6.6**) is still occasionally seen in children with urinary or fecal continence problems. Pseudoverrucous papules have been reported (Loppo & Solomone 2002).

Management is directed at re-education and behavior modification. The irritants mentioned above and in **Table 6.8** should be identified and eliminated or reduced. Advice must be given about soap substitutes, moisturizers, towels and toilet paper. Topical corticosteroid ointments, with or without antibiotic and anticandidal agents, are reasonably employed to get the situation under control. Antihistamines by mouth (but not topically) are useful. Topical local anesthetics should be avoided because of the risk of sensitization. Occasionally secondary infection may be so severe that a swab should be taken and oral antibiotics prescribed. Coffee consumption might usefully be curtailed (Veien et al 1987).

The discussion above has centered on chronic irritation. A more *acute* picture characterized by itch, burning or pain, swelling, erythema and even vesiculation may occur if chemicals of high irritancy or in high concentration are accidentally or deliberately used on the genitalia. Patients with a rash and especially afraid of a sexually transmitted disease will sometimes ill advisedly employ the most inappropriate of agents. Treatment is with soaks of potassium permanganate, very potent corticosteroid creams (sometimes systemic corticosteroids) and systemic antibiotics. Occasionally, what is in effect a caustic burn may supervene and then specialized (plastic surgical) help may be sought.

Allergic contact dermatitis

Immunological hypersensitivity to some chemicals occurs as a Type IV allergic reaction involving cell-mediated immunity after prior sensitization to the agent concerned. There are common allergens (lanolin, perfume, nickel, rubber, etc.) that cause a significant prevalence of disease.

The risks to the anogenital area come about from: (i) direct contact with the allergen, for example, medicaments – even coal tar allergy has been reported (Cusano et al 1992), toiletries, contraceptive usage, prosthetic limbs (Lyon et al 2000) in amputees and urushiol as in poison oak, poison ivy and poison sumac phytodermatitis (Gamulka 2000) or with subsequent exposure to sunlight (e.g. psoralens from fig or citrus plants) as in phytophotodermatitis; in the United States phyto- and phytophotodermatitis may be more common than in Europe but genital involvement is rarely seen; (ii) transfer of allergen, for example, from another part of the anatomy e.g. the hands: saw dust and epoxy resins or from a sexual partner: contraceptive jellies, hygiene sprays, douches; and (iii) involvement in a more generalized eczematous response (e.g. to a medicament or dressing used on venous eczema or ulceration, as in the autosensitization/secondary spread/secondary generalization syndrome).

Symptoms are pain, burning or itching and signs of erythema, swelling, vesiculation and exudation or erythema scale and lichenification, depending on acuity, appearing about one week after first contact with the allergen (if previously unsensitized) or within 1–2 days, possibly a few hours, if already allergic. The patient may present with pruritus ani or paraphimosis (Farina et al 1999).

The principles of management are the identification of the potential allergen (**Tables 6.7–6.9**) and its likely source and then its elimination. There may be clues to these factors at presentation but subsequent patch testing is required (**Fig. 6.7**). Following patch testing, Bauer et al (2000) made a final diagnosis of allergic contact dermatitis in 35% of patients with anogenital skin problems. Allergic contact dermatitis can persist even with the withdrawal of the trigger allergen. Soap

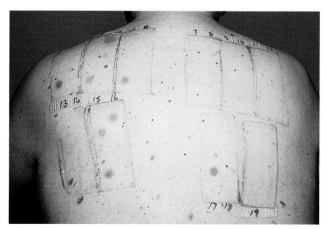

Fig. 6.7 Patch tests. Back. Several positive results are visible as circular erythematous plaques.

Table 6.7 Potential sensitizers in emollients

Beeswax

Benzyl alcohol

Benzyl cinnamate

Butylated hydroxyanisole

Butylated hydroxytoluene

Cetostearyl alcohol

Chlorocresol

Disodium edetate

Hydantoin

Fragrances

Parabens (hydroxybenzoates)

Imidazolidinyl urea

Oxybenzone

Phenyl ethyl alcohol

Phenoxyethanol

Propylene glycol

Sorbic acid/sorbates

Triethanolamine

Lanolin (wool, fats and derivatives)

Benzalkonium chloride

Chlorhexidine

Crotamiton

Chamomile

Triclosan

Quatenium-15

Table 6.8 Potential sensitizers in topical corticosteroids

Butylated hydroxyanisole

Butylated hydroxytoluene

Cetostearyl alcohol

Chlorocresol

Triethanolamine

Ethylenediamine

Fragrances

Parabens (hydroxybenzoates)

Propylene glycol

Sorbic acid

Sorbitan sesquioleate

Lanolin (wool, fats and derivatives)

Steroid moieties

Table 6.9 Allergens of particular relevance to anogenital contact dermatitis

Rubber allergens – thiuramdisulphide, mercapto thiabendazole

Fragrance (perfume)

Balsam of Peru (myroxylon pereirae)

Local anesthetics – benzocaine, lignocaine

Parabens

Hydroxy quinolones

Ethylenediamine

Methyldibromoglutaronitrile — Euxyl K 400

Methylchloroisothiazolinone/methylisothiazolinone — Kathon CG

Antifungals — nystatin

Antibiotics — neomycin

Steroid moieties

Latex condoms

Powder/lubricants in condoms

Spermicides

Mitomycin-C

Clothing dyes

substitutes, moisturizers, and potent topical corticosteroids are required in the acute phase and sometimes oral antihistamines, antibiotics and corticosteroids. Potassium permanganate soaks and wet dressings can be useful.

The commonest relevant sensitivities (**Table 6.9**) are due to rubber accelerators, contraceptives, preservatives and fragrances in toiletries and medicaments as well as the active agents (antibiotics, antifungals, steroids, anesthetics) in the latter.

With rubber dermatitis it is not just young sexually active male condom-users (Hindson 1966; Bircher et al 1993; Shenot et al 1994; Harmon et al 1995) that are at risk but also incontinent men who use external urinary collection devices (Paul's tubing). Anoreceptive homosexual men are susceptible to condom hypersensitivity. For patients who are allergic to rubber condoms alternatives made from lamb cecum are available but they provide less protection against sexually transmitted disease than latex. Creating hypoallergenic condoms by washing in an ammonium solution to remove the residues of the accelerator chemicals that actually cause the hypersensitivity has proved unsuccessful (Rademaker & Forsyth 1989; Harmon et al 1995). Patients may also become sensitized to the spermicide (Hindson 1966).

Biocide preservatives such as methyldibromoglutaronitrile (a component of Euxyl K 400) has been used as a preservative in moistened toilet tissue (Van Ginkel & Rundervort 1995) and caused allergic contact dermatitis, likewise methylchloroisothiazolinone/

methylisothiazolinone-Kathon CG (de Groot et al 1991; Lucker et al 1992). Fragrances in moistened toilet paper (Swinyer 1980) or other toiletries and medicaments may similarly be to blame. Lignocaine (Handfield-Jones & Cronin 1993; Hardwick & King 1994) and tetracaine (amethocaine) hydrochloride (Sanchez-Perez et al 1998) used in topical antipruritics for piles can be incriminated. Benzocaine also causes allergic contact dermatitis.

A burgeoning problem for dermatologists has been the development of sensitivity not only to preservatives and antibiotics in dermatologically approved topicals but also to the corticosteroid moiety itself (Miranda-Romero et al 1998).

Mitomycin-C (Fisher 1991), celandine juice (Farina et al 1999) and clothing dye dermatitis of the scrotum (Lucke et al 1998) have also been reported.

Whether foods can cause perianal symptoms through an allergic mechanism is debatable (Aki 1993; Sapan 1993). Cow's milk protein allergy with signs resembling perianal wheal, excoriation and fissuring have been described.

Anogenital symptoms and signs may also be due to immediate-type hypersensitivity to natural rubber latex (Wakelin & White 1999). Individuals may be exposed through latex condom usage and repeated catheterization as occurs in patients with spina bifida or spinal cord injury. Symptoms may be localized and include pruritus, erythema and urticaria. Localized eczema can also occur (Taylor & Pradiswan 1996; Turjanmaa et al 1996). Less commonly systemic symptoms and anaphylactic shock may develop (Taylor et al 1989; Shenot et al 1994). Prick tests can be used to confirm the diagnosis of type-1 latex hypersensitivity or RAST test if the former is not feasible. Natural rubber latex avoidance is obviously necessary in allergic individuals and latex-free condoms made of polyurethane are available.

Atopic dermatitis

Atopic dermatitis (AD) is a common dermatosis and associated with a personal and familial predisposition to dry skin (xerosis or ichthyosis) and other atopic (Greek: strange disease) diseases such as rhinitis, asthma and conjunctivitis. Although undoubtedly linked with high IgE levels, including specific allergens, and although patients have positive prick tests to these allergens the skin signs (and other immunopathological features) of AD are not those of classical Type I allergic reactions due to mast cell activation (of which the cutaneous model is actually urticaria) but Type IV, mediated by Th 2 CD4 T lymphocytes. The classical model for this cell mediated immunological reaction is in fact allergic contact dermatitis.

In AD many of the immunological changes that have been described may be epiphenomena but most dermatologists believe that hypersensitivity to the house dust mite is pivotal to the complex pathophysiology.

Twenty percent of the population may be atopic and up to 10% of children may get atopic eczema presenting as itchy, red scaly lesions on the face and flexures from the age of about two months. It can be the cause of considerable morbidity. However, the majority of children do grow out of the disease (95% or more by the age of 15). If persistent into adulthood then the prognosis for remission is poor. Very rarely eczema in childhood may point to an underlying immunodeficiency disease such as Wiskott-Aldrich syndrome (**Figs 6.8, 6.9**), characterized by the triad of severe eczema (face, flexures and napkin area), infections and thrombocytopenia.

Anogenital disease due to AD is not uncommon (**Fig. 6.10**) but rarely occurs in isolation (unlike the other common chronic dermatoses such as seborrhoic dermatitis and psoriasis). Itching at night, uncomplicated patchy eczema (**Fig. 6.11**), lichenification, excoriations with secondary impetiginization (**Figs 6.12, 6.13**), lichen simplex (see below and **Figs 6.14–6.21**) and even nodular prurigo may occur.

It is not known how anogenital AD is related to circumcision, sexual activity and sexually transmitted disease. Birley et al (1993) found evidence of atopy in a possible 67% of a total of 72% of patients diagnosed as having irritant dermatitis from a consecutive series of all men presenting to a GU clinic with balanitis (they probably meant balanoposthitis). Atopic patients have to be careful about irritation and allergy from condoms and chemical contraceptives.

It has been my impression that AD or an AD-like condition occurs in HIV-positive individuals. AD or an AD-like condition appears to be common especially in

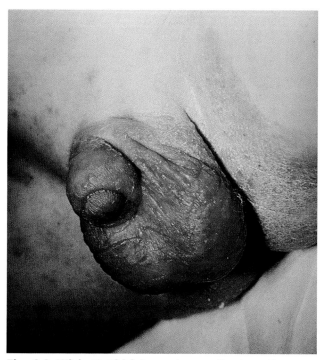

Fig. 6.8 Wiskott-Aldrich syndrome. Scrotum. Eczema. (Courtesy of Dr Peter Copeman, London, UK).

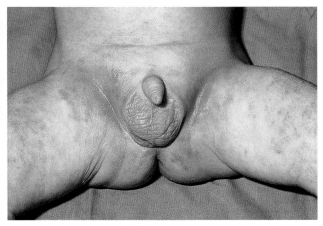

Fig. 6.9 Wiskott-Aldrich syndrome. Anterior pelvic girdle. Flexural and napkin eczema.

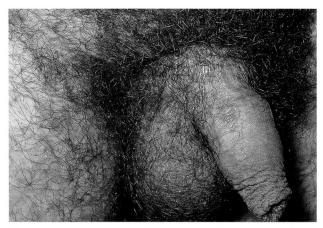

Fig. 6.12 Atopic dermatitis. Penis and scrotum. Lightly impetiginized.

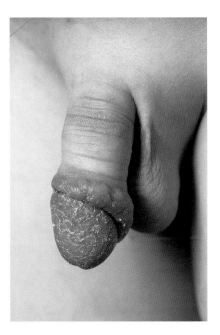

Fig. 6.10 Atopic dermatitis. Glans, prepuce and shaft, penis. Prepubescent boy.

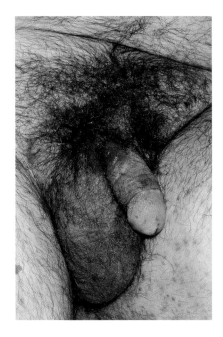

Fig. 6.13 Atopic dermatitis. Penis and scrotum. Impetiginized.

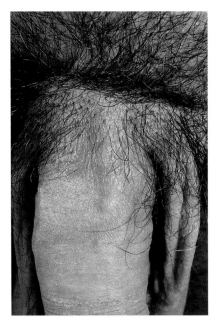

Fig. 6.11 Atopic dermatitis. Penis.

HIV-infected children (Prose 1991). In adults there have been reports of patients whose atopic eczema recurred or worsened during the course of HIV infection (Ball & Harper 1987) and a case of the hyper-IgE syndrome has been described (Lin & Smith 1988). But other commentators have not agreed (Cockerell 1991; Duvic 1991; Staughton & Goldsmith; personal communication). Ring et al (1986) found a decreased frequency of atopic diseases, fewer positive RAST tests and lower average levels of IgE in HIV-positive compared to HIV-negative homosexual individuals.

AD is a clinical diagnosis. A biopsy is not often necessary. Estimation of the serum IgE level strengthens clinical suspicion of the presence of the atopic tendency.

Attention to personal hygiene to avoid irritants such as found in soap and some medicaments is vital (see above) and by using suitable substitutes and skin moisturizers. Similarly, common allergens should be avoided and suspected (see above) in cases of regional

Table 6.10 Treatments for atopic dermatitis

Moisturizers and soap substitutes

Topical corticosteroids (+/– antibiotic/anti-candidal)

Topical tacrolimus/pimecrolimus

Oral antibiotics

Oral antihistamines

Systemic corticosteroids (oral, im ACTH)

UVB phototherapy

Psoralens + UVA (PUVA) phototherapy

Azathioprine

Cyclosporin A

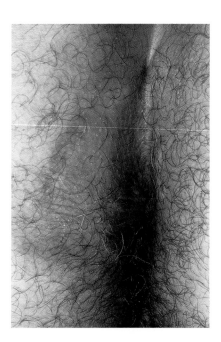

Fig. 6.14 Lichen simplex. Perianal skin.

unexplained exacerbation. Treatment depends on using the lowest-potency topical corticosteroid capable of containing disease. Combinations containing antibiotic and anti-candidal agents are popular at anogenital sites and systemic antibiotics are needed frequently for generalized flares or localized (e.g. anogenital) complications. Oral antihistamines may be useful at night. Systemic corticosteroids (including intramuscular depot synthetic ACTH) are avoided unless at times of real crisis, either medical or social (e.g. weddings and honeymoons).

Other treatments are listed in **Table 6.10** but some are reserved for severe chronic disease. Phototherapy is not routinely used for genital skin disease because of the increased risk of skin cancer at this site.

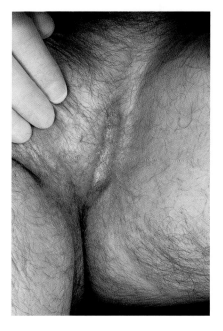

Fig. 6.15 Lichen simplex. Groin.

Lichen simplex

Lichen simplex (Pautrier 1936) presents as itchy red patches or plaques of lichenified (like the bark of a tree) skin and is common around the male genitalia and anus (**Fig. 6.14–6.17**, see also **Fig. 6.2**). It is not usually a flexural condition but can be seen on the penile shaft (**Figs 6.18, 6.19**) and scrotum (**Fig. 6.20**): giant forms (of Pautrier) occur, e.g. on the scrotum giving a pineapple appearance (**Fig. 6.21**). The skin may be broken by excoriations and become secondarily impetiginized or colonized by candida.

Histologically, lichenification is characterized by hyperkeratosis, uniform acanthosis and an unremarkable low-grade perivascular infiltrate of mononuclear leucocytes in the superficial dermis. At mucosal sites hyper- and orthokeratosis create a cornified layer resulting in the clinical appearances of leucoplakia.

Treatment is directed at any underlying cause and the relief of scratching. Soap should be banned, a soap substitute and moisturizer recommended and the area occluded if possible with a bland dressing – wet if the skin is fiercely eczematized. A potent topical corticosteroid ointment can be used for a few days and then

tailed off. Preparations also containing tar or combinations of antibacterial and anti-candidal and antifungal agents are also useful. Two of my cases of extensive giant lichen simplex of the scrotum (**Fig. 6.21**) have been successfully treated by hemiscrotectomy (Porter et al 2001).

Inflammatory linear verrucous epidermal nevus

This rare eczematous lesion is as it is described. Sometimes it is referred to by its acronym, ILVEN. Genital lesions have not been encountered to my knowledge but upper thigh and buttocks may be involved (**Fig. 6.22**).

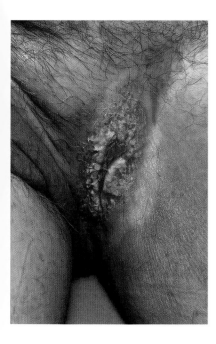

Fig. 6.16 Lichen simplex. Left groin. Erosion from excoriation. Maceration and candidosis.

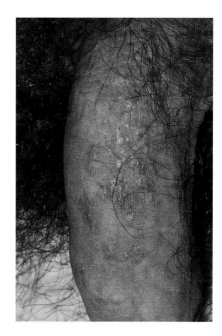

Fig. 6.19 Lichen simplex. Penis shaft, lateral.

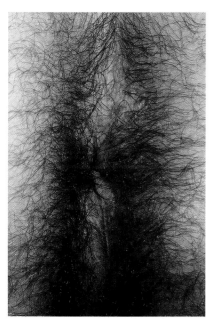

Fig. 6.17 Lichen simplex. Perianal skin. This patient had genital lichen sclerosus (see Fig. 6.141) but histology of the perianal skin showed lichen simplex.

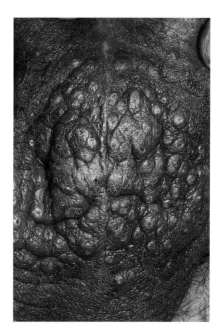

Fig. 6.20 Lichen simplex. Scrotum.

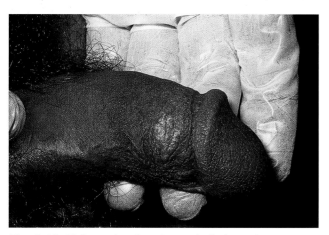

Fig. 6.18 Lichen simplex. Penis shaft, lateral.

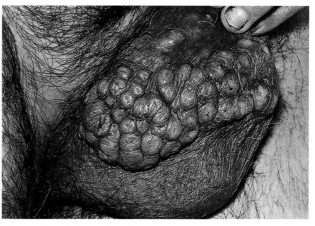

Fig. 6.21 Lichen simplex. Scrotum. Giant 'pineapple' lesion.

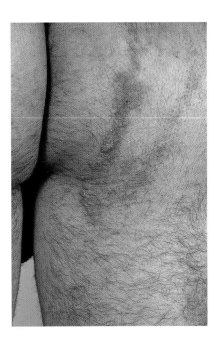

Fig. 6.22 ILVEN (inflammatory linear verrucous epidermal nevus). Buttock.

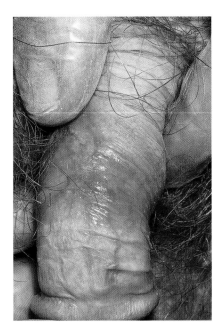

Fig. 6.24 Seborrheic dermatitis. Penis and prepuce. Non-specific proximal posthitis. Patient with seborrheic capititis and seborrheic dermatitis of face and chest.

Seborrheic dermatitis

This is a very common pattern of eczematous disease that probably results from a diathesis that confers on the subject an abnormal hypersensitivity to the normal commensal cutaneous yeast, *Pityrosporum ovale*. The epithet is a partial misnomer because the eruption is commonly found at hairy sites rather than in the truly sebum rich areas.

Patients complain of the cosmetic insult rather than of itch, which may be mild. There is slight erythema, slight to moderate scaling and often perifollicular or frank folliculitis involvement. The scalp (pityriasis capitis, dandruff), ears, glabella and brows, nasolabial folds, axillae, chest and back are commonly involved, as are the groins and penis (**Figs 6.23–6.27**). Indeed these

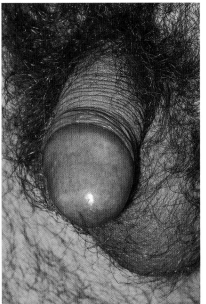

Fig. 6.25 Seborrheic dermatitis. Glans penis and distal prepuce. Non-specific balanoposthitis. The patient had the characteristic rash affecting his glabella and chest.

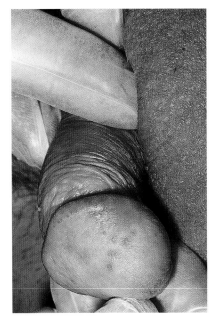

Fig. 6.23 Seborrheic dermatitis. Balanoposthitis in sebopsoriasis/ seboriasis (same case as Fig. 6.28).

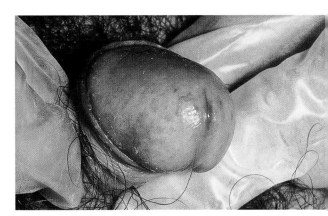

Fig. 6.26 Seborrheic dermatitis. Penis. Non-specific balanoposthitis, but this patient had classical facial seborrheic dermatitis.

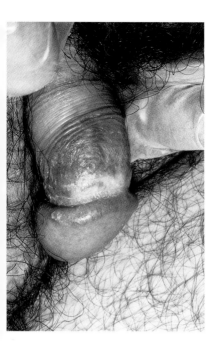

Fig. 6.27 Seborrheic dermatitis. Glans penis and prepuce. Psoriasiform eruption in a patient with classical facial seborrheic dermatitis.

may be the only sites overtly involved and lead to the patient presenting with an anogenital problem, such as pruritus ani or balanoposthitis, to a dermatologist or venereologist. A family history and careful examination of other sites assists the diagnosis inordinately: there may be slight dandruff, mild scaling of the eyebrows or a few spots in an axilla or on the chest. The manifestations of the tendency may vary chronically for many years.

Some patients may also have a tendency to psoriasis ('sebopsoriasis', 'seboriasis'). In the scalp, on the face, in the flexures and at anogenital sites seborrheic dermatitis and psoriasis may be indistinguishable. In sebopsoriasis/ seboriasis the signs will be that little more florid but there will also be a family history or physical signs of subtle or overt psoriasis on careful assessment (**Fig. 6.28**).

Seborrheic dermatitis is common in the later stages of HIV infection when it can be very severe and generalized, even amounting to erythroderma (Duvic

1991). It has been established that seborrheic dermatitis is more common in seropositive homosexual men than seronegative homosexuals. Whilst it is a common diagnosis amongst seropositive individuals who are otherwise well, its severity is increased with CD4 counts below $100/\mu l^3$. Some clinicians have noticed an association of erythroderma, xerosis and seborrheic dermatitis with the development of dementia and spinal cord disease. Extensive refractory seborrheic dermatitis appears to occur in particular conjunction with pulmonary tuberculosis and AIDS in Zambia (Hira et al 1988). The differential diagnosis depends upon the particular clinical presentation but usually comprises other causes of widespread dermatitis; erythroderma, psoriasis and tinea corporis, and seborrheic dermatitis may co-exist with all. It has been my experience and apparently that of others that a more mild seborrheic dermatitis of the scalp, face, trunk or genitalia is a common diagnosis amongst seropositive individuals who are otherwise well.

Diagnosis is achieved on clinical grounds including response to therapy and it is not usually necessary to do a biopsy. However, scrapings can be examined for fungi to exclude tinea. *Pityrosporum* sp. will be seen in large numbers.

Histology shows hyperkeratosis, thickened Malpighian layer (epidermal acanthosis), epidermal edema (spongiosis) and accumulation of neutrophils under the stratum corneum: a deeper lymphocytic infiltration of sebaceous glands and a more perivascular neutrophilic infiltrate is seen in HIV patients than in classical seborrheic dermatitis (Kaplan et al 1987). The findings may be very similar to psoriasis. However, Soeprono et al (1987) describing 25 biopsied cases of seborrheic dermatitis list the following features: spotty keratinocyte necrosis, leukoexocytosis and a superficial perivascular infiltrate of plasma cells and neutrophils with occasional leukocytoclasis that are not commonly found in non-HIV-associated seborrheic dermatitis or psoriasis.

No treatment may be needed. Some men require reassurance that the intermittent penile rash has neither been transmitted to them nor can be given to others and that it is not a sign of poor hygiene; they are relieved to learn that it is just another manifestation of the dandruff their father had badly, or the rash they get spasmodically on their chest, or the 'cradle cap' that affected their infant son.

However, treatments that diminish the commensal *Pityrosporum* load and reduce irritation and eczematization can be very successfully and safely used long term. These include topical antifungals (such as clioquinol, nystatin and imidazoles) as ointments, creams, lotions or shampoos, mixtures of the same agents with mild and moderately potent topical corticosteroids used alongside emollients and soap substitutes. In severe cases, such as with concomitant seborrheic folliculitis or in HIV, then treatment with an oral imidazole and/or an oral tetracycline might be indicated.

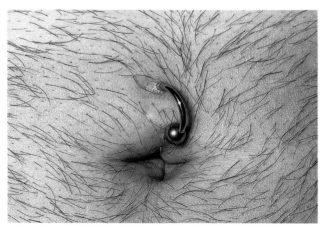

Fig. 6.28 Psoriasis. Umbilicus. Koebnerizing piercing site (same case as Fig. 6.23).

Asteatotic eczema

This pattern of eczema is due to endogenous and exogenous desiccation of the skin. It is dry, red glazed, slightly scaly (crazy paving pattern, eczema craquelé) and itchy. It occurs in elderly, institutionalized or hospitalized patients who are over-washing or over-washed, but an important contribution is the gradual attritional loss of number and function of cutaneous appendageal secretions (sweat and sebum) with age. It may be seen in HIV where there is accelerated skin ageing and in patients who have had radiotherapy or chemotherapy (where presumably the rapidly proliferating cells of the glandular tissues are selectively affected). It can focalize to the anogenital area because this is a common site for over-washing.

PITYRIASIS ROSEA

This is a benign self-limiting dermatosis of unknown etiology, but possibly viral. It consists of an itchy, symmetrical, centripetal (centered on the torso and upper limbs rather than on the extremities and face) eruption of oval, red, scaly patches. The classical disease presents with a single larger petaloid lesion about one week before the other patches declare themselves. It is not unusual for this so called 'herald patch' to appear on suprapubic skin or in the groin. Nor are *formes frustes* (incomplete patterns) rare and the rash can affect the pelvic girdle solely (although careful examination may elicit another patch on the neck or in the axilla). The spots last about eight weeks. Topical emollients, topical corticosteroids and oral antihistamines help the itching. It is customary for dermatologists to exclude secondary syphilis and request the luetic serology tests in this, as in other, papulosquamous eruptions.

PSORIASIS

Approximately 2% of the population are said to have psoriasis but the diathesis may be much more widespread depending on the clinical weight that may be given to hesitant and uncertain family histories (not everyone knows what it is and how to recognize it – including some doctors – and people did not necessarily seek medical attention for mild skin problems in previous generations) and vaguely recalled and undocumented prior rashes, hair and nail problems. There is also the differing interpretation of mild scaling of the scalp, ears, elbows, knees and hyperkeratosis of the palms and soles and nail dystrophy and pitting that is inevitable amongst dermatologists, as well as the overlap that occurs with seborrheic dermatitis and even atopic eczema in some subjects. If ever evaluated precisely it is possible that many more than 2% of men

may have or have had anogenital psoriasis at some time: it is certainly a common anogenital diagnosis in isolation, or supported by 'soft' clinical clues, among the cognoscenti.

The cause of psoriasis is unknown. Genetic factors certainly are important although not well understood. HLA Cw 0602 is associated with 90% of HIV-associated psoriasis (Mallon et al 1998) and 100% of guttate psoriasis (Mallon et al 2000). Environmental precipitants are recognized, for example streptococcal sore throat preceding acute guttate psoriasis. Currently psoriasis is regarded as a disorder of primary immuno-dysregulation determined both by a genetic predisposition and environmental triggers (perhaps streptococcal or other superantigens) that results in the pathological hallmarks of the disease – vascular changes, leukocyte infiltration and epidermal hyperproliferation.

The clinical manifestations of psoriasis (Figs 6.29–6.31; see also Figs 2.1b, j, k, l, m, p, r) are of variably

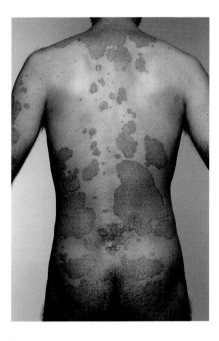

Fig. 6.29 **Psoriasis.** Back and buttocks.

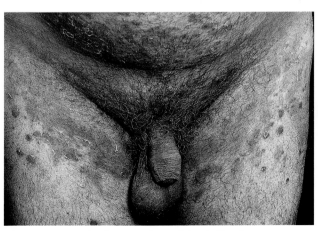

Fig. 6.30 **Psoriasis.** Anterior pelvic girdle. Severe involvement.

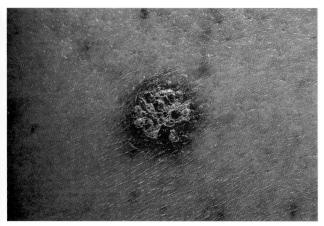

Fig. 6.31 Psoriasis. Salmon-pink, silvery scaled patch. Extragenital site.

itchy, silvery-scaled, erythematous (salmon-pink) patches or plaques (thick or thin), which may be guttate or nummular (drop or coin-sized), separate or confluent, occurring in a symmetrical pattern but especially on extensor surfaces. Sometimes a pustular type is seen, especially on the palms and soles. Palmar plantar keratoderma may occur. The nail changes that accompany psoriasis are listed in the **Table 6.11** (see **Figs 2.1l, 6.32, 6.42, 6.44**). Pitting can also occur in alopecia areata. Onychomycosis can usually be differentiated from psoriatic nail dystrophy but sometimes even experts are mistaken and the two can coincide.

Table 6.11 Nail changes in psoriasis

Pits

Irregular yellow onycholysis

Subungual oil drop lesions

Subungual hyperkeratosis

(see Figs 2.1k, 2.1l, 6.32)

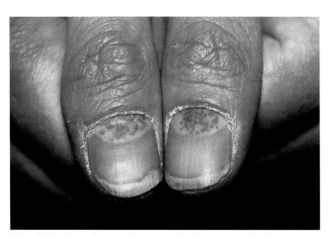

Fig. 6.32 Psoriasis. Thumbnails. Subungual 'oil drop' lesions (same patient as Fig. 6.33).

The scalp (**Fig. 6.33** subtle, **Fig. 6.34** florid, see also Fig. 2.1i, page 24), ears, umbilicus (see Fig. 2.1r, page 25) and face (in sebopsoriasis) are involved, as is anogenital skin (Farber & Nall 1992), especially the sacrum, buttocks (**Figs 6.35, 6.36**), natal cleft (**Figs 6.37–6.39**), pubic mound and groins (**Fig. 6.40**), perianal skin and shaft, glans and prepuce of the penis and less commonly the scrotum (**Figs 6.41–6.43**). The Koebner phenomenon (the appearance of a skin disease at the site of trauma or of another skin disorder) may contribute to this distribution.

To repeat, anogenital sites may be the only sites of psoriasis. However, careful clinical assessment is often very rewarding providing diagnostic pointers at other sites, for example the nails. The penile appearances (**Figs 6.45–6.61**) may be difficult to interpret especially in the uncircumcised patient because a mucosal site is affected rather than keratinized skin. The diagnosis is usually easier in the circumcised male where the morphology is similar to extragenital lesions.

Inverse pattern psoriasis (**Figs 6.62, 6.63**) refers to the manifestation of the disease on intertriginous skin in the axillae, the natal cleft, the gluteal folds, and the groins and under the dependent, flaccid penis (where its

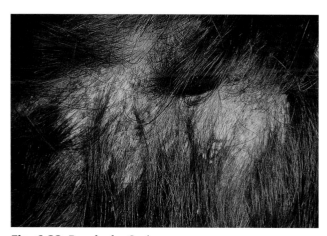

Fig. 6.33 Psoriasis. Scalp.

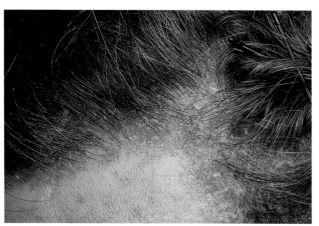

Fig. 6.34 Psoriasis. Scalp.

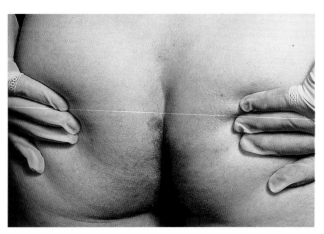

Fig. 6.35 Psoriasis. Buttock.

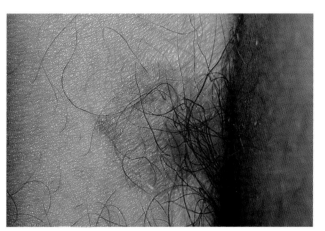

Fig. 6.36 Psoriasis. Buttock. Close-up of Fig. 6.35.

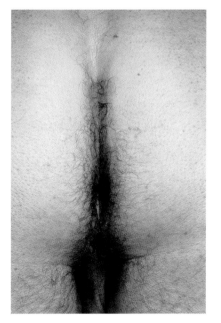

Fig. 6.37 Psoriasis. Natal cleft.

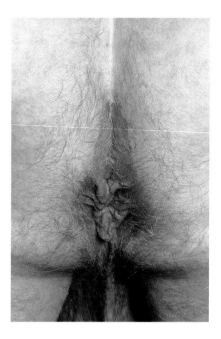

Fig. 6.38 Psoriasis. Natal cleft, perianal. Note: post-hemorrhoidal perianal skin tags.

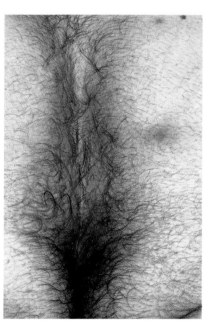

Fig. 6.39 Psoriasis. Natal cleft.

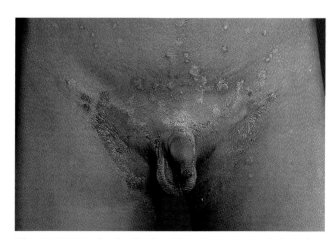

Fig. 6.40 Psoriasis. Groins. Boy. Severe superinfected erosive intertrigo.

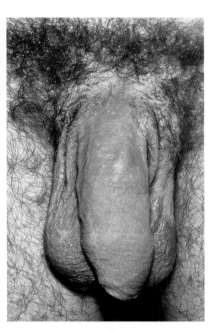

Fig. 6.41 Psoriasis. Thighs, pubis, penis root, scrotum.

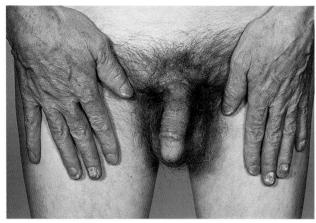

Fig. 6.44 Psoriasis. Fingernails and penis. Psoriatic nail dystrophy and involvement of penis.

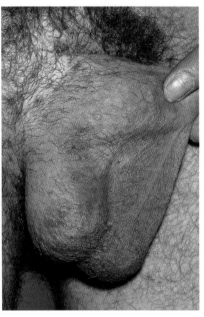

Fig. 6.42 Psoriasis. Scrotum.

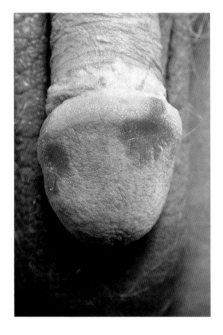

Fig. 6.45 Psoriasis. Dorsal glans penis. Circumcised.

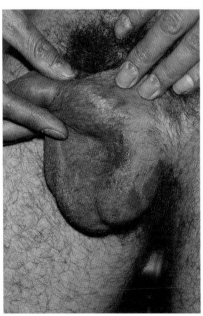

Fig. 6.43 Psoriasis. Scrotum. Note nail involvement. Same patient as Fig. 6.42.

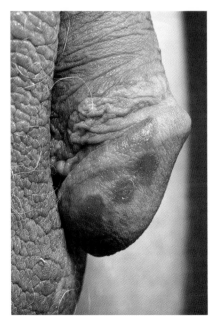

Fig. 6.46 Psoriasis. Lateral glans penis. Circumcised. Same patient as Fig. 6.45.

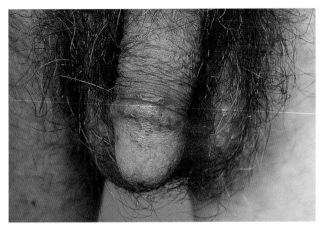

Fig. 6.47 Psoriasis. Glans and prepuce, penis. Same patient as Fig. 6.44.

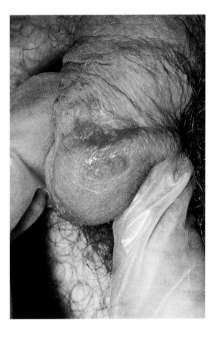

Fig. 6.48 Psoriasis. Glans and coronal sulcus, penis.

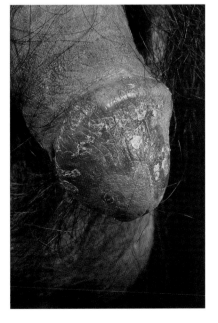

Fig. 6.49 Psoriasis. Glans penis.

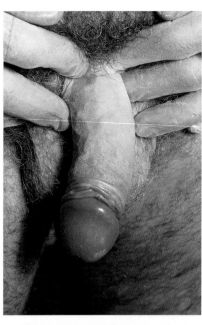

Fig. 6.50 Psoriasis. Glans and prepuce, penis. Uncircumcised.

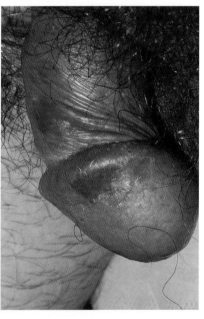

Fig. 6.51 Psoriasis. Glans and prepuce, penis. Uncircumcised.

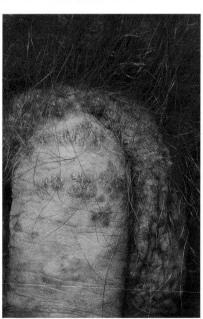

Fig. 6.52 Psoriasis. Proximal shaft, penis. HIV.

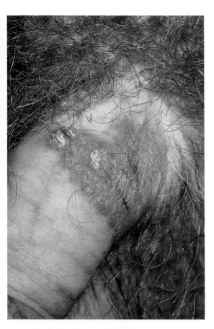

**Fig. 6.53
Psoriasis.**
Proximal shaft,
penis. Compare
with Figs 6.226
(Bowen's
disease), 6.245
(extramammary
Paget's disease).

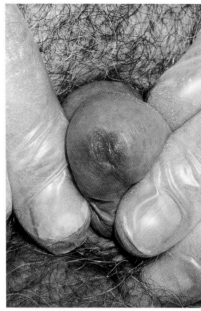

**Fig. 6.56
Psoriasis.** Glans
penis.

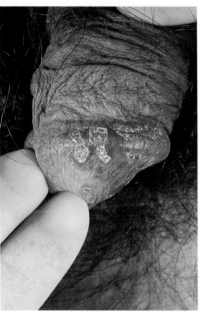

**Fig. 6.54
Psoriasis.** Lateral
glans penis.

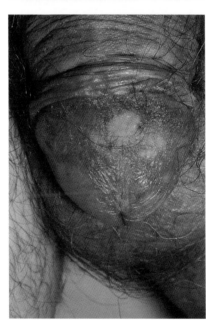

**Fig. 6.57
Psoriasis.** Glans
penis.

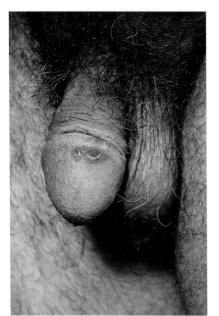

**Fig. 6.55
Psoriasis.** Glans
penis.

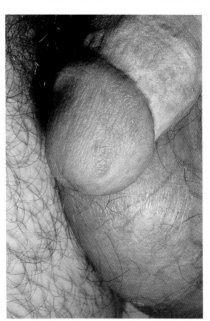

**Fig. 6.58
Psoriasis.** Glans
penis.

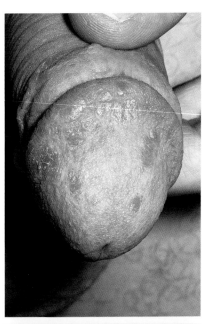

Fig. 6.59 Psoriasis. Glans penis. Reproduced by kind permission of The Royal Society of Medicine Press from Porter and Bunker, 2001.

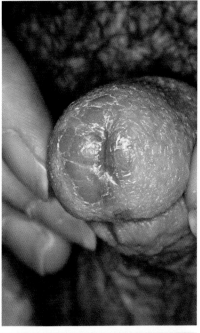

Fig. 6.60 Psoriasis. Glans penis. Peri meatal plaque.

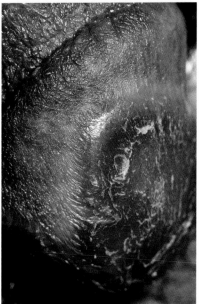

Fig. 6.61 Psoriasis. Glans penis. Rupioid lesions Koebnerizing circumcision (for PIN) in a patient on lithium.

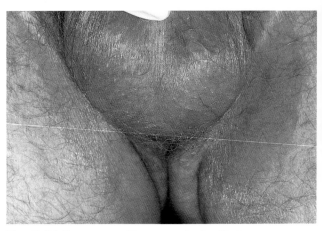

Fig. 6.62 Inverse pattern psoriasis. Groins.

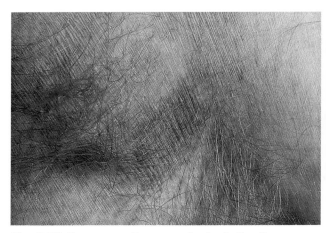

Fig. 6.63 Inverse pattern psoriasis. Axilla. Same patient as Fig. 6.62.

occurrence probably owes something to the Koebner phenomenon) and in the preputial sac and on the glans of the uncircumcised male. It is not usually itchy. Inordinate itch would make one suspect another dermatosis such as an eczematized dermatitis or tinea. A biopsy may need to be done and a scraping examined and cultured for fungi. Soreness supervenes with superinfection, especially with candida.

Interestingly, there is no analogous oral mucosal manifestation of psoriasis recognizably associated with the tendency to develop inverse psoriasis. Geographical tongue (thought by many to be a mucosal expression of psoriasis), which is seen sporadically, seems to occur independently.

Some drugs may trigger or worsen psoriasis, including: lithium, beta-blockers, antimalarials and angiotensin converting enzyme (ACE) inhibitors. Discontinuing the drugs may not always be possible but their potential implication in a new or worsening psoriatic situation should not be ignored.

Psoriasis may worsen or appear for the first time in the HIV-infected patient (Duvic et al 1987). Often it is very severe but curiously may regress in the preterminal phase (Colebunders et al 1992). Pustulosis may predominate and occasionally psoriasis is the cause of an erythroderma. Again anogenital lesions are common and frequently disabling (**Figs 6.64–6.66**). Chronic herpetic infection may complicate perianal psoriasis and elude diagnosis unless thought of.

Usually the diagnosis of psoriasis is clinical but sometimes a biopsy is necessary, for example for solitary mucosal lesions in the uncircumcised to exclude Zoon's balanitis, lichen planus, erythroplasia of Queyrat or Kaposi's sarcoma. Bowen's disease and extramammary Paget's disease may be misdiagnosed as psoriasis when there are single or several foci on the penile shaft and/or in the groins.

On histology (see **Fig. 2.45**, page 36) psoriasis is characterized by a pattern of epidermal thickening consisting of hyperkeratosis thickened rete ridges with thinning of the Malpighian layer over the dermal

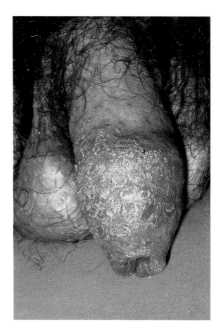

Fig. 6.66 Psoriasis. Penis shaft. Severe involvement in HIV.

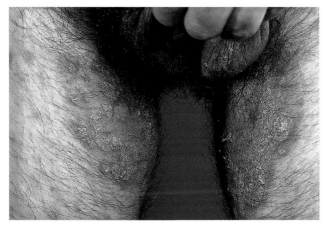

Fig. 6.64 Psoriasis. Upper thighs. Severe involvement in HIV. Note the importance of taking a specimen for mycology to exclude tinea.

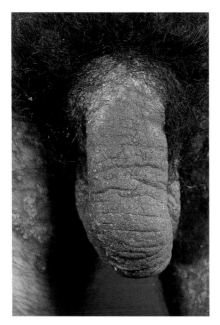

Fig. 6.65 Psoriasis. Penis shaft (and thighs). Severe involvement in HIV. Same patient as Fig. 6.64. Beware missing crusted Norwegian/ scabies.

papillae. There is parakeratosis in the stratum corneum, loss of the granular layer and often collections of degenerating neutrophils just under the stratum corneum. Sometimes these neutrophils accumulate to form epidermal microabscesses. The dermal papillary capillaries are dilated and tortuous and there is an infiltrate of lymphocytes and macrophages found in the dermis.

With a confident clinical diagnosis, which is the norm, adequate reassurance is as effective as in other situations in relieving anxiety about sexually transmitted disease or cancerous or precancerous conditions.

Topical treatment is based around emollients, soap substitutes, corticosteroids combined with antibiotic and antifungal agents or weak tar solutions. Strong, crude tar preparations should be avoided at this site given the propensity of anogenital skin to show a heightened tendency to absorb topical agents and because of the risk of genital cancer: one of the first occupational diseases described was scrotal carcinoma in chimney sweeps. Dithranol may be easily smeared on normal skin leading to burning so is usually avoided in this region. The vitamin D analogue calcipotriol can be helpful. Topical cyclosporin (100mg/ml in wet dressings three times daily have been advocated (Jemek & Baadasgard 1998).

Other more powerful treatments are listed in **Table 6.12**.

Severe anogenital, inverse psoriasis can be an indication for systemic treatment (say, with methotrexate or cyclosporin) in its own right but more often is a relative indication taken with severe and/or widespread extra-genital disease and/or arthritis.

Phototherapy is conventionally contraindicated because of the risk of anogenital cancer. In fact it is suspected that chronic anogenital psoriasis and its treatment creates a risk for anogenital squamous cancer.

Table 6.12 Treatments for psoriasis

Topical	Emollients
	Tar
	Dithranol
	Steroids
	Calcipotriol
	Cyclosporin
Phototherapy	UVB
	PUVA
	Re-PUVA (retinoid + PUVA)
Systemic	Acitretin
	Sulphasalazine
	Cyclosporin
	Hydroxyurea
	Methotrexate

Table 6.14 Radiological features of Reiter's disease

Erosions

Periostitis

Plantar spurs

Sacroiliitis (Figs 6.69, 6.70)

Obliteration of sacroiliac joints

Periostitis of symphysis pubis

Lumbar interspinous calcification (like ankylosing spondylitis)

Lateral subluxation of phalanges on metatarsals

Hammer toe deformities

(After Catterall 1983)

Reiter's disease

Reiter's disease or syndrome is part of the same continuum as psoriasis in genetically predisposed individuals. Reiter's syndrome is defined as arthritis, urethritis and conjunctivitis.

This disease was recognized by Hans Reiter (1916) while he served in the German army in the Kaiser's War but it had been described by Launois in 1899, Fournier in 1868, Sir Benjamin Brodie in 1818 and Stoll in 1776 (Catterall 1983).

It is precipitated by non-specific urethritis or bacillary or amoebic dysentery and associated with HLA B27.

The clinical features and radiological signs are listed in **Tables 6.13** and **6.14** (**Figs 6.67–6.70**).

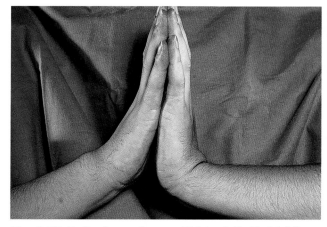

Fig. 6.67 Reiter's syndrome. Wrists. Arthritis (right).

Table 6.13 Clinical features of Reiter's disease

Diarrhea

Non-specific urethritis

Polyarticular arthritis (Figs 6.67, 6.68)

Conjunctivitis

Uveitis/iritis/conjunctivitis (Fig. 2.1a)

Circinate balanitis

Oral erosions/ulcers

Erythema nodosum

Keratoderma blenorrhagica

Neurological lesions

Nephritis

Myositis

Amyloidosis

Aortic valve disease

Electrocardiographic carditis

(After Willkens et al 1981; Catterall 1983; Keat 1983)

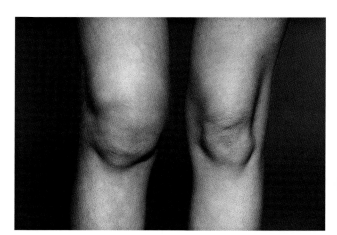

Fig. 6.68 Reiter's syndrome. Knees. Arthritis (right). (Courtesy of Dr Andrew Keat, London, UK).

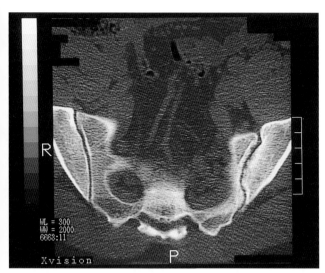

Fig. 6.69 Reiter's syndrome. Sacroiliitis (left). Axial CT showing joint space widening and sclerosis. Note that the right side is normal. (Courtesy of Dr Andrew Keat, London, UK).

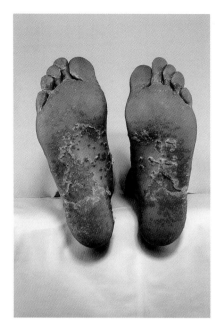

Fig. 6.71 Reiter's syndrome. Keratoderma blenorrhagica.

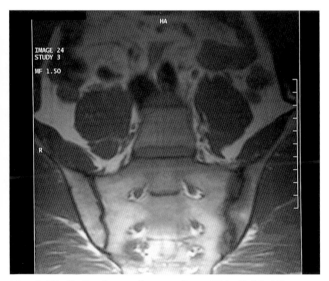

Fig. 6.70 Reiter's syndrome. Sacroiliitis (left). T1-weighted coronal image demonstrating peri-articular low signal of left SI joint. Note that the right side is normal. (Courtesy of Dr Andrew Keat, London, UK).

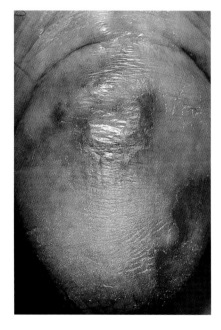

Fig. 6.72 Circinate balanitis. Glans penis. Psoriasiform lesions. This patient was HLA B27 positive.

Skin lesions in Reiter's syndrome may be similar to those of psoriasis. Patients have long been recognized with features of both psoriasis and Reiter's syndrome. Classically, Reiter's patients may have thickened yellow palms and soles with a cobblestone appearance with or without pustular lesions (keratoderma blenorrhagica, **Fig. 6.71**) and characteristic sometimes severe involvement of the penis (circinate balanitis, **Figs 6.72–6.76**; but they may also have any of the features of psoriasis described above (**Fig. 6.77**). The penile lesions have the same histopathology and ultrastructure as psoriasis (Kanerva et al 1982). Oral lesions (**Fig. 6.78**) are classically painless.

Reiter's disease has been reported in AIDS and the earlier stages of HIV infection in its classical or incomplete form (Duvic et al 1987).

The treatment of the skin disease is similar to that for psoriasis. Oral retinoids can be particularly useful especially in HIV.

LICHEN SCLEROSUS

Lichen sclerosus is a curious, uncommon, chronic, inflammatory and scarring dermatosis with a predilection for the genitalia and a low-grade propensity to progress to squamous carcinoma (Ridley 1987; Meffert et al 1995; Powell & Wojnarowska 1999). In men

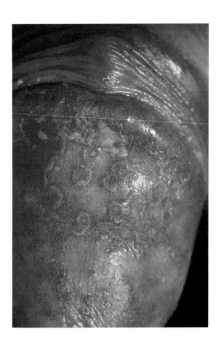

Fig. 6.73 Circinate balanitis. Glans penis. Psoriasiform lesions.

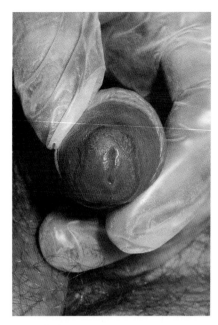

Fig. 6.76 Circinate balanitis. Glans penis. Peri meatal psoriasiform lesion.

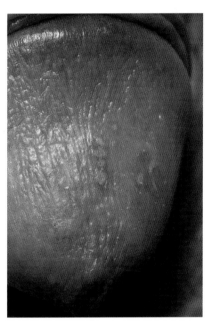

Fig. 6.74 Circinate balanitis. Glans penis. Psoriasiform lesions.

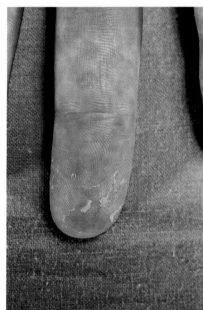

Fig. 6.77 Reiter's syndrome. Digital psoriasiform lesions.

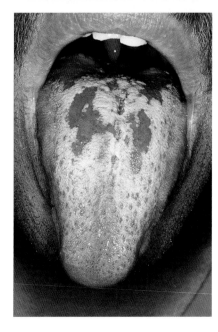

Fig. 6.78 Reiter's syndrome. Tongue. Painless erosions. (Courtesy of Dr Andrew Keat, London, UK).

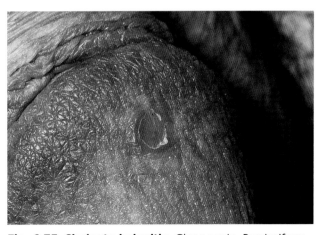

Fig. 6.75 Circinate balanitis. Glans penis. Psoriasiform lesion.

genital disease affects only the uncircumcised (Ledwig & Weigand 1989).

Lichen sclerosus of the penis may be asymptomatic, but diverse, often vague, symptomatology is usually encountered (Riddell et al 2000) (**Table 6.15**). Patients may report and describe itching, burning, bleeding, tearing, splitting, hemorrhagic blisters, any manner of symptoms signifying sexual dysfunction or dyspareunia, discomfort with urination and narrowing of the urinary stream and/or be concerned about the changing anatomy of their genitalia (Pelisse 1987; Feldmann & Harms 1991; Datta et al 1993). Other presentations are non-retractile foreskin (**Figs 6.79–6.82**, i.e. phimosis ['muzzling']), foreskin fixed in retraction, i.e. paraphimosis and urinary retention (even renal failure).

Genital lichen sclerosus (Lipscombe et al 1997), like extragenital disease (**Figs 6.83–6.85**), can manifest as atrophic white patches (leukoderma, **Figs 6.86, 6.87**, see also **Fig. 2.28**, page 32) or plaques, sometimes hypertrophic (**Figs 6.88, 6.89**), or lilac, slightly scaly lichenoid patches or plaques (**Fig. 6.90**) with telangiectasia and sparse purpura (**Figs 6.91, 6.92**). Predominant purpura, (Kossard & Shumack 1989; Kossard 1997 — personal

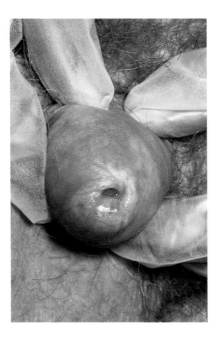

Fig. 6.79 Lichen sclerosus. Phimosis.

Table 6.15 Clinical presentations of male genital lichen sclerosus

Asymptomatic

Spontaneous
  Itch
  Burning
  Soreness
  Pain
  Adhesions
  Blisters
  White patches
  Tight foreskin
  Effacement of normal architectural features
    Narrow meatus
    Dissolution of frenulum
    Loss of pearly penile papules

Dyspareunia
  Itch
  Burning
  Soreness
  Pain
  Bleeding
  Tearing
  Splitting
  Blisters
  Raw patches
  Tight foreskin

Phimosis

Paraphimosis

Dysuria

Urinary retention

Renal failure

Cancer (see page 208)

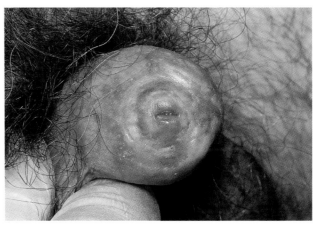

Fig. 6.80 Lichen sclerosus. Phimosis.

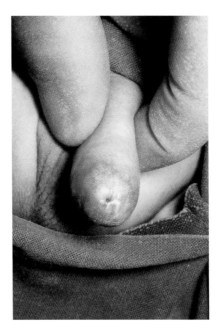

Fig. 6.81 Lichen sclerosus. Child. Penis and distal prepuce. Phimosis and posthitis xerotica obliterans. (Courtesy of Mr Nick Madden, London, UK).

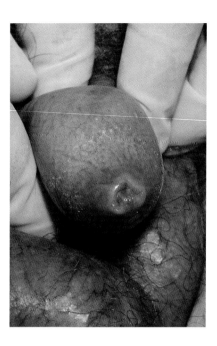

**Fig. 6.82
Phimosis.** Penis.
Probable lichen
sclerosus.

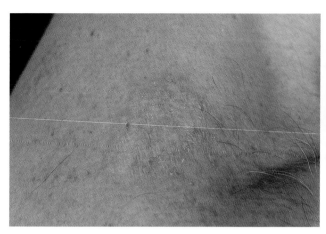

Fig. 6.85 Lichen sclerosus. Neck. This patient denied
genital symptomatology but on examination had a
sclerotic preputial band (Fig. 6.142).

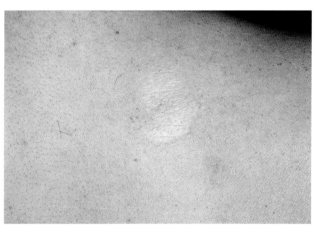

Fig. 6.83 Extragenital lichen sclerosus. Back. Lilac,
scaly patch. This patient had involvement of the penis.

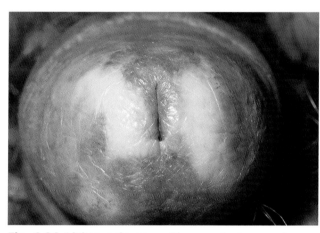

Fig. 6.86 Lichen sclerosus. Glans penis. Low grade
balanitis and peri meatal leukoderma due to mild sclerosis
and atrophy.

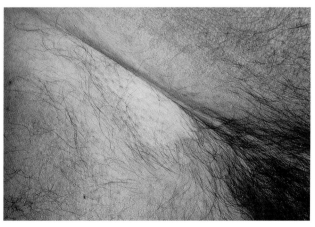

Fig. 6.84 Extragenital lichen sclerosus. Groin.

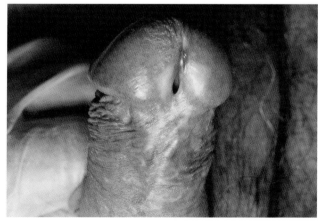

**Fig. 6.87 Lichen sclerosus and congenital
hypospadias.** Ventral glans and distal shaft penis.

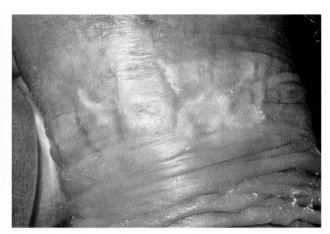

Fig. 6.88 Lichen sclerosus. Proximal prepuce. Low-grade posthitis. Slight lilac erythema with mild, shallow-fissured, slightly hypertrophic plaques.

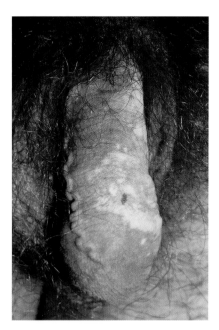

Fig. 6.91 Lichen sclerosus. Penis shaft. Slightly scaly, slightly lilac, scaly patches with atrophy.

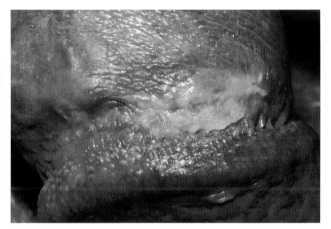

Fig. 6.89 Lichen sclerosus. Dorsal coronal sulcus. Hypertrophic plaque.

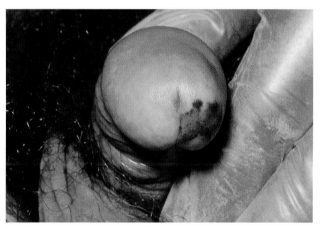

Fig. 6.92 Lichen sclerosus. Glans penis. Purpura and vitiligo. 'Pin hole' meatus.

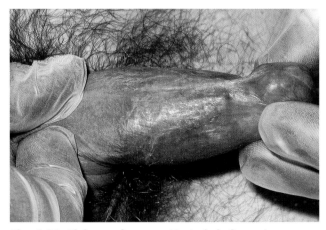

Fig. 6.90 Lichen sclerosus. Ventral shaft, penis. Lichenoid plaque.

communication, **Figs 4.27, 4.28**; Barton et al 1993, see also **Figs 4.25, 4.26**) and hemorrhage (Zderkiewicz 1972), bullae, erosions and ulceration may be encountered (Wallace 1971). Post-inflammatory hyper- and hypopigmentation is uncommon (**Figs 6.104, 6.129**, see also **Figs 4.4, 4.5**): some patients may be diagnosed as having penile melanosis (see page 52).

The signs (**Table 6.15**) may be subtle with meatal 'pin hole' narrowing (**Figs 6.92, 6.99**), slight tightening (due to sclerotic plaques and bands, **Fig. 6.95**) of the retracted prepuce associated with slight difficulty or no difficulty in retraction (some authors refer to this as paraphimosis but I have termed it 'waisting' (see **Figs 6.95, 6.96, 6.98, 6.100, 6.102, 6.103, 6.117**), and also **Figs 2.26, 2.27**), or florid with severe changes due to the lichen sclerosus and associated non-specific or Zoonoid balanoposthitis, adhesions, loss of anatomical definition and dissolution or effacement of the normally sharply defined architectural features such as the frenulum and

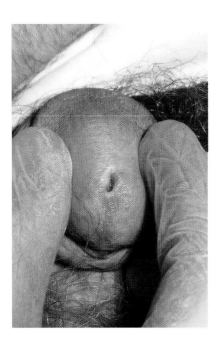

Fig. 6.93 Lichen sclerosus. Glans penis. Meatal narrowing and peri meatal sclerosis.

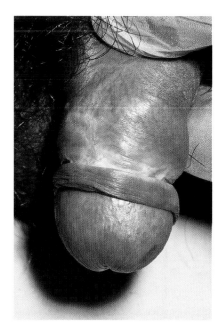

Fig. 6.96 Lichen sclerosus. Low-grade posthitis, moderate waisting due to sclerotic band.

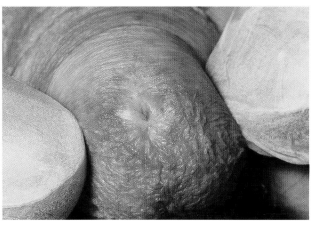

Fig. 6.94 Lichen sclerosus. Glans penis. Low-grade peri meatal disease and 'pin hole' meatus.

the coronal sulcus (**Figs 6.97–6.99**). Overt changes of Zoon's balanitis (**Figs 6.100–6.103**) or post-inflammatory hyperpigmentation (**Fig. 6.104**) may be more florid than the underlying lichen sclerosus. Further examples of the clinical manifestations of lichen sclerosus are demonstrated in **Figs 6.105–6.141**. See also **Table 6.15**.

Whereas posthitis xerotica obliterans refers to chronic damage to the prepuce by lichen sclerosus, balanitis xerotica obliterans (BXO) is a more frequently encountered term describing severe damage from long-standing, sometimes undiagnosed, unchecked disease. Dermatologists teach that BXO can be a consequence of other scarring dermatoses such as lichen planus and cicatricial pemphigoid (Ridley & Neill 1993).

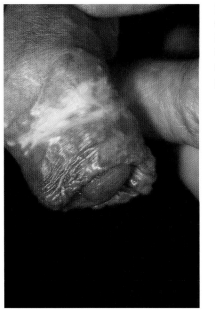

Fig. 6.95 Lichen sclerosus. Proximal prepuce. Constrictive band due to sclerotic plaque.

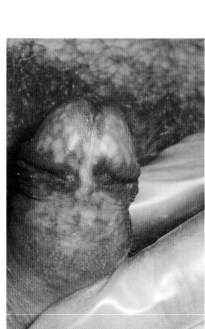

Fig. 6.97 Lichen sclerosus. Ventral glans penis and distal prepuce. Multiple white patches, destruction of frenulum, low-grade posthitis.

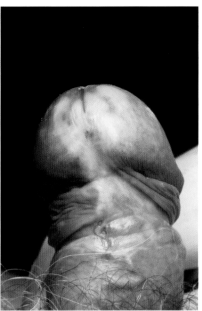

Fig. 6.98 Lichen sclerosus. Glans and distal prepuce. Posthitis, waisting and obliteration of the frenulum.

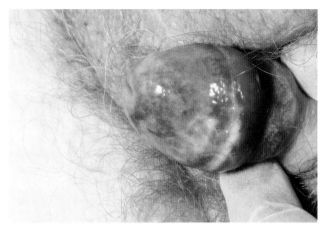

Fig. 6.101 Zoonoid inflammation/presumed lichen sclerosus. Glans penis and prepuce. Zoonoid inflammation and waisting. Loss of coronal definition. Signs of balanitis xerotica on the glans. Circumcision histology showed eroded Zoon's posthitis. At five-year follow-up the glans was quiet but with clinical signs of burn-out lichen sclerosus (BXO).

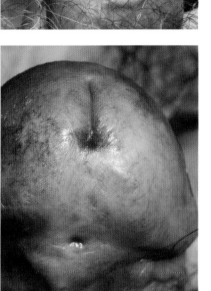

Fig. 6.99 Lichen sclerosus and acquired fistula. Ventral glans penis and coronal sulcus. Chronic disease: grossly abnormal anatomy with loss of frenulum and self-induced fistula.

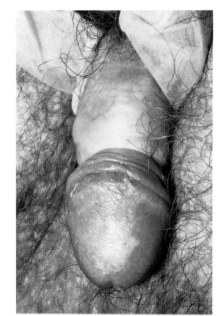

Fig. 6.102 Zoonoid inflammation/ lichen sclerosus. Dorsal glans and prepuce, penis. Zoon's balanitis and posthitis, posthitis xerotica, balanitis xerotica and waisting.

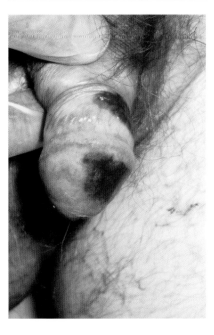

Fig. 6.100 Lichen sclerosis and Zoon's balanitis. Glans and prepuce, penis. Note waisting and concomitant lichen sclerosus.

Anogenital lichen sclerosus is more common than extragenital or oral disease but there may (rarely) be concomitant involvement of these sites. In adults anogenital lichen sclerosus is said to be about ten times more common in women than in men. In my experience, perianal disease is very rare in the male.

The involvement of the anterior urethra can be devastating. Barbagli et al (1999) found that 29% of patients undergoing urethroplasty for urethral stricture had pathological evidence of lichen sclerosus.

Surprisingly, the first report of genital lichen sclerosus in *boys* appeared only in 1977 (Götz et al) but lichen sclerosus may be much more frequent than is generally

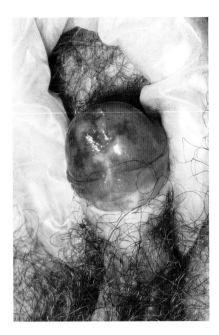

Fig. 6.103 Lichen sclerosus/ zoonoid inflammation. Ventral glans and prepuce. Eroded Zoon's balanitis and posthitis, PXO and waisting. Same patient as Fig. 6.102.

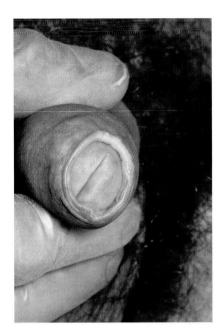

Fig. 6.106 Lichen sclerosus. Glans and preputial orifice, penis. Partial phimosis; 'muzzling'.

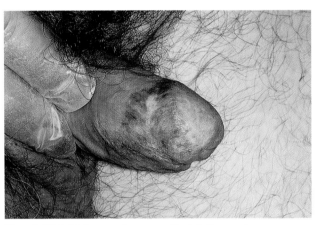

Fig. 6.104 Lichen sclerosus. Post-inflammatory hyperpigmentation. Glans and distal shaft, penis.

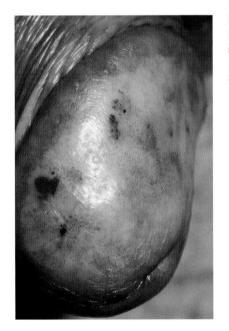

Fig. 6.107 Lichen sclerosus. Glans penis. Atrophy and purpura.

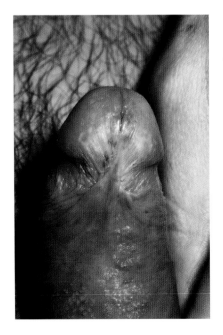

Fig. 6.105 Lichen sclerosus. Ventral shaft and glans, penis. Dissolution of frenulum.

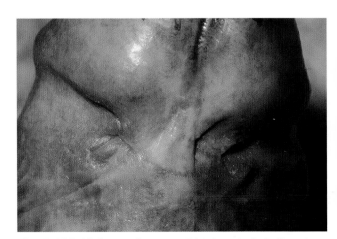

Fig. 6.108 Lichen sclerosus. Distal ventral shaft and glans, penis. Destruction of frenulum.

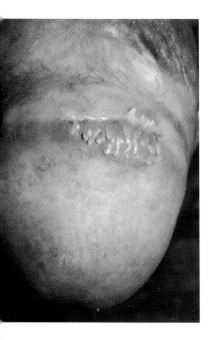

Fig. 6.109 Lichen sclerosus. Dorsal distal shaft and glans penis. Loss of coronal definition and obliteration of pearly penile papules.

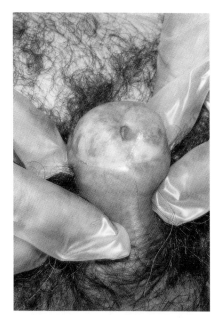

Fig. 6.112 Lichen sclerosus. Ventral shaft and glans, penis. Transcoronal fusion of prepuce, balanitis xerotica and meatal narrowing.

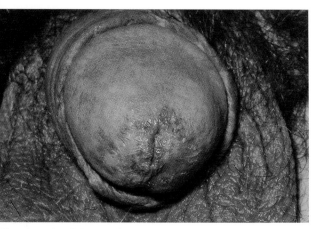

Fig. 6.110 Lichen sclerosus. Glans penis. Peri meatal disease.

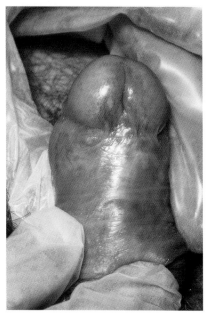

Fig. 6.113 Lichen sclerosus. Ventral shaft and glans, penis. Loss of coronal definition. Meatal slit.

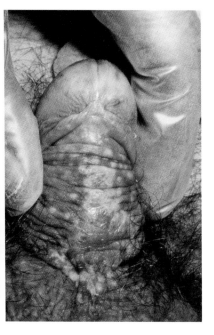

Fig. 6.111 Lichen sclerosus. Ventral shaft and glans, penis.

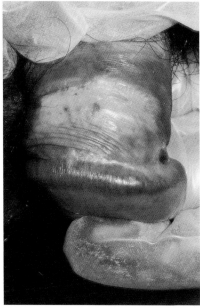

Fig. 6.114 Lichen sclerosus. Lateral shaft, distal prepuce and glans, penis. Sclerotic band, purpura and Zoonoid inflammation.

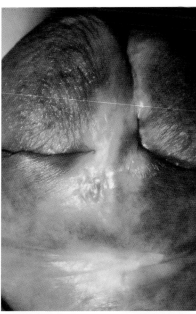

Fig. 6.115 Lichen sclerosus. Distal ventral shaft and glans, penis. Dissolution of architecture of coronal sulcus and frenulum; meatal slit.

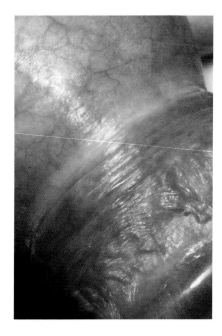

Fig. 6.118 Lichen sclerosus. Mid shaft/prepuce penis. Waisting. Same case as Fig. 6.117.

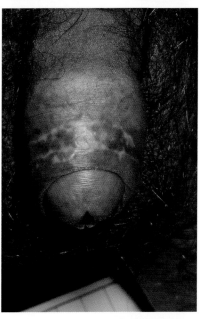

Fig. 6.116 Lichen sclerosus. Distal dorsal prepuce, penis. Sclerotic bands.

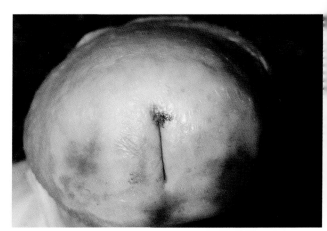

Fig. 6.119 Lichen sclerosus. Glans penis. Subtle balanitis xerotica.

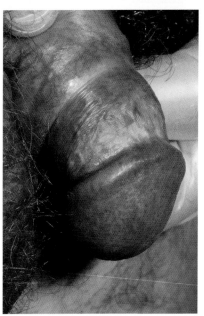

Fig. 6.117 Lichen sclerosus. Mid shaft/prepuce penis. Waisting.

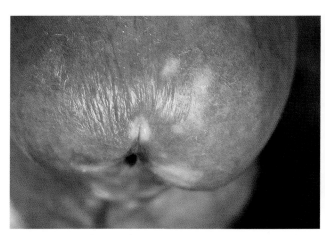

Fig. 6.120 Lichen sclerosus. Glans penis. Hypospadias.

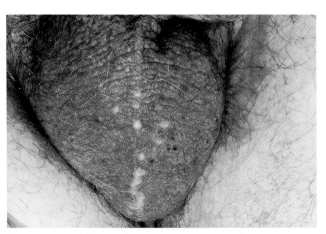

Fig. 6.121 Lichen sclerosus. Scrotum. Sclerotic macules. Patient also has angiokeratomas.

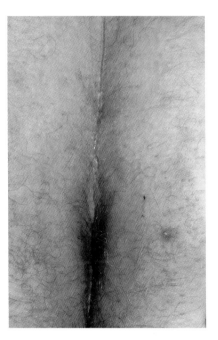

Fig. 6.122 Lichen sclerosus. Natal cleft. Same case as Fig. 6.121.

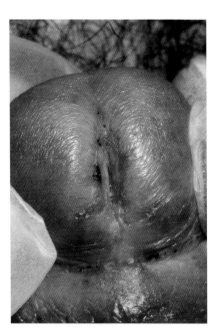

Fig. 6.124 Lichen sclerosus. Ventral glans penis. Meatal narrowing.

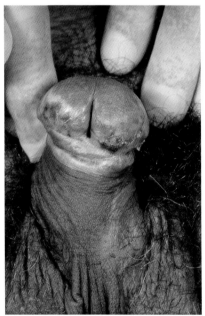

Fig. 6.125 Lichen sclerosus. Ventral glans penis. Balanitis xerotica. Meatal slit.

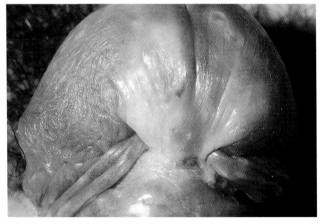

Fig. 6.123 Lichen sclerosus. Ventral glans penis. Sclerosis of frenulum.

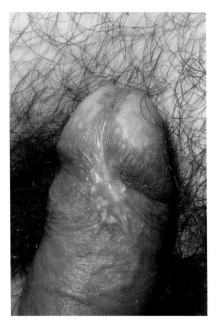

Fig. 6.126 Lichen sclerosus. Ventral glans and distal shaft, penis. Destruction of frenulum.

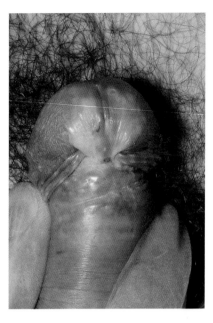

Fig. 6.127 Lichen sclerosus. Ventral glans and distal shaft and prepuce, penis. Sclerosis of frenulum and peri meatal glans.

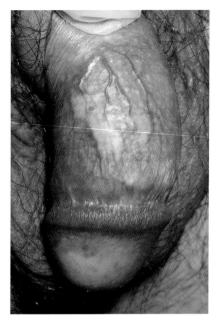

Fig. 6.130 Lichen sclerosus. Lateral prepuce. Plaque of preputial sclerosis. Same case as Fig. 6.126.

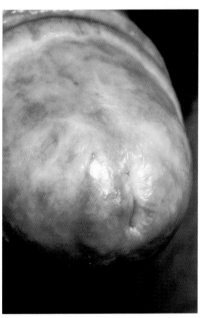

Fig. 6.128 Lichen sclerosus. Glans penis. Balanitis xerotica. Meatal narrowing.

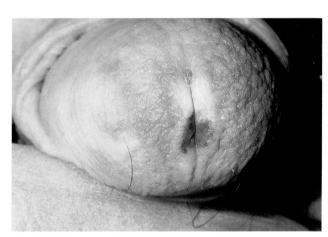

Fig. 6.131 Lichen sclerosus. Glans penis. Meatal narrowing and ecchymosis.

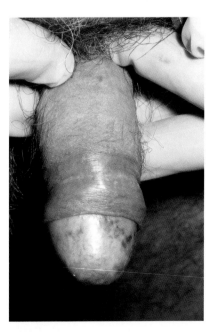

Fig. 6.129 Lichen sclerosus. Dorsal penis, shaft prepuce and glans. Lichenoid posthitis, waisting, balanitis xerotica and penile melanosis or post-inflammatory hyperpigmentation.

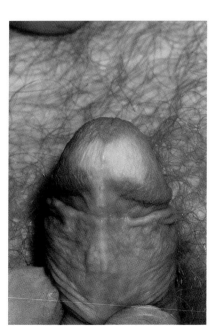

Fig. 6.132 Lichen sclerosus. Ventral glans and distal prepuce, penis. Burnt out posthitis and balanitis xerotica.

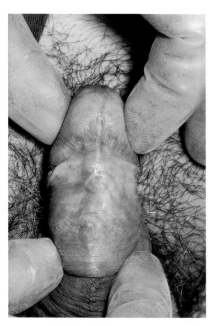

Fig. 6.133 Lichen sclerosus. Ventral glans and distal prepuce and shaft, penis. Frenuloplasty. Burnt-out posthitis and balanitis xerotica.

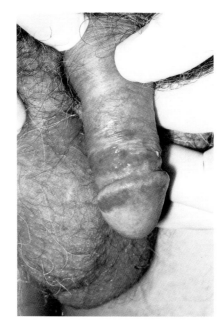

Fig. 6.136 Lichen sclerosus. Lateral shaft, prepuce and glans, penis. Zoon's balanitis. Histology showed lichen sclerosus of the prepuce and Zoon's balanitis of the glans.

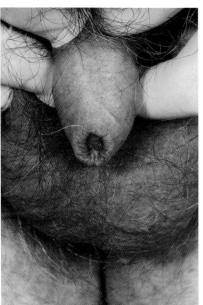

Fig. 6.134 Lichen sclerosus. Preputial orifice, penis. Orificial lichenoid posthitis (lichen sclerosus histologically proven) and incipient phimosis.

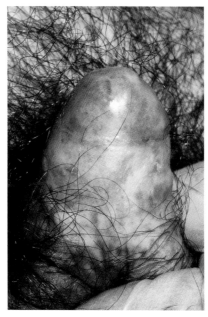

Fig. 6.137 Lichen sclerosus. Ventral glans and shaft, penis. Gross loss of anatomical definition of frenulum and coronal sulcus due to destruction and fusion; balanitis xerotica and meatal narrowing.

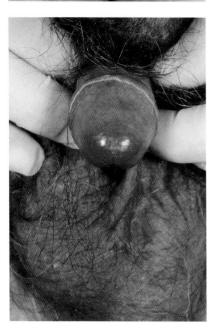

Fig. 6.135 Lichen sclerosus. Dorsal glans penis. Reactive Zoon's balanitis (histologically proven). Same case as Fig. 6.134 with foreskin retracted.

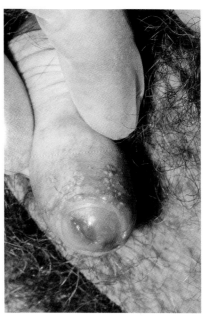

Fig. 6.138 Lichen sclerosus. Penis. Non-specific posthitis, impending phimosis and peri meatal Zoonoid inflammation. Circumcision histology confirmed lichen sclerosus. Note prominent ectopic sebaceous glands of Fordyce.

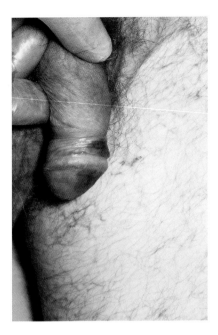

**Fig. 6.139
Lichen
sclerosus.** Penis,
glans shaft and
prepuce.
Prominent Zoon's
balanitis and
waisting with a
sclerotic preputial
band.
Circumcision
showed burnt-out
preputial lichen
sclerosus.

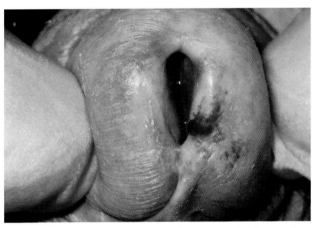

Fig. 6.140 Lichen sclerosus. Glans penis. Wide, pouting
meatus, peri meatal sclerosis and ecchymosis.

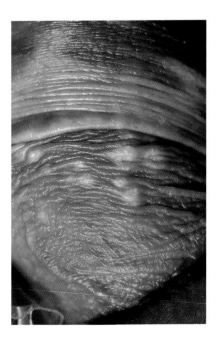

**Fig. 6.141
Lichen
sclerosus.** Distal,
lateral shaft,
penis. Sclerotic
papules and
macules.

supposed in young boys (Fortier-Beaulieu et al 1990).
For example Chu et al (1999) reported that 95% of boys
with phimosis that they treated with potent topical
steroids responded well, without considering that lichen
sclerosus might have been the cause of the phimosis in
some, many, most or even all these cases. This was found
to be the case in 20 out of 21 boys with phimosis
(defined as scarring of the tip of the prepuce) by
Rickwood et al (1980), and in 14 out of 100 prepubertal
boys undergoing elective circumcision for disease of the
foreskin by Chalmers et al (1984). Later figures are
similar (Ridley 1993). The development of secondary
phimosis in school-age boys is highly suggestive of
lichen sclerosus (Meuli et al 1994).

In children lichen sclerosus has been misdiagnosed as
being due to sexual abuse (Jenny et al 1989; Loening-
Baucke 1991) but lichen sclerosus does Koebnerize sites
of trauma so could be provoked by abusive practices
(Berth-Jones et al 1989; Harrington 1990).

Persistent primary phimosis or the secondary development of phimosis in a previously retractable foreskin
should be viewed with suspicion. Some, many or most of
such cases will be due to lichen sclerosus (Höfs &
Quednow 1978; Rickwood et al 1980; Chalmers et al
1984; Clemmensen et al 1988; Ridley 1993; Meuli et al
1994; Shankar & Rickwood 1999). For example,
Flentje et al (1987) found lichen sclerosus in 4.3% of
cases of acquired phimosis that had been circumcised
and analyzed histologically and Aynaud et al (1999)
found histological evidence of lichen sclerosus in
relatively few young adults requiring circumcision for
phimosis, but in 40% of older men.

Most cases of lichen sclerosus can be diagnosed clinically. Sometimes lichen planus is difficult to differentiate
and cicatrizing pemphigoid is rare and likewise hard to
diagnose. Extragenital lichen sclerosus is rarely present
(about 2% of my series **Figs 6.85, 6.142**). If there is

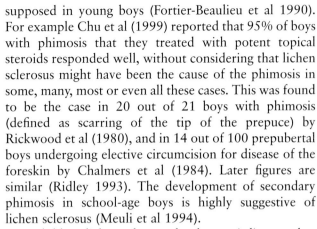

**Fig. 6.142
Lichen
sclerosus.**
Ventral prepuce.
Sclerotic preputial
band. Same
patient as
Fig. 6.85.

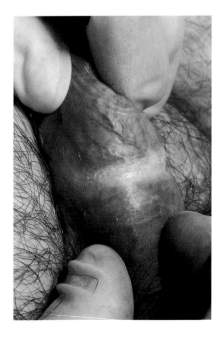

clinical doubt then a biopsy should be done. A biopsy is mandatory if the lesion or part of the lesion is eroded or verrucous.

The histology (**Figs 6.143–6.146**) (Rowell & Goodfield 1998) is classically of variable epidermal thickening (later, thinning), hyperkeratosis and follicular plugging with a band of hyalinization of dermal collagen, featureless but for dilated capillaries, below which there is a band of lymphocytic, T-cell rich (Hinchliffe et al 1994), CD3, CD4, CD8, CD68, HLADR (from vulva studies) positive infiltrate (Farrell et al 1999), also containing increased Langerhans cells (Carli et al 1991).

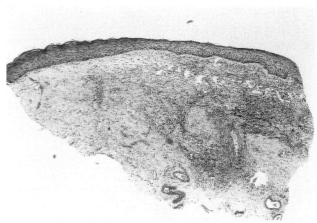

Fig. 6.145 Lichen sclerosus (Zoonoid change). A penile biopsy that to one side (left), where there is no inflammation, shows a degree of hyaline sclerosis of the epidermis, loss of the rete architecture and underlying chronic inflammation. On the other (right), heavily inflamed side, the infiltrate is dominated by plasma cells and the epidermis shows some slight intraepidermal spongiosis. This represents lichen sclerosus with an adjacent area of Zoon's balanitis. (Courtesy of Dr Nick Francis, London, UK).

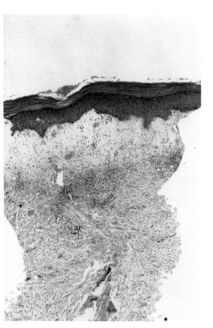

Fig. 6.143 Lichen sclerosus. Low power view of classical lichen sclerosus of the penis showing hyperkeratosis and underlying area of pale hyalinised dermis with some thin-walled dilated capillary sized vessels and a deeper zone of chronic inflammation. (Courtesy of Dr Nick Francis, London, UK).

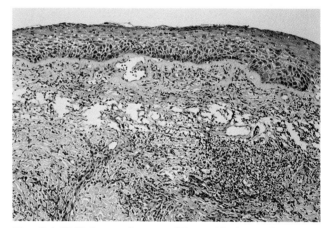

Fig. 6.146 Lichen sclerosus (Zoonoid change). Higher power view of figure 6.145. Shown is the typical small vessel dilatation within the bland and loose edematous hyaline stroma beneath the slightly spongiotic epidermis and then, beneath that, patchy aggregates of chronic Zoonoid inflammation. (Courtesy of Dr Nick Francis, London, UK).

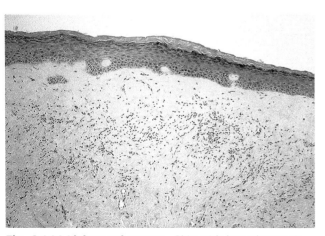

Fig. 6.144 Lichen sclerosus. Skin with hyperkeratosis, some flattening of rete architecture, a dense upper dermal area of sclerosus and an underlying, partly band-like chronic inflammatory cell infiltrate. (Courtesy of Dr Nick Francis, London, UK).

The occasional histological finding of associated endarteritis led originally to the usage of the term 'obliterans' (Das & Tunuguntula 2000). In two cases in boys a dermal lymphohistiocytic and granulomatous phlebitis has been found, one of whom also had evidence of HPV (Cabaleiro et al 2000). A garland-like basal lamina has been found ultrastructurally (Dupré & Viraben 1988). Sometimes lichen sclerosus may be difficult to differentiate from lichen planus and criteria to assist, in the vulva, have been proposed by Fung & LeBoit (1998). Zoonoid inflammation may be present (**Figs 6.145–6.146**).

Guidelines for the management of lichen sclerosus have been published by the British Association of Dermatologists (Neill et al 2002).

Very potent topical corticosteroid (Tremaine & Miller 1989) used under supervision is effective. This appears to induce remodeling of the affected mucosa (testifying to the plasticity of the epithelium at this site), relieve phimosis, improve the histological signs and save the appendage from circumcision (Fortier-Beaulieu et al 1990; Jorgensen & Svensson 1993, 1996; Lindhagen 1996; Dahlman-Ghozlan et al 1999; Riddell et al 2000). It is theoretically possible that this may also mean that the risk of squamous carcinoma is averted.

Confounding secondary candidal and bacterial infection should be treated. Long-term systemic antibiotic therapy (penicillin and dirithromycin) has been claimed to be beneficial (Shelley et al 1999) based on the premise that lichen sclerosus might be due to Borreliosis (Aberer et al 1987; Schempp et al 1993).

Testosterone propionate ointment was advocated at one time (Pasieczny 1977; Heise et al 1984; Skierlo & Heise 1987) but I have no personal experience of this, nor of oral stanozolol (Parsad & Saini 1998) or of freezing with ethyl chloride (Zderkiewicz 1972) or liquid nitrogen cryotherapy, which has been used for lichen sclerosus of the vulva (August & Milward 1980), or ACTH (Di Silverio & Serri 1975). Oral etretinate has been tried with no effect (Neuhofer & Fritsch 1984).

If medical treatment fails then surgery is contemplated. Intervention ranges from circumcision (Meyrick-Thomas et al 1987), frenuloplasty and meatotomy, to sophisticated plastic repair, depending upon the clinical presentation and where the brunt of the disease impacts on the organ (von Happle 1973; Campus et al 1984; Das & Tunuguntula 2000). In boys, complete circumcision is the treatment of choice because all affected tissue is removed and any secondary involvement of the glans probably regresses or resolves (Meuli et al 1994). It is my impression and that of others that this phenomenon pertains in most adult patients with lichen sclerosus. Yet lichen sclerosus can persist or recur including in donor grafts from unrelated sites (Wallace 1971; Lee & Phillips 1994). Carbon dioxide laser treatment for lichen sclerosus and for therapeutic circumcision has been advocated (Aynaud et al 1995; Hrebinko 1996; Kartamaa & Reitamo 1997).

The cause(s) of lichen sclerosus remains obscure: the topic has been well reviewed by Powell & Wojnarowska (1999) whose group has done interesting research, including into the role of proteases (Farrell et al 2000). HPV has been implicated (Ansink et al 1994).

Scant specific enquiry has been made into penile lichen sclerosus. Familial cases occur (Höfs & Quednow 1978). HPV (types 6, 16 and 18) is present in 70% of cases of childhood penile lichen sclerosus (Drut et al 1998). However, the epidemiology and overall tenor of lichen sclerosus as clinically appreciated and experienced (I have seen over 250 cases) is not that of an infectious,

for example, sexually transmitted disease (Farrell et al 1999). One case report exists of sexual partners being afflicted but there was a 10-year interval (Zapolski-Downar et al 1987). The cytokine IL-6 has been implicated in skin diseases characterized by epidermal atrophy, including lichen sclerosus (Romero & Pincus 1992).

Trauma seems to play a role: I have seen cases where the development of the lichen sclerosus was related to injury or surgery and there are such cases reported in the literature (English et al 1998). The presence of the histopathological features of lichen sclerosus in a percentage of acrochordons (skin tags) has led to the suggestion that occlusion of flaccid skin is a pathogenic factor (Weigand 1993). There appears to be an association with anatomical anomaly especially of the urethral meatus (**Figs 6.125, 6.140, 6.147**). Specifically, lichen sclerosus has been related to hypospadias (**Figs 6.87, 6.148**) and its repair (Uemura et al 2000). A case has occurred following edema due presumptively to previous filarial infection (Wille et al 1997).

Patients with lichen sclerosus have an increased incidence of organ-specific autoantibodies (Goolamali et al 1974) and autoimmune disease such as morphea (Wallace 1969), which lichen sclerosus can resemble and with which it can be confused (Tremaine et al 1989) – although morphea of the penis is interestingly very rare (**Fig. 6.149**), vitiligo (**Figs 6.92, 6.150**; Wallace 1971; Meyrick-Thomas et al 1983; Osborne et al 2000), pernicious anemia (Harrington & Dunsmore 1981), and alopecia areata (Meyrick-Thomas et al 1983).

Wojnarowska's group have determined the HLA tissue types of 58 male patients with lichen sclerosus and found an increased frequency of several class II antigens including HLA DQ7, which also occurs more frequently in women with LS (Azurdia et al 1999). Although associ-

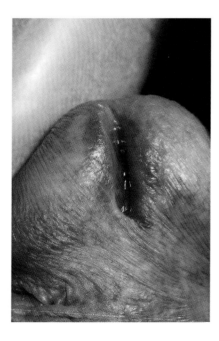

Fig. 6.147 Lichen sclerosus. Ventral glans penis. No frenulum. Elongated 'slit-like' meatus.

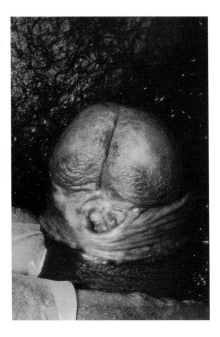

Fig. 6.148 Lichen sclerosus. Glans and ventral shaft penis. Note hypospadias and hyperkeratosis.

ations with autoimmune diseases were found in some male patients these were less common than in women.

Squamous cell carcinoma of the penis is the most serious potential complication of lichen sclerosus (Wallace 1971; Bingham 1978; Weigand 1980; Ridley 1987; Weber et al 1987; Schnitzler et al 1987; Doré et al 1989; Tremaine et al 1989; Doré et al 1990; Pride et al 1993; Simonart et al 1998). In situ change can occur often after long periods (Simonaart et al 1998). In many of the cases of penis cancer I have seen there has been solid or circumstantial, clinical and/or histological evidence of lichen sclerosus.

A risk of 4.0–9.5% has been claimed depending on length of follow-up: indeed the latent period may be one to three decades (Nasca et al 1999; Micali et al 2001). Verrucous carcinoma (Büschke-Lowenstein tumor) has been associated with previous lichen sclerosus (Weber et al 1987; O'Gorman-Lalor et al in press). Carcinoma complicating lichen sclerosus constituted one-third of all cases of penile cancer seen by Campus et al (1992). Involvement of the glans penis constitutes a greater risk (Micali et al 2001). Cancer is possibly a more common complication of *vulval* lichen sclerosus (Wallace 1971). Allelic imbalance has been proposed as the molecular predisposition to atypia and cancer in vulval lichen sclerosus (Pinto et al 2000).

It is not known for certain what impact medical and surgical treatment has on the subsequent incidence of penile cancer (Holly & Palefsky 1993; Maden et al 1993). Patients should be followed up long-term, especially if circumcision has not been performed or if symptoms persist or recur after any modality of treatment. Although describing a small number of patients it is salutary to recount the data of a follow-up study (16 patients followed from 1982 to 1997) from France (Bouyssou-Gauthier et al 1999): preputial disease seemed more readily treatable than disease of the glans, among the nine patients given medical treatment (topical steroids or androgens), lichen sclerosus persisted in seven, one developed a squamous cell carcinoma of the penis and one was considered cured. Liatskos et al (1997) report squamous cell carcinoma of the glans developing in one of eight patients followed up subsequent to circumcision for lichen sclerosus.

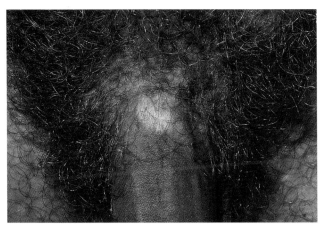

Fig. 6.149 Morphea. Penis base. (Courtesy of Dr Richard Staughton, London, UK).

LICHEN PLANUS

Lichen planus is a common inflammatory dermatosis that has a particular predilection for the mucosae and can indeed involve these sites in isolation (Barnette et al 1993). The etiopathogenesis of lichen planus is not known. Sometimes drugs can precipitate a generalized lichenoid eruption. A case of a lichenoid drug eruption confined to the penis due to propranolol has been reported (Massa et al 1991).

The classical eruption at extragenital sites is often intensely itchy and symmetrical, manifesting flat-

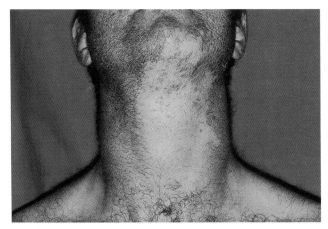

Fig. 6.150 Vitiligo and alopecia areata. Neck and chin. Same case as Fig. 6.92.

topped, polygonal, purple papules coalescing to form annules (**Figs 6.151–6.153**) and plaques and sur-topped by a fine, lacy scale called Wickham's striae. Palms (see Fig. 2.1p), soles, flexor aspects of wrists (**Fig. 6.154**), ankles, scalp, face, trunk; e.g. sacrum (**Figs 6.155–6.157**), axillae (see Fig 2.1s, see also Figs 6.151, 6.152, **6.158**), nails; causing variable patterns of dystrophy (**Figs 6.159, 6.160**), and mouth (**Figs 6.161–6.164**, see also Figs 2.1c, 2.1d, 2.1e, 2.1f, 2.1q) may all be affected. An aggressive form may lead to a scarring alopecia of the scalp (see Fig. 2.1h) and/or a permanent scarring nail dystrophy. Hypertrophic nodular and plaque morphologies are seen. Rarely, the extragenital disease may be erosive, for example, on the palms and soles.

Lichen planus can present in, and remain focalized to, the pelvic girdle (**Fig.6.165**, the genital area (**Figs 6.166– 6.186**) including the groins (**Figs 6.153, 6.187, 6.188**) and perianal skin (**Figs 6.189, 6.190**). Like the classical disease at other sites it presents as itchy, red-purple papules, also as patches or plaques and annular lesions, or as phimosis (Itin et al 1992; Aste et al 1997). Lichen planus manifests the Koebner phenomenon, which may partly explain the orogenital predilection (El-Gadi 1996).

Occasionally an erosive form is encountered (**Figs 6.191–6.195**). A male equivalent to the vulvo-vaginal syndrome of Hewitt with chronic erosive gingival and genital lesions has been proposed (genito-gingival syndrome) and described (Cribier et al 1992). In most cases lichen planus is self-limiting, although some patients relapse and remit. Adhesions can form (**Fig. 6.195**). Post-inflammatory hyperpigmentation (see Figs 6.165, 6.176, see also Figs 4.2, 4.3, 4.6) can persist for months or years.

A case of paraneoplastic lichen planus with orogenital involvement and cicatrizing conjunctivitis in association with thymoma has been described (Hahn et al 2000).

Chronic mucosal erosive lichen planus is associated with a risk of progression to squamous cell carcinoma but most reports concern oral lichen planus. Squamous carcinoma may complicate chronic hypertrophic lichen planus of the lower leg but has also occurred in the context of hypertrophic lichen planus of the glans penis (Worheide et al 1991; Leal-Khouri & Hruza 1994).

The micropapular variant, lichen nitidus (Lapins et al 1978) has an affinity for the penis (**Figs 6.196–6.199**). It can be difficult to diagnose because the signs may be subtle even when the lesions are widespread. Even when itchy the signs due to excoriation and eczematization may eclipse those due to the lichen nitidus.

The differential diagnosis includes psoriasis, Zoon's balanitis, lichen sclerosus, viral warts, Bowenoid papulosis and porokeratosis. Lichen planus is in the differential diagnosis of pruritus ani. A biopsy is frequently necessary for diagnostic purposes but is more importantly done in the follow-up of the rare cases of chronic anogenital disease where the development of ulcero-erosive or verrucous features leads to concern about the development of squamous cell carcinoma.

The classical histology (Daoud & Pittelkow 2003) (**Fig. 6.200**) consists of basal epidermal damage manifest as colloid bodies (degenerating basal epidermal cells), pigmentary incontinence, epidermal acanthosis, hyper-granulosis, compact orthokeratotic hyperkeratosis, a dense 'band-like' lymphohistiocytic inflammatory infiltrate

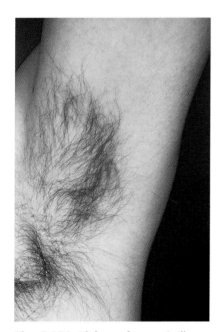

Fig. 6.151 Lichen planus. Axilla. Annular lesion.

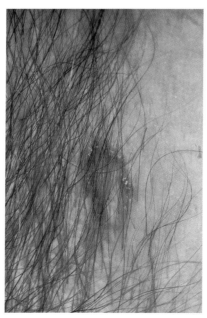

Fig. 6.152 Lichen planus. Axilla. Annular lesion. Same case as Fig. 6.15. Close-up.

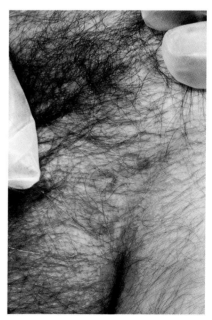

Fig. 6.153 Lichen planus. Groin. Annular lesions. Same case as Figs 6.151, 6.152.

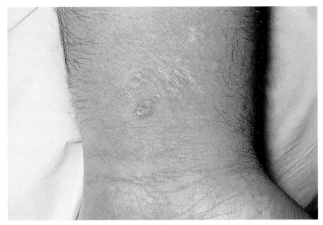

Fig. 6.154 Lichen planus. Flexor aspect of wrist.

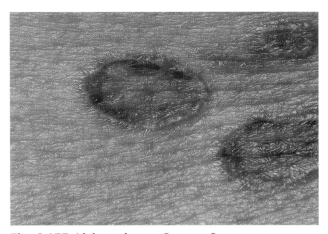

Fig. 6.157 Lichen planus. Sacrum. Same case as Fig. 6.156. Annular lesions. Close-up.

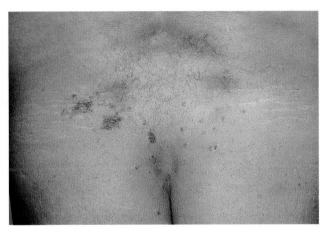

Fig. 6.155 Lichen planus. Sacrum and natal cleft.

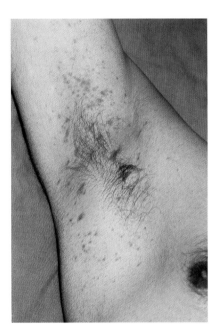

Fig. 6.158 Lichen planus. Axilla.

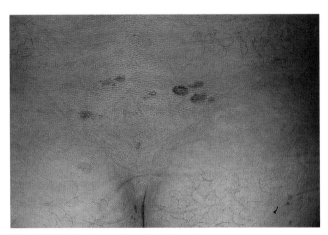

Fig. 6.156 Lichen planus. Sacrum.

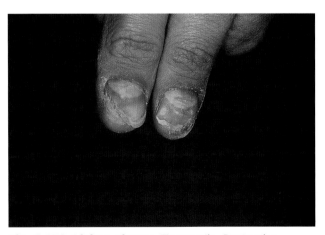

Fig. 6.159 Lichen planus. Fingernails. Dystrophy.

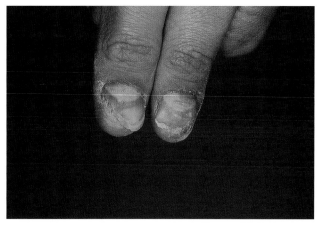

Fig. 6.160 Lichen planus. Nail dystrophy. Same case as Figs 6.164, 6.186.

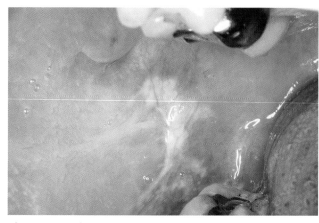

Fig. 6.163 Lichen planus. Buccal mucosa.

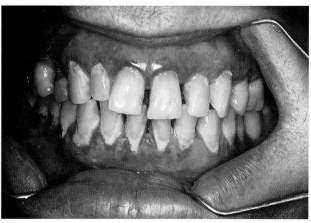

Fig. 6.161 Erosive lichen planus. Gingiva.

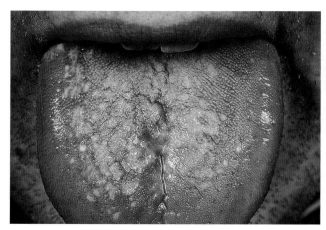

Fig. 6.164 Lichen planus. Tongue. Same case as Figs 6.160, 6.186.

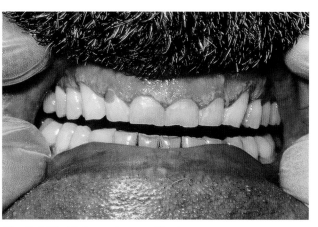

Fig. 6.162 Lichen planus. Gingiva.

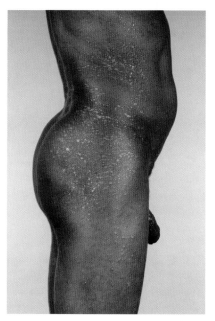

Fig. 6.165 Lichen planus. Pelvic girdle, right. Shiny, lichenoid papules, patches and plaques: post-inflammatory hyperpigmentation.

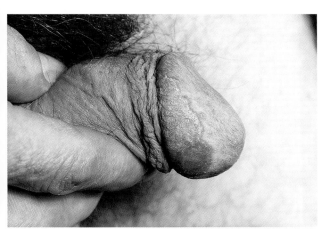

Fig. 6.166 Lichen planus. Glans penis.

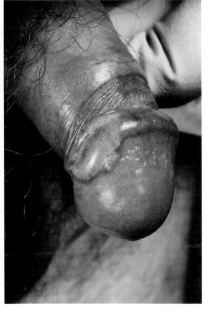

Fig. 6.167
Lichen planus.
Glans penis.

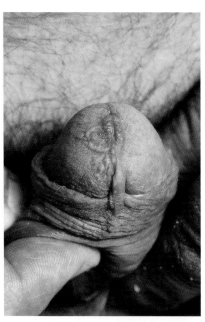

Fig. 6.169
Lichen planus.
Glans penis.

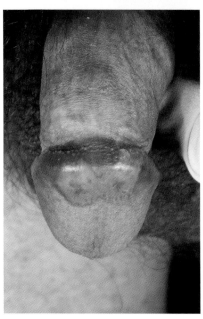

Fig. 6.170
Lichen planus.
Glans penis.

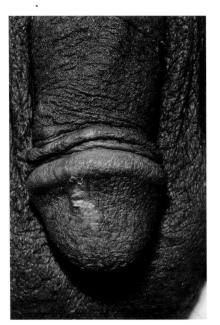

Fig. 6.168
Lichen planus.
Glans penis.

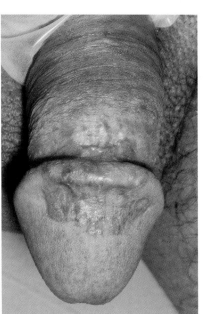

Fig. 6.171
Lichen planus.
Glans penis.
(Reproduced with
permission of the
Royal Society of
Medicine Press
from Porter and
Bunker, 2001.)

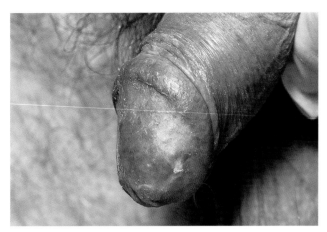

Fig. 6.172 Lichen planus. Penis glans and prepuce.

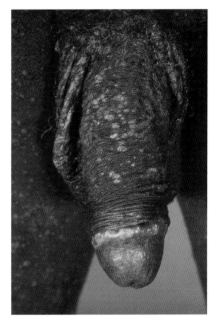

Fig. 6.173 Lichen planus. Penis shaft and glans.

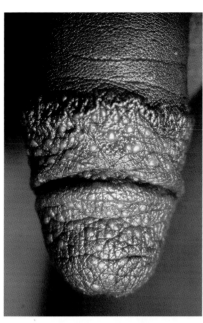

Fig. 6.175 Lichen planus. Penis glans and distal shaft.

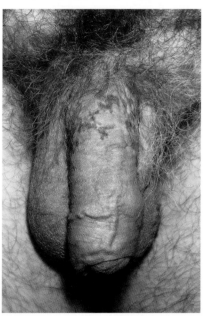

Fig. 6.176 Lichen planus. Penis proximal shaft. Post-inflammatory hyperpigmentation.

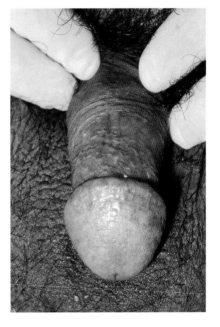

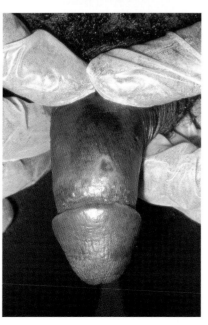

Fig. 6.174 Lichen planus. Penis glans and prepuce.

Fig. 6.177 Lichen planus. Penis shaft. Near-eroded red plaque.

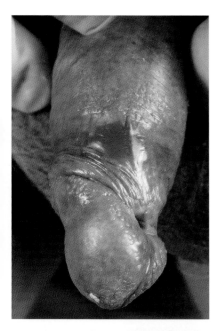

**Fig. 6.178
Lichen planus.**
Penis shaft. Red
plaque.

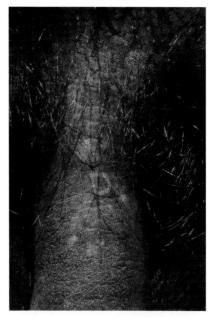

**Fig. 6.181
Lichen planus.**
Penis proximal
shaft. Asian.

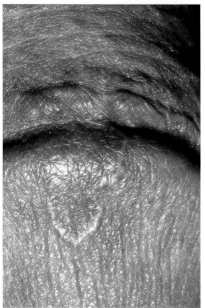

**Fig. 6.179
Lichen planus.**
Glans penis.
Subtle annule.

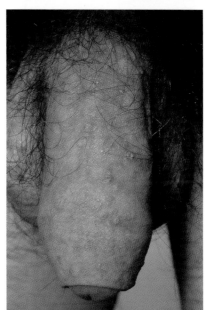

**Fig. 6.182
Lichen planus.**
Penis shaft.

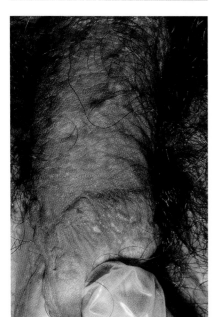

**Fig. 6.180
Lichen planus.**
Penis shaft. Sub-
coronal papules.

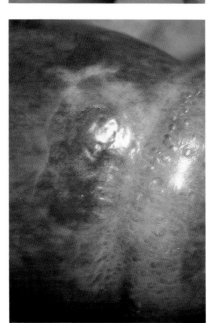

**Fig. 6.183
Lichen planus.**
Distal shaft,
penis. Eroded
lichenoid plaque
with Zoonoid
inflammation.

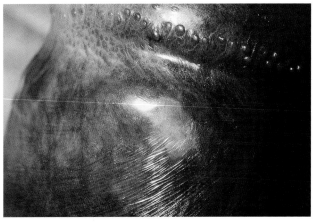

Fig. 6.184 Lichen planus. Distal shaft, penis. Bland lichenoid plaque.

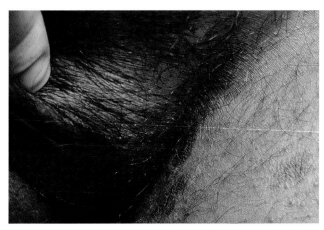

Fig. 6.187 Lichen planus. Groin.

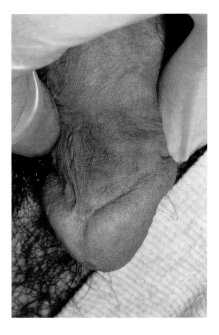

Fig. 6.185 Lichen planus. Distal ventral shaft, penis.

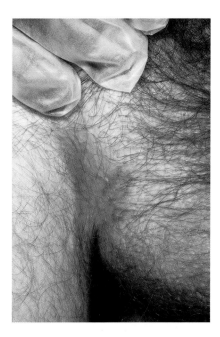

Fig. 6.188 Lichen planus. Groin.

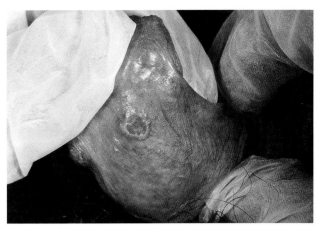

Fig. 6.186 Lichen planus. Ventral shaft, penis. Annular plaque. Same case as Figs 6.160, 6.164.

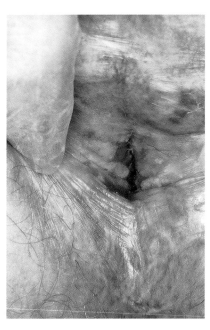

Fig. 6.189 Lichen planus. Anus.

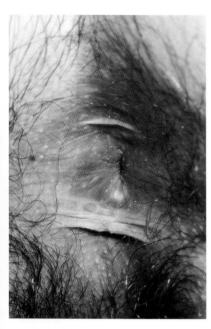

**Fig. 6.190
Lichen planus.**
Anus.

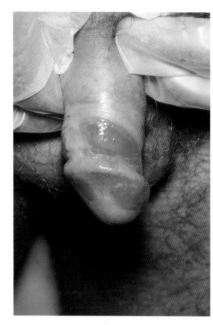

**Fig. 6.193
Erosive lichen
planus.** Penis
glans and
prepuce.
(Reproduced by
kind permission of
Blackwell Science
Ltd from Porter et
al, Erosive penile
lichen planus
responding to
circumcision.
J Eur Acad
Dermatol
Venereol 2001;
15: 266–8.)

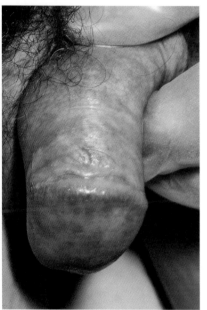

**Fig. 6.191
Erosive lichen
planus.** Penis
glans and
prepuce.

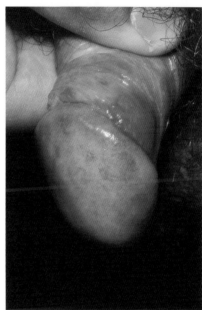

**Fig. 6.194
Lichen planus.**
Lateral glans and
distal shaft, penis.
Erosions.

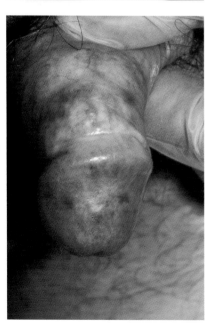

**Fig. 6.192
Erosive lichen
planus.** Penis
glans and
prepuce. This
patient
subsequently
developed
maturity-onset
diabetes.

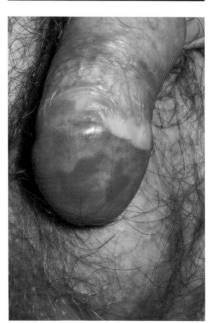

**Fig. 6.195
Erosive lichen
planus.** Glans
and distal
prepuce, penis.
Erosions and
adhesions.

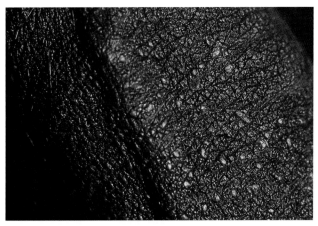

Fig. 6.196 Lichen nitidus. Shaft, penis. Flesh-colored, shiny, micropapules.

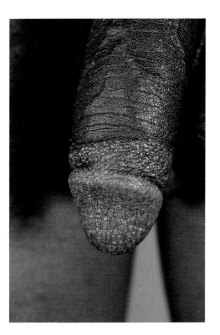

**Fig. 6.197
Lichen nitidus.**
Glans and distal shaft, penis. Flesh-colored, shiny, micro-papules.

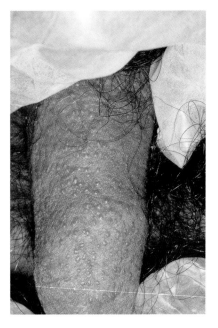

**Fig. 6.198
Lichen nitidus.**
Penis shaft. Flesh-colored micro-papules.

**Fig. 6.199
Lichen nitidus.**
Penis shaft. Flesh-colored micro-papules.

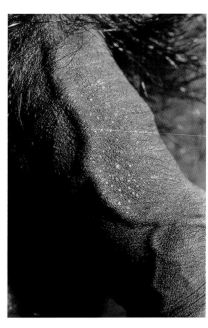

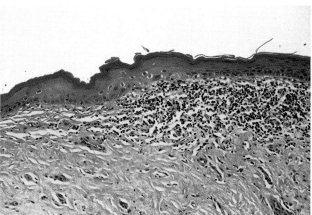

Fig. 6.200 Lichen planus. A medium-power view of penile skin showing flattening of the rete architecture and an underlying chronic lichenoid inflammatory infiltrate with interface inflammation of the basal epidermal layer and associated degeneration. (Courtesy of Dr Nick Francis, London, UK).

and effacement of the rete ridges to produce a 'saw-tooth' effect. Wickham's striae are created by focal hypergranulosis and denser inflammatory infiltrate. Hypertrophic lichen planus may show marked irregular pseudo-epitheliomatous acanthosis, 'cyst-like' follicular expansion and dermal fibrosis. Atrophic lichen planus manifests gross thinning of the epidermis with detect-able compact hyperkeratosis and papillary dermal fibrosis. Mucosal lichen planus shows a thinned epidermis, *parakeratosis* (which is unusual in lichen planus at other sites), significant plasma cells in the infiltrate and mild degrees of epithelial dysplasia.

In lichen nitidus the papules have a parakeratotic 'cap', there is epidermal atrophy, liquefaction degeneration of the basal layer and a dermal infiltrate of lymphocytes, epithelioid cells and occasionally giant cells (Lapins et al 1978).

Potent and very potent topical corticosteroids usually suffice for treatment. Patients are told to continue with the treatment until the lesions are non-itchy and flat. They are warned about post-inflammatory hyper-pigmentation. Topical cyclosporin (100mg/ml wet dressings tds) may be useful (Jemec & Baadasgard 1993). Oral cyclosporin (3mg/kg per day) may be necessary (Schmitt et al 1993). Intralesional and systemic corticosteroids are sometimes exhibited: for severely itchy disease, erosive orogenital involvement and scarring of the scalp and nails.

Circumcision may be necessary for phimosis (Aste et al 1997) and should be considered in refractory erosive disease (Porter et al 2001). The rationale is that the removal of Koebnerizing influences allows the lichen planus to heal. Inadvertently photodynamic therapy was used in one patient with lichen planus of the glans penis to good effect (Kirby et al 1999).

ACRODERMATITIS ENTEROPATHICA

Although a vesicobullous disorder, the principal presenting signs are crusted psoriasiform or eczematous plaques affecting the acral extensor surfaces of the digits and the periorificial sites: mouth, nose, ears and anus (**Fig. 6.201**). There is usually associated diarrhea. The congenital form appears after birth and is therefore a pediatric condition (some cases resolve at puberty) probably due to deficient zinc absorption from the gastrointestinal tract. Until zinc supplementation was recognized as curative therapy most children died.

Acquired forms do occur. In the adult male acrodermatitis enteropathica should be considered in the differential diagnosis of perianal eczema, psoriasis or candidosis in the presence of:

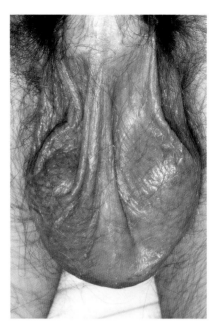

Fig. 6.202 Zinc deficiency. Scrotum. Erythema. Patient with Crohn's disease. (Courtesy of Drs John Cotteril, Leeds, and Walter Bottomley, Blackpool, UK, and reproduced by kind permission of Blackwell Science Ltd from Bottomley WW, Lotterill JA. Acquired zinc deficiency presenting with an acutely tender erythematous scrotum. Br J Dermatol. 1993; 129: 501-2.)

i) Gastrointestinal disease causing malabsorption syndromes, e.g. Crohn's disease;
ii) Extensive gastrointestinal surgery such as small intestinal bypass;
iii) Malnutrition as in alcoholics; and
iv) Recent prolonged parenteral nutrition where zinc supplementation may not have been optimal.

A reticulate eczematous eruption may be found on the extensor aspects of the limbs in alcoholics but has also been reported to affect the perianal and scrotal skin (Ecker & Schroeter 1978; Gaveau et al 1987). Bottomley & Cotterill (1993) have described this and an acutely tender erythematous scrotum in a patient with Crohn's disease (**Fig. 6.202**).

Other deficiency diseases with some clinical (and histological) similarity to acrodermatitis enteropathica are pellagra, migratory necrolytic erythema (**Fig. 6.203**), maple syrup urine disease and neonatal citrullinemia.

Diagnosis is by blood zinc estimation and confirmed by zinc replacement. Biopsy is not usually necessary but the histopathology is characteristic: parakeratosis, psoriasiform hyperplasia of the epidermis, subcorneal pustulosis and large pale and dyskeratotic spinous keratinocytes.

NECROLYTIC MIGRATAORY ERYTHEMA

This is sore or painful annular erythematous eruption with a central glassy appearance and serpiginous border surrounded by scaling. It can be focalized to the genitalia (Bewley et al 1996, **Fig. 6.203**). This is a characteristic cutaneous manifestation of the glucagonoma syndrome: elevated plasma glucagon, weight loss, anemia, diabetes

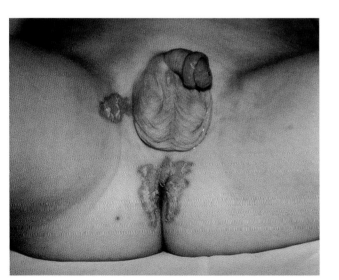

Fig. 6.201 Acrodermatitis enteropathica. Groins and perineum. (Courtesy: Dr Peter Copeman, London, UK).

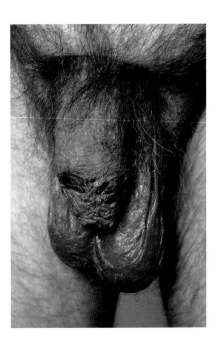

Fig. 6.203 Necrolytic migratory erythema. Scrotum and prepuce, penis.

mellitus and a pancreatic islet of Langerhans tumor (Binnick et al 1977).

HAILEY-HAILEY DISEASE (BENIGN FAMILIAL PEMPHIGUS)

The clinical features of this disease are moist, crusted plaques or scaly patches studded with pustules and warty papules involving the flexures (**Fig. 6.204**). Very occasionally the disease can affect the entire skin (Tanaka et al 1992). Lesions are induced by physical trauma. Very rarely papular plaques similar in appearance to genital warts have been reported.

It is similar in some clinical and histological respects to Darier's disease although they are distinct genetic entities. In Hailey-Hailey disease extra flexural and oral involvement is uncommon although the nails may show longitudinal leukonychia (white streaks) but not increased fragility (Burge 1992). The differential diagnosis in the groins is of an intertrigo, with Darier's disease an important alternative to consider.

Hailey-Hailey disease is an autosomal dominant disorder of keratinocyte adhesion with gradual onset in young adulthood and a tendency to improve with age.

The diagnosis is confirmed histologically, the signs being epidermal hyperplasia, hyperkeratosis and parakeratosis, gross elongation and thinning of the dermal papillae, intact basal membrane and suprabasal clefting due to non-dyskeratotic acantholysis.

The mainstay of treatment is topical corticosteroids and topical antibiotics. Dermabrasion (Kirtschig et al 1993), excision and grafting, CO_2 laser ablation (McElroy et al 1990) are options of last resort. Radiotherapy (Grenz rays and electrons) and etretinate have been used successfully (Kurwa & Vickers 1985).

DARIER'S DISEASE (KERATOSIS FOLICULARIS)

Flexural disease (**Fig. 6.205**) is mild in most patients but does occur in the vast majority. It can be very sore and malodorous. The intertriginous features are similar to those of Hailey-Hailey disease (above). Nearly all patients will have keratotic papules in seborrheic areas and hand involvement (palmar pits) and nail dystrophy (fragility, Union Jack nails: red, white and blue streaks, V-shaped terminal nicks). Sunlight is a known precipitant and bacterial or herpetic superinfection is well recognized. The molecular explanation for the

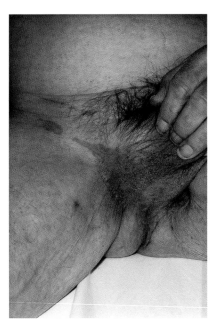

Fig. 6.205 Darier's disease. Groin. Erosive intertrigo.

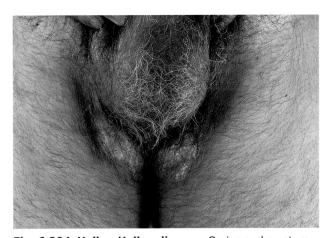

Fig. 6.204 Hailey-Hailey disease. Groins and scrotum. (Courtesy of Dr Nick Soter, New York, NY, USA).

acantholysis that causes the epidermal disruption in Darier's disease has been shown to be mutations in the ATP2A2 gene encoding the SERCA2 calcium pump of the sarco/endoplasmic reticulum (Chao et al 2002; Tavadia et al 2002).

The histology is similar to Hailey-Hailey disease but the acantholysis is dyskeratotic and the elongation of the dermal papillae is not seen.

Topical treatment for Darier's disease follows the same lines as for Hailey-Hailey disease. However, a very useful modality in the former is the use of oral retinoids such as isotretinoin and acitretin. Use of these agents is limited in women of child-bearing potential because of fetal teratogenicity and the benefits of long-term use have to be weighed against the risk of side-effects due to the hypervitaminosis A syndrome, especially DISH (Diffuse Idiopathic (misnomer) Skeletal Hyperostosis). Local radiotherapy to flexural sites has helped some patients in the past and recently CO_2 laser ablation has been advocated (McElroy et al 1990).

One patient with Darier's disease has developed an HPV 16-associated squamous carcinoma of the scrotum during oral isotretinoin treatment. He had not previously had radiotherapy to the genitocrural area (Orihuela et al 1995).

GENITOCRURAL PAPULAR ACANTHOLYTIC DERMATOSIS

Several reports have now appeared of a genital, inguinal and perineal eruption of multiple discreet papules or macerated patches in patients with no rash elsewhere and no family history. Histologically the appearances are similar to Darier's disease and Hailey-Hailey disease and immunofluorescence is negative (Wong & Mihm 1994).

KAWASAKI SYNDROME

An erythematous, desquamating perineal eruption occurring in the first week of the disease may be the first cutaneous feature in as many as two-thirds of children with Kawasaki disease (Friter & Lucky 1988). The setting is of persistent fever (longer than five days), cervical lymphadenopathy and mucocutaneous signs, viz., bilateral conjunctival injection, edema, erythema and desquamation of the hands and feet and a more polymorphic exanthem. Myocarditis and arthritis may occur. Kawasaki disease is usually self limiting but post vasculitic coronary artery aneurysm formation can cause myocardial infarction and a mortality of 1–2%. Early recognition and prompt treatment with intravenous immunoglobulins and oral aspirin are clinical ideals.

PITYRIASIS VERSICOLOR

The penis is rarely affected by this common dermatosis and probably almost never in isolation (Avram et al 1973; Aljabre & Sheikh 1994). Occasionally the anterior pelvic girdle is the site involved (see Fig. 4.8). Red, macular, superficially scaly lesions that progress to patchy macular hypopigmentation occur on the neck, torso and proximal upper limbs. The causative organism is the yeast *Malassezia furfur*. Diagnosis can be confirmed by yellow fluorescence under Wood's light and the presence of short, curved hyphae and groups of spherical yeast organisms (meatballs and spaghetti) on microscopic examination of a potassium hydroxide cleared skin-scraping specimen stained with India ink. Treatment is with topical antifungals (selenium sulphide or imidazole) or oral itraconazole 200mg daily for one week.

TINEA

Tinea (or 'ringworm') refers to superficial dermatophytosis. Tinea is a common disease of the pelvic girdle especially of the groins (**Figs 6.206–6.208**, see also Fig. 2.2) and is usually due to *Trichophyton rubrum*. It is not always spread from the nails or feet although people with tinea manuum or unguium *can* spread it to the groins or perianal skin because they are common sites of chronic itch (**Fig. 6.209**).

Tinea cruris is itchy, and diagnosed in the presence of red-brown, scaly patches with raised, redder edges extending out of the groins and onto the abdomen (**Fig. 6.210**), buttock (**Fig. 6.211**) and down the thighs. Because of the site, annular lesions are not always obvious but can be imagined. Unfortunately, it is not

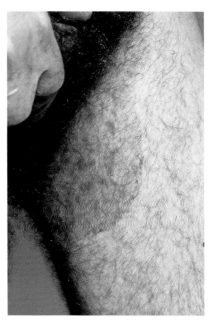

Fig. 6.206 Tinea cruris.

107

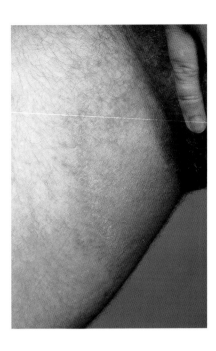

Fig. 6.207 Tinea cruris. Note acute margin.

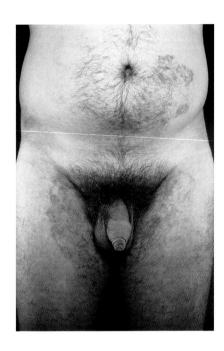

Fig. 6.210 Extensive tinea cruris.

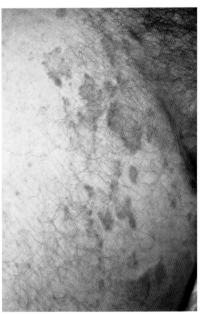

Fig. 6.208 Tinea cruris.

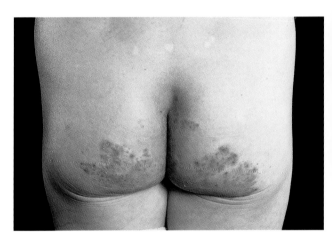

Fig. 6.211 Tinea incognito. Buttocks.

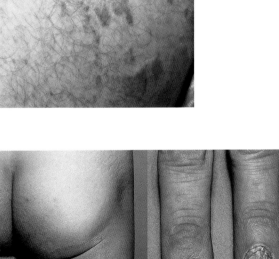

Fig. 6.209 Tinea corporis and unguium. Buttock eruption and finger nail dystrophy. Same patient.

that easy because many patients have previously been misdiagnosed and/or partially treated with topical corticosteroids plus or minus topical antifungal agents.

Tinea incognito (**Figs 6.211, 6.212**) is the name given to the presentation in the previously topical corticosteroid-treated patient where the symptom of itch and the signs of inflammation, including the redness, the scale and the well-demarcated, often scalloped, elevated active margins, have been suppressed, although there is often subtle post-inflammatory hyperpigmentation (Ive & Marks 1968). There will, however, be numerous fungal hyphae and this makes the diagnosis, by microscopy of a potassium hydroxide preparation of a skin scraping, relatively easy. Patients partially treated with topical antifungals are harder to diagnose for two reasons: the signs are attenuated *and* there will be few hyphae making microscopy difficult; also culture may be inhibited by the presence of the drug in the specimen presented to the laboratory. Re-evaluating the patient

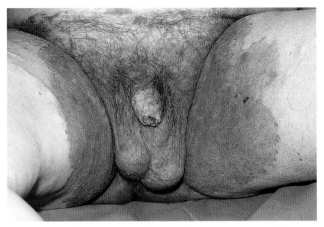

Fig. 6.212 Tinea incognito. Abdomen, groins, thighs and scrotum. Injudicious topical steroid application.

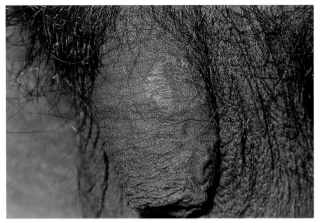

Fig. 6.214 Tinea penis. Penis shaft. (Courtesy of Prof. Bhushan Kumar, Chandigarh, India).

after a few days abstention from topical treatment is often advisable.

A degree of tinea incognito is present in practically all cases now encountered due to the ready availability of topical steroids and antifungals. Other problems are the concomitant presence of erythrasma (Schlappner et al 1979).

Tinea of the penis (**Figs 6.213, 6.214**) or scrotum is not common and when it occurs it is usually associated with crural disease. Rarely encountered is the occurrence of tinea on the glans penis as a seat of itch or pain and producing an erythematous patch or a crop of scaly papules (Pillai et al 1975; Kumar et al 1981; Pandey et al 1981; Dekio & Jidoi 1989; Dekio et al 1990; Pielop & Rosen 2001). Pandey et al (1981) associated penile tinea (in India) with occlusion due to the wearing of a langota – described as a T-shaped bandage tied over the genitalia.

Wood's light examination is sometimes helpful in the diagnosis of more exotic fungal infections and for excluding erythrasma.

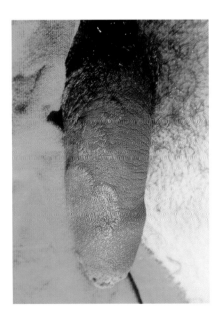

Fig. 6.213 Tinea penis. Penis shaft. (Courtesy of Prof. Bhushan Kumar, Chandigarh, India).

Anogenital dermatophytosis usually requires oral treatment with griseofulvin, terbinafine or itraconazole. Topical treatments often fail because of the anatomical complexity of the area and it is difficult to sustain complete, protracted, regular coverage of the whole area with a cream or ointment and because there may be mycosis of feet or hands, toes or fingernails.

PSEUDO-EPITHELIOMATOUS MICACEOUS AND KERATOTIC BALANITIS

Pseudo-epitheliomatous micaceous and keratotic balanitis (PEMKB) is a rare penile condition that was first described by Lortat-Jacob & Civatte (1961, 1966). It presents as thick, scaly, micaceous patches (Bart & Kopf 1977; Read & Abell 1981; Bargmann 1985; Ganem et al 1999) on the glans penis from which a verrucous (penile horn) or erosive tumor may emerge (**Figs 6.215, 6.216**). It occurs in older men who have not been circumcised. It has been misdiagnosed as Reiter's disease. Histology shows hyperkeratosis, parakeratosis, acanthosis, prolongation of the rete ridges and mild lower epidermal dysplasia. A non-specific inflammatory infiltrate of eosinophils and lymphocytes is seen in the dermis.

Although Ridley (1987) has supposed that it may be a variant or forerunner of lichen sclerosus, PEMKB is probably a form of locally invasive verrucous carcinoma (Beljaards et al 1987). Metastases have not been reported except in association with penile cutaneous horns (Goldstein 1993). One patient developed an aggressive penile soft tissue sarcoma from which he died (Irvine et al 1987).

Treatment can pose a difficult problem with recurrence and chronicity common. Topical 5-FU, radiotherapy (Bart & Kopf 1977) and surgery have all been employed.

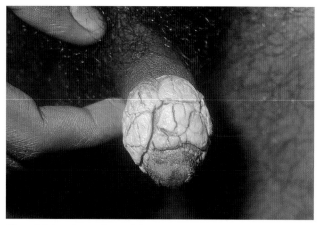

Fig. 6.215 Pseudo-epitheliomatous micaceous and keratotic balanitis. Glans penis. Verrucous plaques. (Courtesy of Prof. Bhushan Kumar, Chandigarh, India).

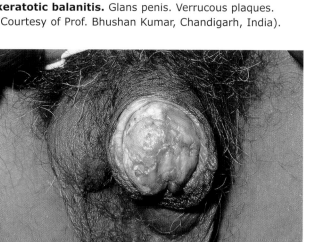

Fig. 6.216 Pseudo-epitheliomatous micaceous and keratotic balanitis. Glans penis. Verrucous plaque. Underlying lichen sclerosus. (Courtesy of Prof. Bhushan Kumar, Chandigarh, India).

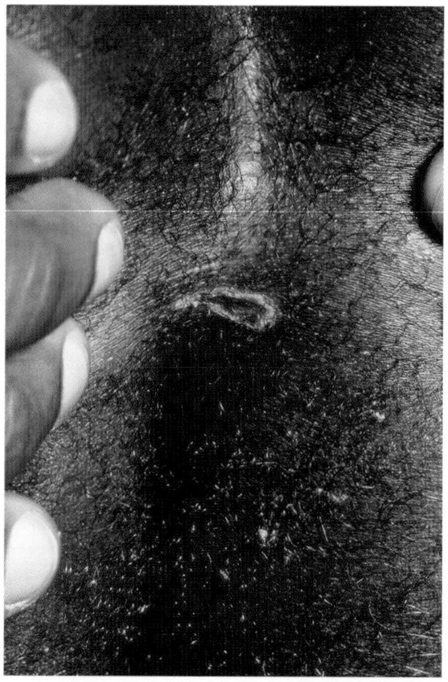

Fig. 6.217 Porokeratosis. Natal cleft. (Courtesy of Dr Nick Levell, Norwich, UK).

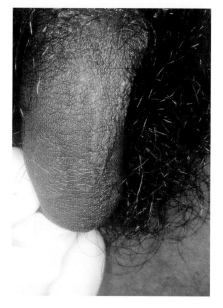

Fig. 6.218 Porokeratosis of Mibelli. Dorsal shaft, penis. (Courtesy of Prof. Bhushan Kumar, Chandigarh, India).

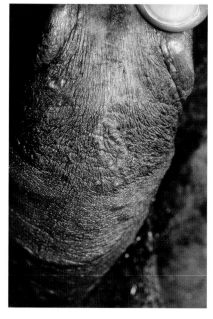

Fig. 6.219 Porokeratosis. Ventral penis shaft. Same case as Fig. 6.217. (Courtesy of Dr Nick Levell, Norwich, UK).

POROKERATOSIS

Genital porokeratosis of Mibelli is rare. Annular raised (double-rimmed) lesions have been found in the natal cleft (**Fig. 6.217**), on the scrotum and on the penis (**Figs 6.218, 6.219**), including the glans (**Fig. 6.220**). Rarely lesions may be ulcerative (Watanabe et al 1998). Porokeratosis may be misdiagnosed clinically as psoriasis, Bowen's diseases, granuloma annulare or lichen planus but histology of the margin shows the characteristic cornoid lamella (Levell et al 1994). I have treated one case successfully with topical 5-FU (Porter et al 2001).

ERYTHROPLASIA OF QUEYRAT AND BOWEN'S DISEASE OF THE PENIS

Erythroplasia of Queyrat (EQ), Bowen's disease of the penis (BDP) and Bowenoid papulosis (BP, see page 203)

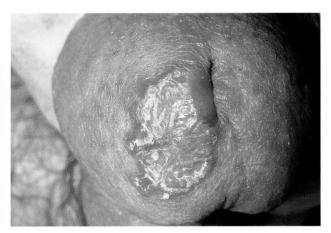

Fig. 6.220 Porokeratosis. Glans penis. Successfully treated with topical 5-FU (Porter et al 2001).

are three clinical variants of carcinoma in situ of the penis (Porter et al 2000; Porter et al 2002). Penile intraepithelial neoplasia (PIN – corresponding to CIN, VIN and AIN) is an increasingly encountered term favored by some (principally pathologists) and may be a convenient umbrella term. However, there is difficulty achieving consensus on clinicopathological classification (particularly 'grade') and clinical utility. An attractive alternative is to use the expression 'squamous intra-epithelial lesion' (SIL) and to qualify it with the descriptor 'high' or 'low' grade (Cubilla et al 2000). EQ, BDP and BP all describe disorders of the penis in predominantly uncircumcised, Caucasian men. Circumcised patients have been recorded (Milstein 1982). Anal intraepithelial neoplasia is an analogous term. It is discussed on page 206.

Although EQ and BDP are synonymous in describing carcinoma in situ of the penis (Graham & Helwig 1959, 1977; Graham et al 1961; Gerber 1994), BD is used to refer to squamous cell carcinoma in situ at other cutaneous sites (as originally described by Bowen in 1912) and in a dermatologist's mind is associated with multifocal disease, prior arsenic ingestion, sunlight exposure and internal malignancy. I think that EQ should be used to describe red, shiny patches or plaques of the mucosal sites (glans and prepuce of the uncircumcised) and BDP for red, scaly patches and plaques of the keratinized sites. This distinction has not always been made in the literature and perhaps not everyone would agree with it.

Bowenoid papulosis (see page 203) is analogous but clinically different from EQ and BDP, presenting as multiple warty lesions, often pigmented in keratinized sites and multiple, more inflamed in less mucosal sites. Lesions are less papillomatous, smoother topped, more polymorphic and more coalescent than common genital viral condylomata acuminata and occur in younger, sexually active men, rather than as the patches or scaly plaques in older men of EQ and BDP, respectively. However, age may not be a clear discriminator (McAninch & Moore 1970). Bowenoid papulosis probably has less malignant potential than EQ and BDP but is associated with local HPV infection (especially HPV 16) and systemic disease, particularly HIV, in my experience (Lloyd 1970; Wade et al 1979; Schwartz & Janniger 1991; Demeter et al 1993; Gerber 1994).

Descriptions of precancerous conditions of the penis date back to Paget (1874), Fournier and Darier (1893), Morestin (1903) and Queyrat (1911). In 1874, Sir James Paget described a premalignant disease of the mammary areola and commented that 'I believe that a similar sequence of events may be observed in other parts. I have seen a persistent "rawness" of the glans penis, like a long-standing balanitis followed after more than a year's duration by cancer of the substance of the glans.' Tarnovsky (1891) is credited with a brief remark about a case. Fournier and Darier (1893) and Morestin (1903) made 'conjectural associations' between penile lesions with similar clinico-pathological features and the eventual development of an intraepithelial malignancy at the same site. It was Queyrat (1911) who coined the term 'erythroplasie' to describe barely raised, well-defined, red, shiny, velvety plaques on the glans penis. But again, the supervention of frank carcinoma, though supposed, was not substantiated.

In 1912, Bowen described two cases of long-standing, non-healing, isolated, erythematous, scaly patches and plaques (e.g. **Fig. 6.221**) occurring on, respectively, the buttock and the calf of two middle-aged men. Only by clinical and histological analogy with known precancerous dermatoses such as senile keratosis, arsenical keratosis, xeroderma pigmentosum, and Paget's disease of the nipple, did he infer that these lesions were precancerous, although 'no signs of malignancy [had] appeared'. Darier later suggested that Bowen's name be attributed to dermatoses fitting his (Bowen's) original clinico-pathological description (Shelley & Crissey 1953).

Blau and Hyman (1955) and Graham and Helwig (1977) represent the contrasting views of those who have either separated or equated the two conditions. Although EQ is similar to Bowen's disease, it has been argued that it may be misleading and confusing to call it

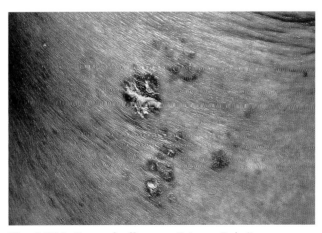

Fig. 6.221 Bowen's disease. Extragenital site. Psoriasiform scaly plaques.

Bowen's disease of the penis. Erythroplasia of Queyrat is neither associated with mucocutaneous lesions at other sites nor with internal malignancy (Graham & Helwig 1959, 1964) or previous arsenic exposure (Graham et al 1961), which are correlates of Bowen's disease occurring at other sites (Graham & Helwig 1959; Graham et al 1961). However, the contemporary presentation of Bowen's disease is of less multifocality and no association with arsenic ingestion or internal malignancy – actinic influences seem now to predominate. So these distinctions from 50 years ago have less resonance now.

The etiology of EQ and BDP is unknown. The natural history as defined by Graham and Helwig (1973) would be consistent with a local carcinogenic influence in uncircumcised men. Smegma has been proposed as that such factor with additional contributions from poor hygiene, trauma, friction, heat, maceration and inflammation (Graham & Helwig 1973). Circumcision protects against penile cancer for which phimosis and balanitis are known risk factors (see page 18). Poor hygiene and phimosis may lead to the retention of smegma but the carcinogenicity of human smegma has not been ascertained (Hellberg et al 1987).

It has not always been and is not always now appreciated that phimosis is a physical sign and not a diagnosis. There may be more in the carcinogenic propensity of phimosis than simply physical retention of smegma. Lichen sclerosus (see page 79) is a common cause of phimosis and is a premalignant condition. The photo dye treatment of herpes simplex ceased in the 1970s because of the occurrence of Bowen's disease of the penis in young men without other risk factors for erythroplasia (Berger & Papa 1977). The role of smoking in the causation of penis cancer is discussed on page 209, likewise the significance of HPV (Griffiths & Mellon 1999).

HPV is found in the majority of lesions of EQ, BDP, BP (principally type 16, but also types 1, 2, 8, 11, 18, 31, 33, 34, 39, 42, 51, 52, 57b, and 67) and in 15–80% of penile cancers (types 6, 16, 18, 31, 33, 35, 45, 52, 68) but there are exceptions (Ikenberg et al 1983; Boshart et al 1984; Durst et al 1985; Villa & Lopes 1986; Loning et al 1988; Guerin-Reverchon et al 1990; Soler et al 1991; Demeter et al 1993; Cupp et al 1995; Gregoire et al 1995; Ranki et al 1995; Majewski & Jablonska 1997; Dianzani et al 1998; Inagaaki et al 1998; Meyer et al 1998; Griffiths & Mellon 1999; Park et al 1998; Ohnishi et al 1999; Salvatore et al 2000; Wieland et al 2000; Yoneta et al 2000; Bezerra et al 2001; Rubin et al 2001). HPVs 16, 18 and 33 are considered the most oncogenic. Recently, cases of erythroplasia of Queyrat have been shown to be associated with *coinfection* with the rare epidermodysplasia verruciformis-asssociated HPV 8 and the genital high-risk HPV 16 (Wieland et al 2000). However, although HPV may be demonstrated in these precancerous clinical situations, the epidemiological characteristics of penile carcinoma are not consistent with those of a sexually transmitted disease (Hellberg et

al 1987), unlike carcinoma of the cervix where HPV (zur Hausen 1985; Keerti 1997) is highly incriminated. How HPV causes anogenital cancer and the role of the host immune response to HPV and the influence of smoking in carcinogenesis are important evolving fields of study (Kadish 2001; Moore et al 2001).

Clinically, therefore, erythroplasia of Queyrat presents as a disorder of the glans or prepuce of the penis in uncircumcised, predominantly Caucasian men. Circumcised patients have been recorded (Milstein 1982). Some patients may be quite young (Mcaninch & Moore 1970). Lesions are barely raised, well-defined, red, shiny, velvety plaques on the glans penis or mucosal prepuce (**Figs 6.222–6.225**, see also Fig. 2.18). BDP presents as a red, possibly slightly pigmented, possibly scaly patch or plaque of the keratinized penile shaft or

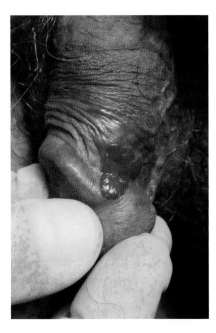

Fig. 6.222 Erythroplasia of Queyrat. Lateral distal penis shaft and glans, coronal rim and sulcus.

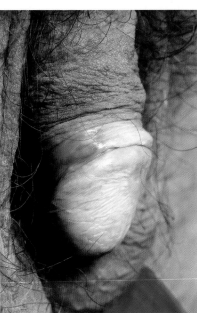

Fig. 6.223 Erythroplasia of Queyrat. Prepuce, lateral penis.

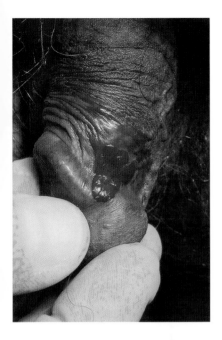

Fig. 6.224 Erythroplasia of Queyrat. Lateral coronal sulcus, penis.

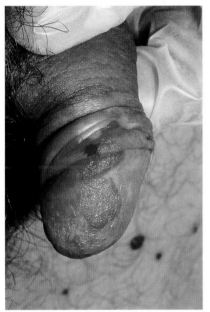

Fig. 6.225 Erythroplasia of Queyrat. Glans and distal prepuce, penis. Patient with systemic lupus erythematosus and long-standing iatrogenic immuno-suppression. Unstable glans with severe intraepithelial neoplasia and previous penile tip carcinoma excised. (Reproduced by kind permission of Blackwell Science Ltd from Porter WM et al. Penile intraepithelial neoplasia: Clinical spectrum and treatment of 35 cases. Br J Dermatol. 2002; 147: 1159–65.)

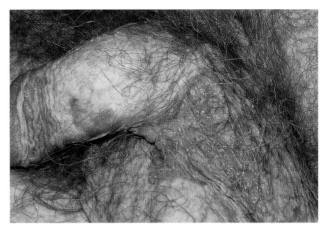

Fig. 6.226 Bowen's disease. Scrotum and shaft penis. Compare with Fig. 6.45 (psoriasis) and 6.245 (extramammary Paget's disease).

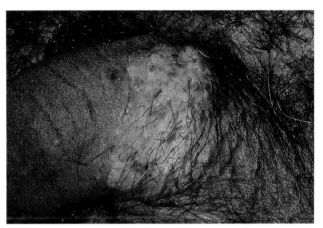

Fig. 6.227 Bowen's disease. Penis shaft, root. Irregular, red, scaly plaque. (Reproduced by kind permission of Blackwell Science Ltd from Porter WM et al. Penile intraepithelial neoplasia: Clinical spectrum and treatment of 35 cases. Br J Dermatol. 2002; 147: 1159–65.)

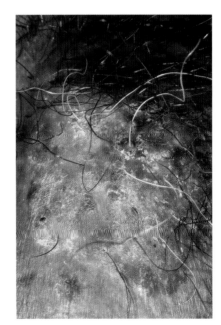

Fig. 6.228 Bowen's disease. Penis shaft, root. Irregular, red, scaly plaque with patchy hyperpigmentation. Same case as Fig. 6.227.

proximal prepuce (**Figs 6.226–6.230**) or occasionally of the circumcised glans (**Fig. 6.231**). It can be found around the anogenital skin including the groins (**Fig. 6.232**) but is rare on the scrotum (Gerber 1985). There may be several foci of either and they may occur concomitantly. The presentations of anal intraepithelial neoplasia are described on page 206. **Figures 6.230, 6.233** and **6.234** show penile, inguinal and perianal intraepithelial

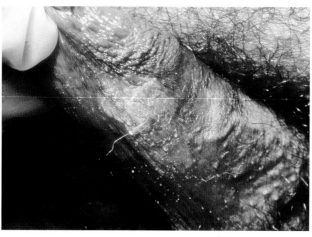

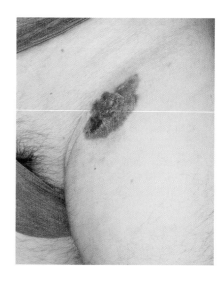

Fig. 6.232 Bowen's disease. Left groin.

Fig. 6.229 Bowen's disease. Lateral penis shaft. Several brown, scaly plaques.

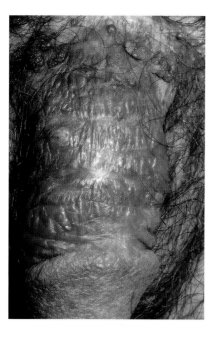

Fig. 6.230 Bowen's disease and Bowenoid papulosis. Penis glans and shaft. Psoriasiform, red, scaly patch and pigmented, warty papules. HIV-positive patient.

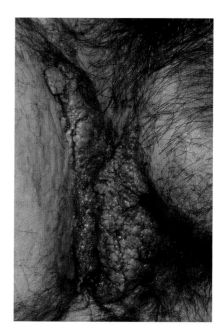

Fig. 6.233 Giant condyloma with PIN. Right groin. HIV-positive patient. Same case as Fig. 6.230 at a later date.

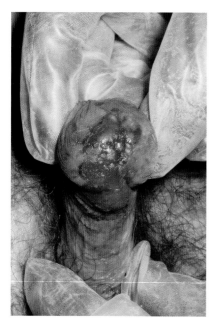

Fig. 6.231 Bowen's disease. Glans penis distal, ventral penis. Elderly, ill, circumcised (in childhood) patient.

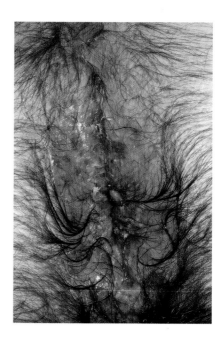

Fig. 6.234 Anal intraepithelial neoplasia. Red, eroded and scaly patches and warty change. HIV-positive patient. Same case as Fig. 6.230.

114

neoplasia in an HIV-positive patient who has responded poorly to HAART.

The non-specificity of the clinical appearances make for an important differential diagnosis which includes inflammatory disorders such as psoriasis, lichen sclerosus, erosive lichen planus and Zoon's balanitis (Davis-Daneshfar & Trueb 2000) and cancerous conditions such as Kaposi's sarcoma.

A biopsy is clearly indicated in instances where the clinical diagnosis is uncertain. Aynaud et al (1994) have suggested that shrewd clinical interpretation predicts which lesions will show intraepithelial neoplasia histologically (and contain oncogenic HPV). Occasionally it may be necessary to perform a second biopsy where the initial histology is inconclusive. It has been suggested that, where glans and shaft are both involved, the glans may be the preferential biopsy site from which to make the microscopic diagnosis.

On histological examination there are the features of an intraepithelial carcinoma (**Figs 6.235–6.237**). Frank squamous cell carcinoma with invasion and metastases may eventuate.

The evidence that has confirmed that EQ/BDP may result in squamous cell carcinoma has been reviewed comprehensively by Blau and Hyman (1955) and Graham and Helwig (1977). The grade of the intraepithelial neoplasia and the development of invasive carcinoma are related to age (Aynaud et al 2000). The risk for progression to invasive cancer is said to be higher for EQ (33%) than BDP (Wieland et al 2000).

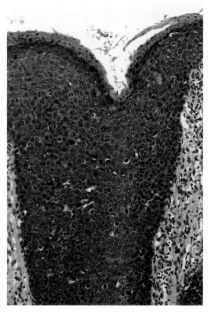

Fig. 6.236 Intraepithelial neoplasia. Full-thickness dysplasia with moderate to marked pleomorphism of the nuclei and increased numbers of mitotic figures throughout the epidermis. The changes extend down and around a follicle: Bowenoid dysplasia of a high grade. (Courtesy of Dr Nick Francis, London, UK).

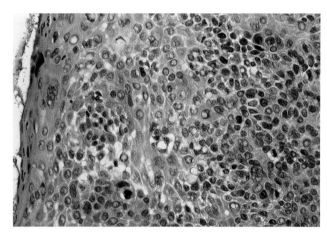

Fig. 6.237 Intraepithelial neoplasia. Dysplasia with displaced mitotic figures and pleomorphism of the cells extending to the level just underneath a thin parakeratotic layer. (Courtesy of Dr Nick Francis, London, UK).

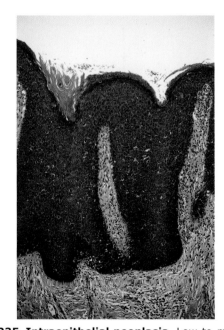

Fig. 6.235 Intraepithelial neoplasia. Low-to-medium-power view showing hyperkeratosis with irregular markedly elongated acanthotic proliferation of epidermis in which there is marked crowding of the epidermal cells with no evidence of ordered maturation toward the surface. These are the appearances of Bowen's disease. (Courtesy of Dr Nick Francis, London, UK).

Treatment depends on many factors. I believe that it should begin with circumcision. At a stroke this removes a major risk factor for cancer, provides extensive tissue for histology and an opportunity, under anesthesia, to examine the whole organ and obtain further biopsies.

5-FU as a 5% cream has long been regarded as a conventional option for the treatment of BD/EQ/BP. Its use developed from the desire to simplify treatment, reduce the morbidity associated with surgery or radiotherapy and reduce the recurrence rate associated with less radical physical modalities such as curettage or electrosurgery.

5-FU was not the first topical chemotherapeutic to be used against premalignant and malignant dermatoses. Neoarsphenamine (Sachs & Sachs 1948), colchicine and methotrexate (Belisario 1965) and mechlorethamine (Madison & Haserick 1962) have been used. After World War 2 some authors particularly recommended neoarsphenamine for the treatment of EQ (Sachs & Sachs 1948) but it is possible that their cases were not true EQ, given that they were all in circumcised Jewish men and that there were no signs of malignancy or pre-malignancy on histology.

5-FU was first used on the skin by Klein et al (1962) and then taken up by Jansen et al (1967) who emphasized the advantages of 5-FU in Bowenoid skin conditions: namely its selective destructivity, lack of scarring and lack of systemic toxicity. They were the first to report its use and efficacy in two cases of EQ. Thereafter, sporadic reporting of the usage of 5-FU occurred until the mid 1970s (Jansen et al 1967; Fulton et al 1968; Huesner & Pugh 1969; Lynch 1969; Lewis & Bendl 1971; Goette et al 1975; Goette & Carson 1976). 5-FU has also been used with success in the treatment of Bowenoid papulosis (Kossow et al 1980).

Thus the earliest advocates regarded the greatest advantages of topical 5-FU to be its applicability at sites where radical excision was not justified because of the low-grade malignant potential of the underlying disease in contrast to the deforming nature of the surgery, for example, the pinna of the ear and the penis (Jansen et al 1967; Fulton et al 1968; Hueser & Pugh 1969; Lynch 1969; Lewis & Bendl 1971; Goette et al 1975; Goette & Carson 1976; Tolia & Castro 1976; Sturm 1979; Kossow et al 1980). Although there have been no clinical trials there have been no reports of unfavorable response or of significant local or systemic side effects. However, most authors comment on, and all exponents are aware of, the pronounced circumlesional irritation that may initially lead the patient to believe the condition is worsening rather than improving. Dermatologists are used to this propensity of 5-FU.

A useful clinical regimen is to use cyclical 5-FU and topical corticosteroid treatment. Different physicians have their own favorite regimens. For example, the patient is told to use 5-FU once daily on the affected part for several days until the area is red and sore. Then, potent topical corticosteroid cream (perhaps containing an antibiotic and antifungal) is used until the area is quiet again and the 5-FU treatment resumed. Patients are monitored closely and even in remission followed up closely.

Other treatments (Gerber 1994) include cryosurgery, curettage and electrocautery, excisional surgery, radio-therapy (Kaplan & Katoh 1973; Boynton & Bjorkman 1991; Tietjen & Malek 1998); Mohs micrographic surgery (Brown et al 1987, 1988; Moritz & Lynch 1991) laser (Boyton & Bjorkman 1991) and topical or systemic photodynamic therapy (Petrelli et al 1992; Stables et al 1995; Harth & Hirshowitz 1998; Harth et al 1998; Stables et al 1999).

Patients (and their sexual partners) presenting with these conditions should be counseled and screened for HPV and other sexually transmitted diseases including HIV infection. Smoking must be discouraged. Treatment should be conservatively ablative. Follow-up should be long-term (Aynaud et al 2000).

MYCOSIS FUNGOIDES

This is cutaneous T-cell lymphoma. It can be difficult to diagnose clinically and histologically and run a long, indolent and variable course. Fixed, red, scaly eczematoid or psoriasiform patches and plaques are the early manifestations. These may be easily misdiagnosed as due to one or other benign inflammatory dermatosis and respond partially and intermittently to topical corti-costeroid treatment. It is usually a widespread eruption but localized perianal disease at presentation (**Fig. 6.238**) has been described (Hill et al 1995) and occasionally disease can be confined to or concentrated in the genital region (**Figs 6.239–6.243**).

EXTRAMAMMARY PAGET'S DISEASE

Extramammary Paget's disease presents as an irritating, itchy, burning, red, scaly patch or plaque and may be multifocal (**Figs 6.244–6.247**). It can be found anywhere around the anogenital area (Redondo et al 1995, Butler et al 1997) including the glans penis (Metcalf et al 1985), and may be multicentric. An 'underpants' pattern of erythema has been described in some patients (Murata et al 1999, **Fig. 6.248**). Extramammary Paget's disease is frequently misdiagnosed as an inflammatory dermatosis, such as psoriasis or eczema (Aldeen & Lau 1999), or Bowen's disease (see also Figs 2.45 and 6.226). Subclinical Paget's disease occurs where the skin looks normal macroscopically but is involved microscopically. The disease behaves indolently, spreading by local extension and metastasis (Helwig & Graham 1963; Gerber 1985).

The combination of genital and extragenital extra-mammary Paget's disease is extremely rare. Overt and latent axillary Paget's disease may coexist (Kawatsu & Miki 1971; Makino et al 1998). Axillary macular lesions that change shape and color daily have been reported in association with penile and pubic Paget's disease in two patients (Imakado et al 1991, **Figs 6.249, 6.250**). Extremely rarely depigmented Paget's disease occurs presenting as a pale patch (including of the root of the penis) and then the differential diagnosis is vitiligo, depigmented mycosis fungoides and lichen sclerosus (Chen et al 2001).

Genital extramammary genital Paget's disease containing an area of cutaneous squamous carcinoma has been reported once (Tanabe et al 2001).

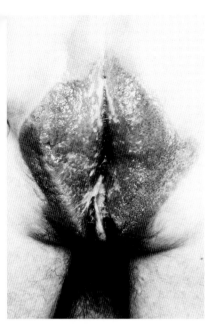

Fig. 6.238 Cutaneous T-cell lymphoma. Anus. (Courtesy of Dr Virginia Hill, Birmingham, UK and reproduced by kind permission of S Karger AG Basel from Hill VA et al. Cutaneous T-cell lymphoma presenting with atypical perianal lesions. Dermatology 1995; 190: 313–316.)

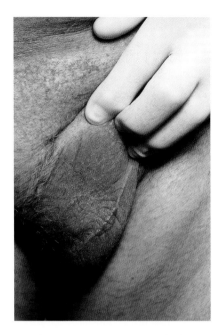

Fig. 6.241 Mycosis fungoides. Inferomedial scrotum and raphe. Infiltrated plaque. Note (a) steroidal rosacea superiorly and (b) radio-dermatitis of pubis.

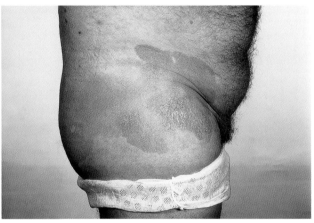

Fig. 6.239 Mycosis fungoides. Pelvic girdle. Patch stage.

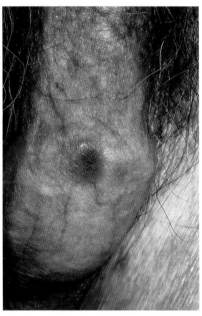

Fig. 6.242 Mycosis fungoides. Dorsal shaft, penis. Infiltrated nodule. Same case as Fig. 6.240.

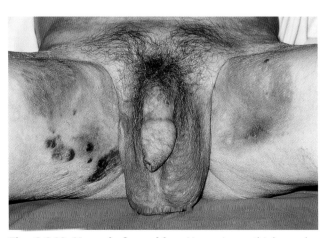

Fig. 6.240 Mycosis fungoides. Upper inner thighs and shaft of penis.

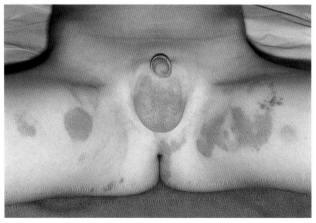

Fig. 6.243 Mycosis fungoides. Genitocrural skin. Involvement of pubis, thighs, scrotum and perianal skin. (Courtesy of Drs Nerys Roberts and Jeff Cream, London, UK).

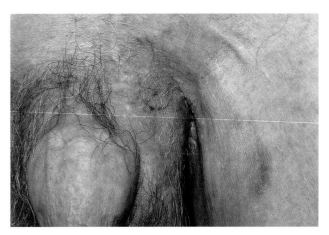

Fig. 6.244 Extramammary Paget's disease. Left groin. Psoriasiform plaque.

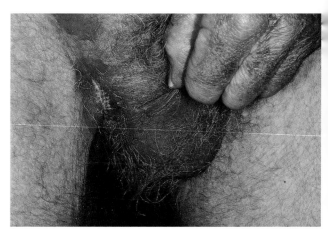

Fig. 6.247 Extramammary Paget's disease. Right groin and scrotum. A nodule in the right groin was excised and shown histologically to be an appendageal neoplasm.

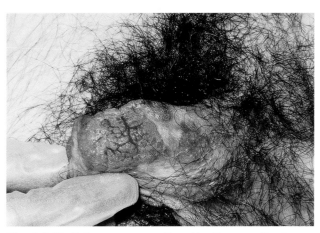

Fig. 6.245 Extramammary Paget's disease. Scrotum and shaft penis. Compare with Fig. 6.45 (psoriasis) and 6.226 (Bowen's disease).

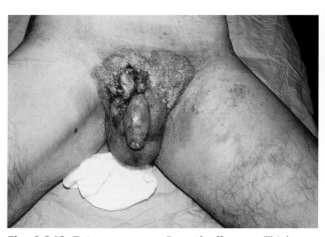

Fig. 6.248 Extramammary Paget's disease. Thighs and genitocrural skin. Well-defined plaques, pubis. Irregularly marginated non-scaly erythema of left thigh. (Courtesy of Dr Yozo Murata, Akashi, Japan).

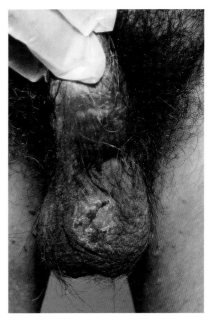

Fig. 6.246 Extramammary Paget's disease. Scrotum and ventral base, penis. Same case as Fig. 6.245.

Histologically, large nests of big vacuolated cells with circular nuclei and foamy pale cytoplasm are found in the epidermis – Paget's cells. If dermal involvement occurs the prognosis is poor. A caveat is that Pagetoid dyskeratosis can be found in a number of benign lesions such as nevi, skin tags, lentigines, occurring on the buttocks, intertriginous areas and elsewhere (Tschen et al 1988). Anogenital Paget's disease can be accompanied by epidermal hyperplasia reminiscent of fibroepithelioma of Pinkus according to Ishida-Yamamoto et al (2002).

Val-Bernal & Garijo (2000) make the point that pale cells resembling Paget's cells can be seen incidentally in benign papular, intertriginous conditions (Tschen et al 1988; Kohler et al 1998) and, in their work, 37% of prepuces sent to the histology laboratory following circumcision for phimosis.

Immunohistochemical and enzyme histochemical evidence points to sweat gland epithelium as the source of Paget's cells in extramammary Paget's disease (Hamm

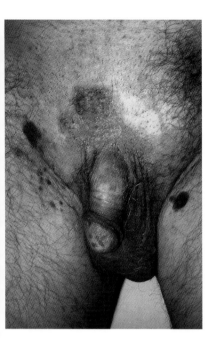

Fig. 6.249 Extramammary Paget's disease. Pubis. 72-year-old Japanese male. (Courtesy of Dr Sumihisa, Tokyo, Japan, and reproduced from Imakado S et al. Archives of Dermatology, 1991; 127: 1243. Copyright 1991, American Medical Association.)

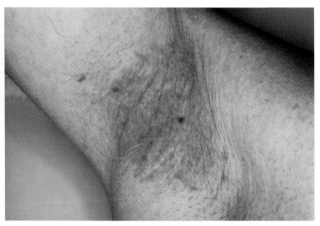

Fig. 6.250 Extramammary Paget's disease. Axilla. 72-year-old Japanese male. Ill-defined erythematous plaques, bilaterally, changing daily occasionally to reveal normal-looking skin. Same case as Fig. 6.249. (Courtesy of Dr Sumihisa, Tokyo, Japan and reproduced from Imakado S et al. Archives of Dermatology, 1991; 127: 1243. Copyright 1991, American Medical Association.)

et al 1986). The occurrence along the milk line has led to the suggestion that the so-called clear cells of Toker are possibly the histiogenic precursors of both clear cell papulosis and mammary and extramammary Paget's disease, respectively (Chen et al 2001). HPV is not present (Snow et al 1992) but the c-erbB-2 oncoprotein may play a role in the pathogenesis of extramammary Paget's disease (Wolber et al 1991).

It is generally agreed that mammary Paget's disease is an epidermal manifestation of an underlying breast adenocarcinoma (Paget 1874). Extramammary Paget's disease is found in areas rich in apocrine sweat glands such as the axillae and anogenital region. Extramammary Paget's disease can be associated with an underlying malignancy. In a large series (Helwig &

Graham 1963) 24% of patients had a proximate cutaneous adnexal adenocarcinoma, 12% were found to have a concurrent and another 17% to have a non-concurrent internal malignancy (Chanda 1985). Therefore, when extramammary Paget's disease is diagnosed a search for a synchronous or metachronous malignancy is necessary.

While considered to represent a form of carcinoma in situ, extramammary Paget's may itself become invasive and metastatic (Jensen et al 1988; Iwamura et al 1999; Khoubehi et al 2001) and there may be subjacent carcinoma, as stated, for example, in peri-urethral glands (Jenkins & Conroy 1989) or distant carcinoma, for example, prostate (Koh & Nazarina 1995) or bladder (Turner 1980), or both, for example, periurethral glands and bladder (Tomaszewski et al 1986). Pagetoid epidermal invasion of inguinal cutaneous metastatic mesothelioma of the tunica vaginalis of the testes has been reported (Cartwright & Steinman 1987).

Paget's disease has been treated with cryotherapy and topical 5-FU (Arensmeier et al 1994). Widespread excisional surgery (plastic repair may be needed) is probably the treatment of choice (Jensen et al 1988). It may be treated successfully by micrographic surgery (Mohs & Blanchard 1979; Brown et al 1988). Radiotherapy is regarded as ineffective (Gerber 1985) but this may not always be the case (Rosin 1984). Photodynamic therapy may hold promise (Petrelli et al 1992).

KAPOSI'S SARCOMA

Solitary Kaposi's sarcoma (KS) of the penis was recognized, if rarely, before the HIV epidemic (Dehner & Smith 1970) and cases are still occasionally seen in HIV-negative patients (Maiche et al 1986; Marquart et al 1986; Bayne & Wise 1988; Marquart et al 1991; Myslovaty et al 1993; Grunwald et al 1994; Guy et al 1994; Koyuncuoglu et al 1996; Berkmen & Celebioglu 1997; Kavak et al 2001). In HIV infection the penis, like the mouth, is a common (20%) site to find Kaposi's sarcoma either as part of disseminated multifocal disease or as a solitary lesion (Lowe et al 1989).

KS in HIV can present as a dull red patch or plaque on the glans penis (**Figs 6.251–6.256**) or preputial sac (**Figs 6.257, 6.258**) as well as affecting the penile shaft (**Figs 6.259–6.261**), scrotum and perianal skin in one its more classical manifestations namely purple, slightly scaly patches or plaques, nodules and ulcerative lesions (Conger & Sporer 1985; Schwartz et al 1991; Yuhan et al 1998). An engorged, 'hypervascular' presentation has been described (Bayne & Wise 1988) as has penile lymphoedema (Schwartz et al 2000) and acute phimosis (associated with laryngeal involvement necessitating emergency circumcision and tracheostomy (Morris-Jones et al 2000). Rectourethral fistula caused by Kaposi's sarcoma has been reported (Teichman et al 1991). Odd morphology may mean mixed pathology (Bunker & Staughton 2002).

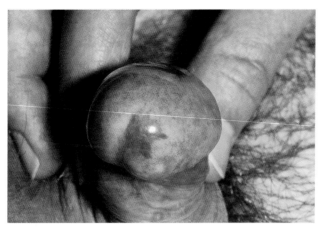

Fig. 6.251 Kaposi's sarcoma. Glans penis. Dull red patch.

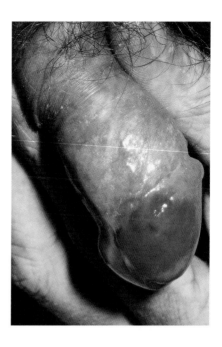

Fig. 6.254 Kaposi's sarcoma. Glans penis.

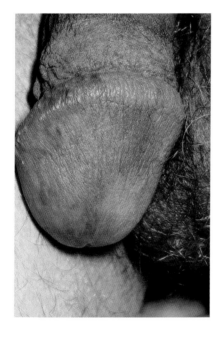

Fig. 6.252 Kaposi's sarcoma. Glans penis.

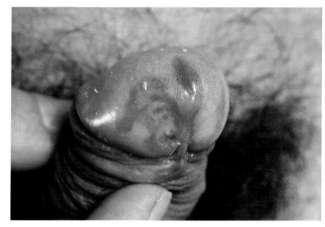

Fig. 6.255 Kaposi's sarcoma. Glans penis.

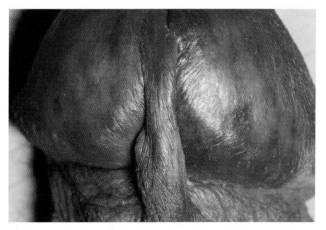

Fig. 6.253 Kaposi's sarcoma. Glans penis. Same case as Fig. 6.252.

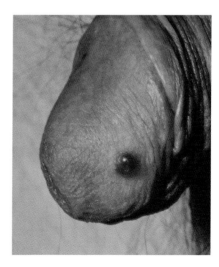

Fig. 6.256 Kaposi's sarcoma. Glans penis. (Courtesy of Dr Peter Copeman, London, UK).

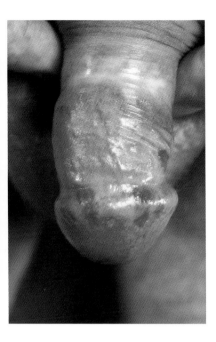

Fig. 6.257 Kaposi's sarcoma. Glans and prepuce, penis.

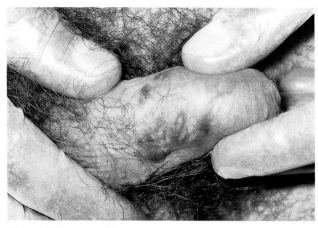

Fig. 6.260 Kaposi's sarcoma. Lateral penis shaft.

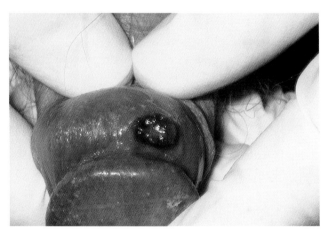

Fig. 6.258 Kaposi's sarcoma. Preputial sac.

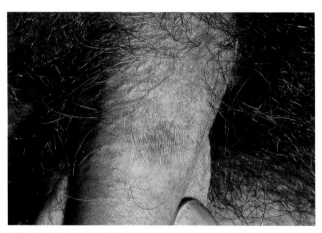

Fig. 6.261 Kaposi's sarcoma. Mid-shaft, penis. distal shaft, penis.

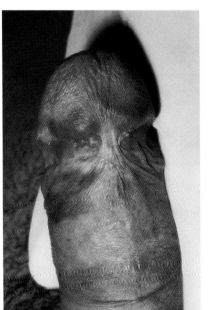

Fig. 6.259 Kaposi's sarcoma. Glans coronal sulcus and distal shaft, penis.

The prevalence of KS amongst the first 1000 homosexual men with AIDS reported to the Centers for Disease Control in the USA was 45% whereas it was 23.5% in the fourteenth group. The prevalence amongst intravenous drug abusers has remained at about 5% and in hemophiliacs at 1% (Schwartz et al 1991; Fine 1992; Tappero et al 1993).

Classical KS was first described in 1872 (Philippson 1902). It occurs in elderly male central Europeans, Italians or Jews and is solitary and acral and may involve the penis. An affected father and son have been reported (Invernizzi et al 1993). A familial endemic KS occurs in black Africans and is florid and aggressive. There has been a report of a Greek form of KS with Peloponnese clustering (Rappersberger et al 1989). A third group of KS occurs in patients with iatrogenic immunosuppression (Roszkiewicz et al 1998). AIDS-related KS is multicentric and often involves the face, oral mucosa, palate and genitalia.

Pseudo-Kaposi's sarcoma is a complication of long-standing vascular malformations such as the Klippel-Trenaunay-Weber syndrome (Stewart-Blufarb type) or chronic venous insufficiency and stasis dermatitis (Mali type). It is usually found on the leg but may involve the penis (Kapdagli et al 1998).

There may be diagnostic difficulty with morphologically non-diagnostic lesions in at-risk or worried individuals and the importance of index of suspicion and skin biopsy. Rapidly progressive ulceration of KS may mimic infection (Schmidt et al 1992). The conventional differential diagnosis includes nevi and histiocytoma but cryptococcosis (Blauvelt & Kerdel 1992), histoplasmosis (Cole et al 1992), leishmaniasis (Romeu et al 1991), lesions due to pneumoocystis (Litwin & Williams 1992) and dermatophytosis (Crosby et al 1991) may also mimic and/or complicate KS. KS masquerading as pyogenic granuloma has become a well-recognized clinical presentation.

Epithelioid angiomatosis/hemangiomatosis which has some clinical similarity to KS was first described in the context of HIV infection by Cockerell (1988) but this has been shown now to be the consequence of infection with the cat-scratch organism (bacillary angiomatosis, see page 182).

The differential frequency of occurrence of KS in risk groups for HIV has been mentioned (Schwartz et al 1991; Tappero et al 1993). The sex ratios for classical sporadic KS appear to have changed during the 20th century from about 10:1 (male:female) to 2:1. KS was first observed in a renal transplant patient in 1968 after many such operations had been performed and after an increased risk of lymphoma was already evident in these patients. The incidence of KS in immunosuppressed patients post-transplant is about 4%. Previously, KS in children was almost unheard of, but children with AIDS (non-hemophiliacs) have a prevalence of KS of about 4%. Congenital non-AIDS immunodeficiency states do not predispose to KS as they do to lymphoma. The

incidence of KS in post-transfusion AIDS patients is about 3%.

There are epidemiological studies that suggest Kaposi's sarcoma is acquired during particular types of sexual activity (receptive fellatio and frequent anal douching) and susceptibility is determined by immunogenetics, being strongly associated with HLA-DR1 and DQw1 (Goedert 1990). A homosexual man with benign, long-standing (10 years), multicentric, non-classical KS with evidence of multiple previous infections but *not* HIV has been reported, in whom the only evidence of immune dysfunction was slight impairment of monocyte phagocytosis and evidence of cutaneous anergy (Archer et al 1990).

Observations like those above were put forward to support the idea that KS is caused by an infectious agent with a pattern of transmission that overlaps with HIV. A virus rarely present in infected blood could be responsible for KS in the presence of immunodeficiency in patients who abuse intravenous drugs or who have transfusions (renal patients have frequently had multiple transfusions), but could also, like HIV, be transmitted sexually. CMV and HPV (16) were incriminated.

The similarity of KS to avian hemangiomatosis has been noted; this condition is due to an avian retrovirus. The appreciation that the unusual vascular proliferation of bacillary angiomatosis in HIV-infected patients seems to result from cat-scratch disease suggests also that the similar KS may be a consequence of a separate infection and that the organism may not be a virus but a bacterium. There is now compelling evidence that KS is due to human herpes virus (HHV) 8 (Antman & Chang 2000).

The histological features of Kaposi's sarcoma are well described (Smith et al 1991) and consist of dilated, irregular shaped, vascular structures which are typically slit-like in a fully developed nodular lesion. The differential diagnosis may be clarified by immunohistochemical and other techniques that identify endothelial cells (factor VIII related antigen and *Ulex europeus* lectin), which have been thought to be the cells of origin of KS, and HHV 8. Mixed pathologies have been described (Bunker 1996; Bunker & Staughton 2002). For example, an HIV-positive man with HHV 8-positive penile lesions with overlying Bowenoid epithelial dysplasia and HPV 16 also present has been reported. Absence of viral DNA from uninvolved skin in this patient suggests more than coincidental coinfection and that the two viruses may be synergistic (Simonart et al 1999). A staging classification of KS is given by Tappero et al (1993).

Treatments used in KS are listed in **Table 6.16**. There has been no cure for KS (Tappero et al 1993) but generally highly active antiretroviral treatment (HAART) and specifically intravenous cidofovir have improved the clinical situation in recent years. Radiotherapy (Lands et al 1992; Ruszczak et al 1996) and local and systemic chemotherapy have their places in management.

Table 6.16 Treatment for Kaposi's sarcoma

Local treatment		Systemic treatment
Cryotherapy		HAART
Radiotherapy		Isotretinoin
Topical retinoids	Alitretinoin	Cidofovir
Topical antivirals	Cidofovir Docosanol	Aggressive chemotherapy, e.g. daunorubicin, doxorubicin, bleomycin, paclitaxel, vincristine, etoposide
Intralesional e.g. TNFα, interferon α, vinca alkaloids		Human chorionic gonadotrophin
Surgery, e.g. curettage, cautery, infra red, excision, laser		Interleukin-4
Photodynamic therapy		
Cosmetic camouflage		

(After Bunker & Staughton 2002; Esdaile et al 2002; Gill et al 1997; Langtry et al 1994; Tulpule et al 1997; Duvic et al 2000; Scolaro et al 2001; Tulpule et al 2002).

The dermatologist has a role to play in the diagnosis and management of the clinically less overt, more banal lesion. In patients with scarce lesions or with focal, unsightly skin involvement then excision may be suitable. Occasionally cryotherapy with liquid nitrogen is successful, as may be laser treatment (Chun et al 1999). Radiotherapy can be effective (Vapnek et al 1991). Cosmetic camouflage may be offered; Kaposi's lesions on the face tend to offend more by their coloration than by their bulk or obtruberance. Spontaneous resolution has been documented (Casado et al 1988).

These general remarks have only limited usefulness for genital lesions. Each case should be considered on its merits.

FIXED DRUG ERUPTION

Clinically, fixed drug eruption is characterized by the acute eruption of swollen plaques, sometimes with central blister formation, erosion and ulceration. Ulcerative drug reactions are also discussed on page 169. The symptoms are itch or burning. The genitalia are classical sites of predilection as are the face and extremities. Lesions heal with post-inflammatory hyperpigmentation. On first exposure the eruption can take 1–2 weeks to appear but subsequently appears just a few hours after ingestion. Recurrence occurs at the same site each time the drug is exhibited and such re-challenge (provocation) can be used as a diagnostic test (Kanwar et al 1988). Gruber et al (1997) describe the case of a man with known sensitivity to co-trimoxazole who developed a penile fixed drug eruption after coitus with his wife whilst she was taking the drug for a sore throat.

Causes are phenolphthalein in laxatives (**Fig. 6.262**), non-steroidal anti-inflammatory drugs and salicylates as listed, paracetamol (**Fig. 6.263**), sulphonamides, co-trimoxazole (Cherian 2001), tetracyclines (Sehgal & Gangwani 1986; Coldiron & Jacobson 1988) including doxycycline and minocycline (Correia et al 1999), papaverine (Kirby et al 1993), erythromycin (Mutalik 1991), oxyphenbutazone (Sehgal & Gangwani 1986), methylphenidate (scrotum, Cohen et al 1992), acetaminophen (Cohen et al 1992), acetyl salicylic acid (Sehgal & Gangwani 1986; Kanwar et al 1988), amoxicillin (Gil García et al 1994; Jimenez et al 1997), propanolol (Massa et al 1991), betalactams and ciprofloxacin (Saenz de San Pedro Morera et al 1999). Litt (2001) lists all possible causes of a fixed drug eruption. See also **Table 6.17**.

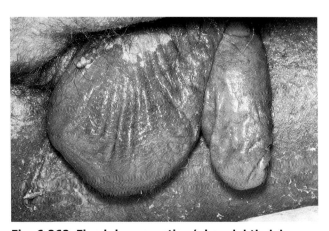

Fig. 6.262 Fixed drug eruption/phenolphthalein. Penis, scrotum and thigh. (Courtesy of Dr Sallie Neil, London, UK).

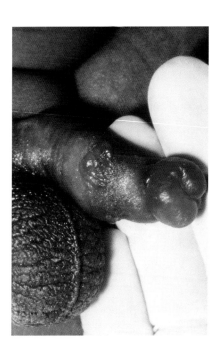

Fig. 6.263 Fixed drug eruption (bullous). Penis. Neonate.

Table 6.17 Causes of genital fixed drug eruption

Tetracyclines

Phenolphthalein (in laxatives)

Sulphonamides

Co-trimoxazole

Barbiturates

Oxyphenbutazone

Acetylsalicylic acid

Quinine

Papaverine

Amoxicillin

Acetaminophen

Methylphenidate

Paracetamol

Propranolol

The histopathology is distinctive. There is a mixed perivascular infiltrate of lymphocytes, neutrophils and eosinophils that may extend into the epidermis and abut onto necrotic keratinocytes. Melanophages appear in the dermis more chronically.

Treatment obviously centers on identification and withdrawal of the offending agent. Very potent topical corticosteroid treatment used in the acute phase may attenuate the symptomatology.

Intertrigo, balanitis and posthitis

Intertrigo (**Table 7.1**) is the name given to any dermatosis occurring in skin folds. Any scale is usually rapidly removed by frictional abrasion and a degree of epithelial loss may result in erosion that renders the site especially susceptible to secondary infection, e.g. with candida (see below).

Balanitis describes inflammation of the glans penis, *posthitis*, inflammation of the prepuce (Waugh 1998). *Balanoposthitis* means inflammation of the glans and prepuce and can be regarded as a special form of intertrigo. By definition, therefore, balanoposthitis cannot occur in the circumcised male, but balanitis might.

Generally, dermatologists feel that balanitis, posthitis and balanoposthitis (**Table 7.2**) are probably more commonly due to inflammatory and precancerous dermatoses than genitourinary physicians who teach that most cases are due to infection – usually with candida (Edwards 1996; English et al 1997). Yet Birley et al (1993) write 'in our patients it is far from clear whether the isolates from preputial swabs were involved in the inflammatory process or were merely incidental to it. The latter seems likely since although bacterial pathogens were isolated from four of the 18 patients with non-specific dermatitis, recovery swiftly followed the use of emollient creams only.' Only one of their 43 cases had candida.

However, candida is a ready opportunist so its presence may not always indicate primary infection and does not prove that it is the prime cause of the symptoms and signs of the genital inflammation (see page 133).

Table 7.1 Causes of genitocrural intertrigo

Common causes	Rare causes
Eczema	Eczema
Exogenous	Exogenous
Irritant contact	Allergic contact
Endogenous	Endogenous
Seborrheic	Atopic
Psoriasis (inverse	Reiter's syndrome
pattern)	Lichen sclerosus
Erythrasma	Hailey-Hailey disease
Candidosis	Darier's disease
Tinea	Streptococcal dermatitis
Trichosporosis (in India)	Gonorrhea
Pseudo-acanthosis	Secondary syphilis
nigricans	Part of a syphilide
	Mucous patch
	Acute primary HIV
	infection
	Trichosporosis (in the
	developed world)
	Extramammary Paget's
	disease
	Langerhans cell
	histiocytosis

Table 7.2 Causes of balanoposthitis

Common causes	Rare causes
Eczema	Crohn's disease
Exogenous	Streptococcal dermatitis
Allergic contact	Staphylococcal cellulitis
Irritant contact	Syphilis
Endogenous	Chancre with balanitis
Seborrheic	of Follman
Psoriasis	Mucous patch
Reiter's disease	*Mycoplasma*
Zoon's balanitis	Lymphogranuloma
Non-specific	venereum
balanoposthitis	Non-syphilitic, spirochetal,
Lichen sclerosus	ulcerative balanoposthitis
Gonorrhea	Tinea
HPV	Trichomoniasis
Herpes simplex	Amoebiasis
Candidosis	Myiasis
	Scabies
	Eccrine syringofibro-
	adenomatosis
	Erythroplasia of Queyrat
	Kaposi's sarcoma
	Chronic lymphatic leukemia
	Fixed drug eruption

Diabetes may be an important predisposing factor to candidosis and other infective causes or complications of balanoposthitis. Chopra et al (1982) reported that diabetes was diagnosed in 36% of men between 17 and 59 years of age presenting with phimosis of less than two years' duration. On histology no specific preputial pathology was identified.

ZOON'S BALANITIS

Zoon's plasma cell balanitis is a disorder of the middle-aged and older uncircumcised male (Zoon 1950, 1952). Although an analogous condition has been reported to afflict the vulva (Davis et al 1983; Woodruff et al 1989; Yoganathan et al 1994) and mouth, lips (Baughman et al 1974) and epiglottis (Baughman et al 1974). Since Zoon's (1950, 1952) original reports of the persistent balanitis (which he originally termed balanoposthitis chronica circumscripta plasmacellularis) there have been many accounts in the literature but the etiology remains uncertain.

The evidence suggests that Zoon's balanitis is a chronic, reactive, principally irritant mucositis related to a *dysfunctional* prepuce. Retention of urine and squames between two tightly apposed and infrequently and inadequately separated and/or inappropriately bathed, commensally hyper-colonized, desquamative, secretory epithelial surfaces leads to a disturbed 'preputial ecology' (Altmeyer et al 1998; Bunker 1999).

Chronic infection with *Mycobacterium smegmatis* has been postulated but the case is not convincing (Yoganathan et al 1994). HPV is not involved (Kiene & Folster-Holst 1995). HSV2 has been incriminated in a patient with vulval disease (Kuniyuki et al 1998). Trauma (Zoon's is often located on the dorsal aspect of the glans and/or the adjacent prepuce; sites of maximal friction on foreskin retraction) and irritation by urine (Yoganathan et al 1994) are probably important factors.

The lower incidence in women might be because it is relatively asymptomatic and therefore fewer females are aware they have the condition. However, it might be that in both sexes one of the contributing factors is low-grade chronic irritant exposure to urine, which is more common in men by accumulation under the foreskin. It is of note that the one female in this series had a long-standing history of urinary incontinence.

Immunohistochemical findings can be variable (Dupre et al 1981) but overall a tenable interpretation is that Zoon's balanitis represents a non-specific poly-clonal reaction in the tissues (Nishimura et al 1990; Farrell et al 1996), consistent therefore with an irritant mucositis. In the largest immunohistochemical study on Zoon's balanitis to date, we found predominant IgG and less IgA as did Toonstra and van Wichen (1986) but we found very little IgD, which they did. Nishimura et al (1990) reported one case where IgE staining was predominant and suggested that IgE-mediated hypersensitivity may play a role but in our study IgE was not a significant finding.

The presentation is often indolent and asymptomatic (Murray et al 1986). Staining of the underclothes with blood is documented (Jolly et al 1993) but many patients are indifferent to the problem. Well demarcated, glistening, moist, shiny, bright red or autumn brown patches involve the glans and mucosal prepuce (**Figs 7.1–7.14, see also** Figs 2.17, 4.27, 6.103), (Zoon 1952; Brodin 1980; Kumar et al 1995). There is no involvement of the keratinized penile shaft or keratinized foreskin. The urethra (fossa navicularis) may be involved (Merot & Harms 1983). Other signs include dark red stippling – 'cayenne pepper spots' – and purpura with hemosiderin deposition (Jonquieres 1971; Jonquieres & de Lutzky 1980) including a resemblance to lichen aureus (see Figs 4.27, 4.28) as reported by Kossard and Shumack (1989), although this patient subsequently developed lichen sclerosus of the glans (Kossard & Shumack 1989; Kumar et al 1995; Kossard 1997, personal communication). Also solitary or multiple lesions of differing sizes (guttate or nummular), characteristically 'kissing' and, rarely, erosive, vegetative and nodular presentations (Bureau et al 1962; Amerio et al 1973; Dupre et al 1976; Dupre & Schnitzler 1977; Crudeli et al 1986), but atypical or unusual morphology should be viewed with suspicion and biopsied.

The classical histology (Ive 1968) is of epidermal attenuation (absent granular and horny layers), diamond-/lozenge-shaped basal cell keratinocytes with sparse dyskeratosis and spongiosis. There may be erosion or ulceration. There is a band of dermal infiltration with plasma cells of variable density and arguable specificity (Souteyrand et al 1981). Extravasated erythrocytes, hemosiderin and vascular proliferation are also found. Although Zoon stressed the presence of the plasma cell infiltrate in this condition, Souteyrand et al (1981) noted that the plasma cell numbers could be widely variable and suggested that their presence might be a relatively non-specific feature (**Fig. 7.15**).

The differential diagnosis includes psoriasis, seborrheic dermatitis, contact dermatitis, erosive lichen planus, fixed drug eruption, secondary syphilis, erythroplasia of Queyrat (Davis-Daneshfar & Trueb 2000) and Kaposi's sarcoma – even histoplasmosis has been cited (Shelley & Shelley 1992). Screening for sexually transmitted disease is usually mandatory with penile presenting symptomatology. Although most of the above can usually be excluded with some confidence on clinical grounds, this is not always so (Altmeyer et al 1998). A properly targeted biopsy is advised and the pathologist should be encouraged to look for *concomitant* disease (e.g. lichen sclerosus, PIN) especially in the eventual whole preputial specimen following circumcision.

Although the condition may improve with altered washing habits and the intermittent application of mild

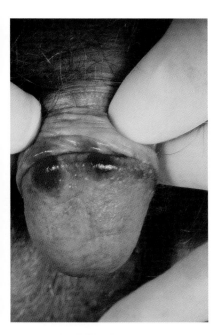

Fig. 7.1 Zoon's balanitis. Glans and prepuce, penis. 'Butterfly' or 'kissing' lesions.

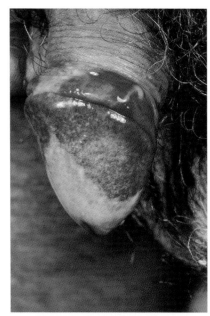

Fig. 7.4 Zoon's balanitis. Glans and prepuce, penis.

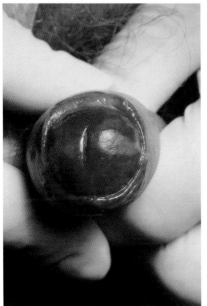

Fig. 7.2 Zoon's balanitis. Glans and prepuce, penis

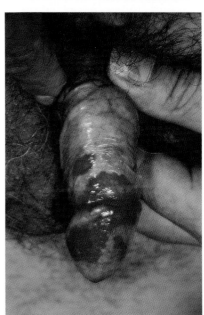

Fig. 7.5 Zoon's balanitis. Glans and prepuce, penis.

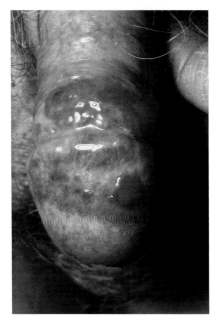

Fig. 7.3 Zoon's balanitis. Glans and prepuce, penis.

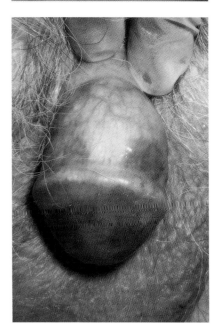

Fig. 7.6 Zoon's balanitis. Glans and prepuce, penis. Note waisting.

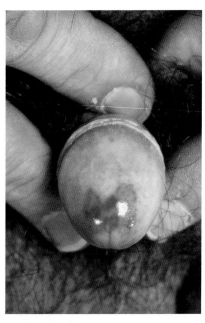

Fig. 7.7 Zoon's balanitis. Perimeatal glans penis.

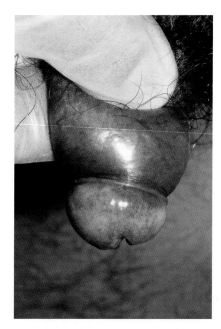

Fig. 7.10 Zoon's balanitis. Glans penis. Note incipient phimosis.

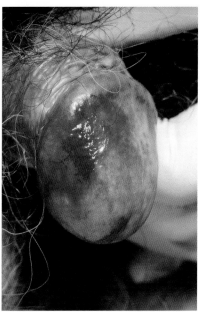

Fig. 7.8 Zoon's balanitis. Glans penis.

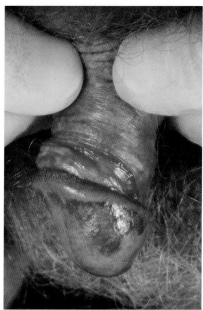

Fig. 7.11 Zoon's balanitis. Glans and prepuce, penis.

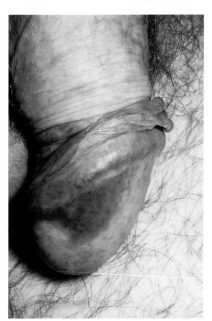

Fig. 7.9 Zoon's balanitis. Glans penis. Hemosiderin deposition. Same case as Fig. 7.8. Post-topical treatment.

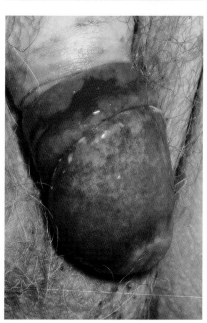

Fig. 7.12 Zoon's balanitis. Glans and prepuce, penis. Note waisting.

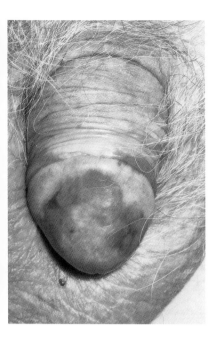

Fig. 7.13 Zoon's balanitis. Glans and prepuce, penis.

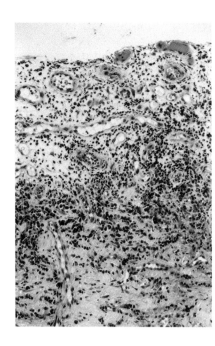

Fig. 7.15 Zoon's balanitis. The key features are erosion, ulceration, vascular ectasia and congestion with no intact epidermis on the surface. Beneath this there is edema and a band-like chronic inflammatory infiltrate, which is heavily infiltrated by plasma cells and beneath this there is some fibrosis. (Courtesy of Dr Nick Francis, London, UK.)

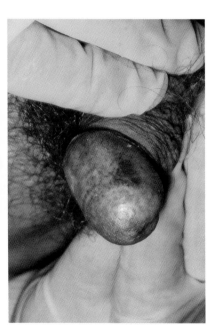

Fig. 7.14 Zoon's balanitis. Glans penis.

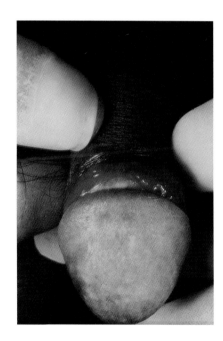

Fig. 7.16 Secondary Zoonoid inflammation. Biopsy showed an underlying foreign body granulomatous reaction for which an explanatory history was not forthcoming.

or potent topical corticosteroid (+/– antibiotics and anti-candidals), Zoon's balanitis usually persists or relapses. Definitive curative treatment is surgical circumcision (Sonnex et al 1982; Fernandez Vozmediano et al 1984; Ferrandiz & Ribera 1984; Arango Toro et al 1990; Kumar et al 1995; Altmeyer et al 1998; Pellice i Vilalta

et al 1999). The CO_2 laser has been deployed to good effect (Baldwin & Geronemus 1989; Aynaud et al 1995).

The florid signs of Zoon's may be secondary (Fig. 7.16), thereby concealing more subtle evidence of underlying preputial disease, such as lichen sclerosus (see Fig. 6.100–6.103), representing the actual primary cause of the disruption of the normal delicate anatomical arrangements and physiological dynamics of the parts. Frank cases of lichen sclerosus, lichen planus, Bowenoid papulosis and penile cancer often appear to have Zoonoid changes on clinical examination and on histology (see Figs 6.145–6.146).

Jonquieres (1971) has proposed that there is a separate entity, purpuric and lichenoid balanitis, not dissimilar clinically from Zoon's balanitis (or erythroplasia of Queyrat) but with a more lichenoid band-like infiltrate, telangiectatic and spongiotic histology. He has also described a vulval corollary (Jonquieres & Lutzky 1980).

It is possible that some of the clinical and histological variants that have been reported (Bureau et al 1962; Jonquieres 1971; Dupre et al 1976) and a recent ill-substantiated claim that Zoon's per se is a premalignant condition (Joshi 1999) are a consequence of this phenomenon. My own view is that Zoon's balanitis indicates a dysfunctional foreskin.

NON-SPECIFIC BALANOPOSTHITIS

Every attempt should be made to make a precise diagnosis when patients present with signs of balanoposthitis. Sexually transmitted disease, immunosuppression and diabetes must be excluded. A primary dermatosis is often present: psoriasis, seborrheic dermatitis (see Fig. 6.25), Zoon's balanitis, lichen sclerosus, lichen planus, warts, carcinoma in situ. A suitably targeted biopsy can be helpful. The histology may be non-specific too (Fig. 7.17).

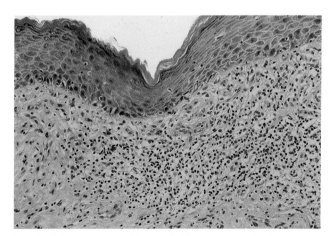

Fig. 7.17 Non-specific posthitis. Hyperkeratosis, a relatively normal thickness of epidermis (although there might be some slight thickening) and underlying that, chronic inflammation that is part lichenoid in pattern but shows no features of interface change nor hyaline sclerosus. (Courtesy of Dr Nick Francis, London, UK.)

Non-specific balanoposthitis is a diagnosis of exclusion and probably not common. Candidosis may be present, I believe, as a secondary opportunistic phenomenon rather than as a primary cause of disease, in most if not all cases. Preputial *dysfunction* is probably the cause in all cases and many will probably have lichen sclerosus as the underlying morbid state.

Treatment can be very difficult, with failure to respond to local toilet, soap substitution, topical steroids, and topical and systemic antibiotics. At one time topical carbenoxolone gel was under evaluation (Csonka & Murray 1971).

The ultimate recourse is to circumcision, which is curative in most instances and provides further tissue for histological substantiation of the presumed underlying genital dermatosis. However, in a significant number of patients the histology will be non-specific (even if there had been either hard or soft signs of an underlying dermatosis, such as lichen sclerosus, on clinical evaluation on one or more occasions) and the only rational conclusion is that such patients have had non-specific preputial dysfunction due to non-specific irritation, trauma and secondary candidosis such that a genuine non-specific balanoposthitis ensued, the pace of normal preputial repair and regeneration being exceeded by the pace of day-to-day attrition or wear and tear (**Figs 7.18–7.22**).

ERYTHRASMA

In this condition velvety, red, superficially scaly plaques are found extending symmetrically from the groins onto the upper thighs (**Figs 7.23–7.25**). In the inguinal folds erythrasma is an intertrigo and may be macerated and eroded. It is not usually very itchy but can be slightly sore in the groins and may have been present for years. However, erythrasma has been identified as the cause of pruritus ani (Bowyer & McColl 1971). Other sites of predisposition include the axillae and toe web spaces. The causative organism is a Gram-negative organism, *Corynebacterium minutissimum*.

Erythrasma is a clinical diagnosis clinched by coral-pink fluorescence (due to the elaboration by the micro-organism of protoporphyrinogen III) under a 360nm ultra-violet source: Wood's light, (see Figs 2.30, 2.31,) bacteriology and exclusion of tinea cruris. Tinea may coexist (Schlappner et al 1979) as can candida. Topical treatment with clindamycin, erythromycin or an imidazole is effective but a course of oral erythromycin is definitive and effective at several sites simultaneously. However effective these treatments may be, erythrasma is prone to recur.

GONORRHEA

This sexually transmitted disease usually presents as urethritis (with purulent semen-like discharge) and

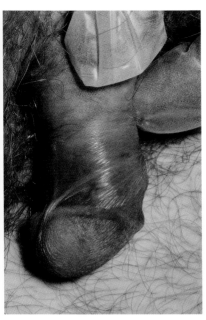

Fig. 7.18 Non-specific (balano)posthitis. Glans penis and distal prepuce. Significant non-specific posthitis (to a much lesser extent, balanitis). No specific clinical diagnosis could be made. Circumcision was curative but the histology was non-specific.

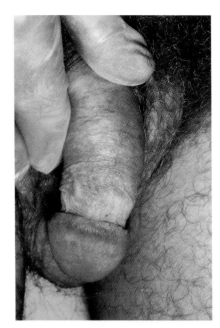

Fig. 7.21 Non-specific posthitis. Glans and shaft, penis. Low-grade proximal posthitis. No specific clinical diagnosis suggested itself. Medical treatment failed. Circumcision was curative but the foreskin histology was non-specific.

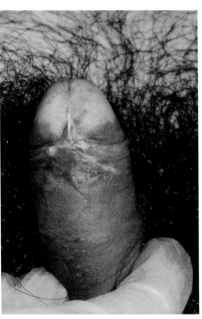

Fig. 7.19 Non-specific posthitis. Glans and ventral distal prepuce. Clinically this patient was diagnosed as having lichen sclerosus but the circumcision histology was non-specific. Circumcision was curative and the condition of the glans has normalized with time.

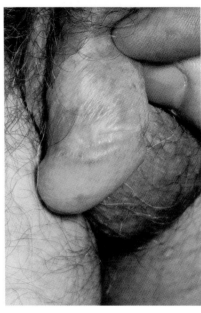

Fig. 7.22 Non-specific balanoposthitis. Glans and shaft, penis. Low-grade distal posthitis. No specific clinical diagnosis suggested itself. Medical treatment failed. Circumcision was curative but the foreskin histology was non-specific.

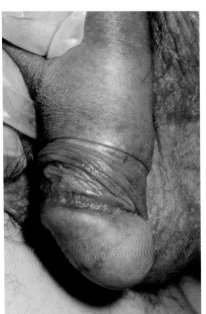

Fig. 7.20 Non-specific balanoposthitis. Lateral glans and shaft, penis. Patchy balanitis and posthitis with waisting. The clinical diagnosis was lichen sclerosus. The patient did not respond to medical treatment. Circumcision was curative but the foreskin histology was non-specific.

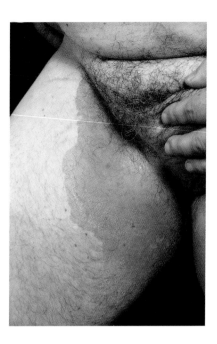

**Fig. 7.23
Erythrasma.**
Groin.

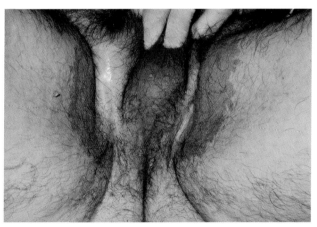

Fig. 7.24 Erythrasma. Groins.

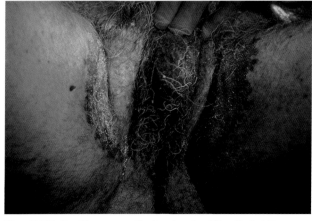

Fig. 7.25 Erythrasma. Groins (under Wood's light).
Same case as Fig. 7.24.

rarely as pharyngitis or conjunctivitis about 4–7 days after infection. Unlike women, only a few men have asymptomatic disease. Sometimes there is urinary retention. Anogenital skin manifestations commonly include balanoposthitis (the erythematous patch may be well demarcated and look very much like Zoon's balanitis) and meatal, preputial and penile edema and less commonly painful lymphadenopathy. Very rarely an ulcer has been reported (Landergren 1961; Haim & Merzbach 1970). It can be confusing if an anatomically anomalous penile structure is the primary site of infection (e.g. para-urethral or median raphe sinuses, Johnson & Thin 1972; Quiles et al 1987). Occasionally patients develop appendageal glandular infection (of Tyson's sebaceous glands, Cowper's glands, Littre's glands, Morgagni's lacunae), prostatitis or epididymitis. Even more rarely there is thrombosis of the dorsal vein of the penis and lymphangitis. Gonococcal pus can cause a secondary folliculitis or cellulitis of the skin of the abdomen or thighs.

If gonorrhea causes a systemic infection then bacteremic skin lesions in the form of erythematous vesicopustules (usually on the distal limbs) may be discovered on clinical examination – the gonococcal dermatitis syndrome. Rarer but more serious are the complications of endocarditis, septic arthritis and meningitis.

Gonorrhea is caused by *Neisseria gonorrhoeae*. It is a Gram-negative organism and diagnosed by that feature on staining smears where the bacteria appear as intracellular diplococci.

Treatment is with amoxicillin and probenecid. Patients (and partners) should be rigorously evaluated and excluded of other sexually transmitted diseases.

CANDIDOSIS

Candidosis (thrush) presents as an intertrigo. Burning and soreness are more likely than itch. Coalescent red patches or plaques involve the folds, often with superficial erosions. Pustulosis extends out onto the skin of the abdomen or buttocks, or thighs from the irregularly marginated, intertriginous lesions.

Genitourinary physicians hold that candida can be the cause of urethritis and balanoposthitis (Catterall 1966). The glans may be eroded. Candidosis of the penis, which appears to have a prevalence of about 10% of that of vaginal candidosis, has attracted very little research interest (Odds 1982).

Probably candida can frequently be found as a secondary pathogen in anogenital dermatoses. Eliciting the signs of candidosis or proving the presence of the organism should evince a thoughtful clinical search for an underlying dermatological or medical cause. This remark has particular resonance because the signs due to candida may be more florid than the underlying cause.

It is not an overgeneralization to say that the tables that accompany this chapter (causes of red scaly patches, of intertrigo and of balanoposthitis) contain all of the possible dermatological causes of secondary candidosis.

Obesity predisposes to candidal intertrigo (**Fig. 7.26**) but medical causes (**Table 7.3**) include diabetes mellitus, iatrogenic immunosuppression and systemic antibiotic treatment. Although it is indisputable that oropharyngeal candidosis is almost invariably found in HIV infection, anogenital disease is not frequently alluded to. It may be overlooked in the face of more pressing symptomatology in other sites or systems: in any case many patients take long-term imidazole antifungals orally.

The reason why *Candida albicans* is such a ready opportunist is that, although it is not regarded as a normal cutaneous commensal, it is a part of the resident flora of the gastrointestinal tract and may be retrieved from intertriginous areas including the preputial folds in the absence of symptoms and signs. Candidal balanoposthitis could be a sexually transmitted disease that may have an affinity for the anatomically abnormal penis or to those so predisposed by other factors or disease and where there is chronic vaginal or anal carriage in a partner. Screening should occur for other sexually transmitted diseases.

Diagnosis is clinical and supported by direct demonstration of the budding forms of the yeast and pseudohyphae (visualization is enhanced in a potassium hydroxide preparation by a drop of India ink under the cover slip) and microbiological culture.

Table 7.3 Medical causes of candidosis
Obesity
Diabetes mellitus
HIV infection
Iron deficiency
Cushing's syndrome
Iatrogenic immunosuppression
Debilitating infection or cancer
Incontinence
Systemic antibiotic treatment

Underlying disease should be identified and treated and predisposing factors rectified. Treatment (Goldstein 1993) includes topical nystatin, clioquinol or an imidazole, often very usefully combined with hydrocortisone or a moderately potent corticosteroid. Under certain severe circumstances an oral imidazole may be indicated.

TRICHOSPOROSIS

Trichosporosis is a common form of genitocrural and perianal intertrigo in India (Kamalam et al 1988). Predominant symptoms are itching or burning. Accompanying the intertrigo may be scaly papules. Coexisting dermatophyte, candida, trichomycosis and erythrasma infection may be found. Topical dequalinium chloride is used for treatment.

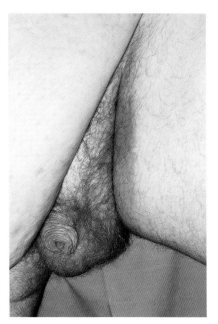

Fig. 7.26 Candidal intertrigo. Groin. Gross obesity, dependent abdomen (left).

ECCRINE SYRINGO-FIBROADENOMATOSIS (OF MASCARO)

This is a rare benign cutaneous lesion resulting from proliferation of the eccrine acrosyringium. Clinical features range from a solitary papule or nodule to multiple lesions with a linear arrangement or palmoplantar distribution with hyperhidrosis. One case with penile involvement manifesting as a balanoposthitis (**Figs 7.27–7.29**) has appeared in the literature (Ochonisky et al 1994). It may be complicated by insulin dependent diabetes, otitis media, sinusitis and pancreatitis.

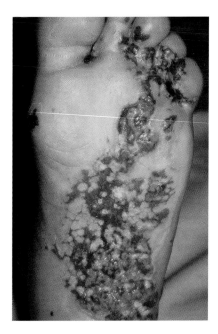

Fig. 7.27 Eccrine syringofibro-adenomatosis (of Mascaro). Foot. Hyper-hidrosis. Boggy erythematous plaque. (Courtesy of Dr Sophie Ochonisky, Paris, France, and reproduced from Ochonisky S et al. Arch Dermatol. 1994; 130: 933–4. Copyright 1994, American Medical Association.)

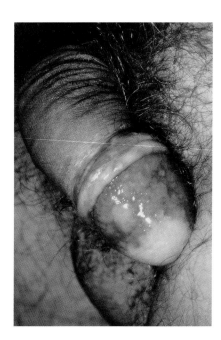

Fig. 7.28 Eccrine syringofibro-adenomatosis (of Mascaro). Glans and distal prepuce. Glossy and erythematous balanoposthitis with tiny white papules of punctuate hyperkeratosis. Same case as Fig 7.27. (Courtesy of Dr Sophie Ochonisky, Paris, France, and reproduced from Ochonisky S et al. Arch Dermatol. 1994; 130: 933–4. Copyright 1994, American Medical Association.)

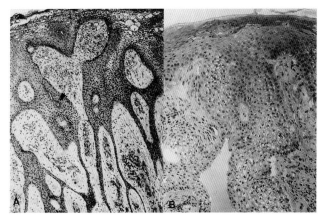

Fig. 7.29 Eccrine syringofibroadenomatosis (of Mascaro). Histology, H&E ×40 (left) ×100 (right). Foot (left), penis (right). Same case as Figs 7.27 and 7.28. (Courtesy of Dr Sophie Ochonisky, Paris, France, and reproduced from Ochonisky S et al. Arch Dermatol. 1994; 130: 933–4. Copyright 1994, American Medical Association.)

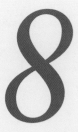

Erosions, ulcers and blisters

An *erosion* is defined as an area of loss of the epithelial surface: it will heal without scarring.

An *ulcer* represents full-thickness loss of epithelium and deeper tissue damage: it cannot heal without fibrosis and scarring. Some erosions may be non-specific because excoriation due to pruritus causes epithelial disruption. Intertrigos are frequently eroded because of friction and maceration.

Bullae and *vesicles* (blisters – fluid-filled spaces in the skin) burst to leave erosions. The causes of ulceration and erosion may overlap because an erosion may become secondarily traumatized or infected and so become an ulcer. The causes of erosions, ulcers, blisters and vesicles are listed in **Tables 8.1–8.6**.

Table 8.1 Causes of anogenital erosions

Common causes	Rare causes
Trauma	Child abuse
Intertrigo	Hailey-Hailey disease
Excoriated eczema and	Darier's disease
other pruritic	Autoimmune bullous
dermatoses,	diseases
e.g. Scabies	Pemphigus
Inverse pattern psoriasis	Bullous pemphigoid
Zoon's balanitis	Cicatricial pemphigoid
Lichen sclerosus	Linear IgA disease
Lichen planus	Dermatitis herpetiformis
Herpes simplex	Erythrasma
Candidosis	Streptococcal dermatitis
	Gonorrhea
	Secondary syphilis
	Mucous patch
	(herpetiform)
	Herpes zoster
	Acute primary HIV infection
	Cytomegalovirus in HIV
	Tinea
	Paracoccidioidomycosis
	Erythroplasia of Queyrat
	Kaposi's sarcoma
	Langerhans cell histiocytosis
	Topical steroids
	Fixed drug eruption

Table 8.2 Causes of anogenital vesicles and blisters

Common causes	Rare causes
Erythema	Acute contact
multiforme/Stevens-	dermatitis, e.g.
Johnson syndrome	phytophotodermatitis
Lichen sclerosus	Lichen planus
Bullous impetigo	Autoimmune bullous
Herpes simplex	diseases
Fixed drug eruption	Bullous pemphigoid
	Cicatricial pemphigoid
	Linear IgA disease
	Dermatitis
	herpetiformis
	Herpes zoster

Table 8.3 Causes of anogenital ulcers

Common causes	Rare causes
Trauma	Child abuse
Pressure sores	Extrusion of testicular prosthesis
Aphthae	Embolization
Pilonidal sinus	Dermatitis artefacta
Anal fistula	Penile necrosis
Erythema	Spontaneous scrotal ulceration
multiforme/	Sarcoid
Stevens-Johnson	Behçet's disease
syndrome	Autoimmune bullous diseases
Hidradenitis	Bullous pemphigoid
suppurativa	Cicatricial pemphigoid
Crohn's disease	Linear IgA disease
Chancroid	Necrobiosis lipoidica
Granuloma inguinale	Pyoderma gangrenosum
Lymphogranuloma	Necrotizing vasculitis
venereum	Wegener's granulomatosis
Syphilis-primary	Systemic lupus erythematosus
chancre	Polyarteritis nodosa
Squamous	Idiopathic systemic vasculitis
carcinoma	Hereditary spherocytosis with
	vascular necrosis
	Degos' malignant atrophic
	papulosis

Table 8.3 (*Cont'd*) Causes of anogenital ulcers

Rare causes (*cont'd*)

Calciphylaxis
Hypereosinophilic syndrome
Pseudomonas
  Ecthyma gangrenosum
  Necrotizing anorectal ulcer in leukemia
Gonorrhea
Fournier's gangrene
Tuberculosis and tuberculids
Leprosy
Syphilis: snail track ulcers
Yaws
Non-syphilitic spirochetal ulcerative
  balanoposthitis
Herpes simplex
HIV (primary infection and established
  disease)
Deep fungal infections
  Histoplasmosis
  Blastomycosis
  Paracoccidioidomycosis (South American
    blastomycosis)
  Cryptococcosis
Actinomycosis
Leishmaniasis
Amoebiasis
Filariasis
Langerhans cell histiocytosis
Extramammary Paget's disease
Basal cell carcinoma
Verrucous carcinoma
Sweat gland carcinoma
Kaposi's sarcoma
Leukemia
Lymphoma
Drug reaction

Table 8.5 Causes of dorsal perforation of the prepuce

Hidradenitis suppurativa
Pyoderma gangrenosum
Florid condylomata
Podophyllin
Chancroid
Herpes simplex
Squamous carcinoma

Table 8.6 Causes of penile necrosis

Decubitus ulcer
Spider bite
Priapism
Embolism
Strangulation and tourniquet syndromes
Vacuum erection device
Chronic renal failure
Diabetes mellitus
Thrombocytopenia
Polycythemia
Cryoglobulinemia
Coagulopathy
Vasculitis
Pyoderma gangrenosum
Calciphylaxis
Ecthyma gangrenosum
Fournier's gangrene
Herpes simplex
Mucormycosis (with acute myeloblastic leukemia)
Leukemia
Warfarin

Table 8.4 Diagnosis of genital ulcers

	Duration	Recurrence	Pain	Pruritus	Induration	Size	Destruction	Adenopathy
Herpes simplex	Short	Yes	Yes	Possible	No	Small	No	Yes
Syphilis	Short	No	No	No	Yes	Small	Rarely	Yes
Chancroid	Short	No	Yes	No	No	Small	No	Yes
GI	Long	No	No	No	Mild	Large	Yes	No
LGV	Short	No	Yes (nodes)	Rarely	No	Small	No	Massive
Leishmaniasis	Long	No	No	No	Yes	Small	Mild	Possible
Amebiasis	Long	No	Yes	No	Yes	Variable	No	Yes
Behçet's	Variable	Yes	Yes	No	Yes	Variable	No	No
Crohn's	Variable	Possible	Possible	No	Mild	Variable	No	No
Lichen planus	Variable	Possible	Yes	No	No	Variable	No	No
Pyoderma gangrenosum	Short	Yes	Yes	Possible	Yes	Variable	Yes	If infected
Cancer	Long	No	No	Possible	Yes	Variable	Yes	Possible (poor prognosis)
Factitial	Variable	No	No	Possible	If infected	Variable	Possible	If infected

Courtesy of Rosen & Brown 1998 by kind permission of Prof. Theodore Rosen, Houston, Texas, USA.

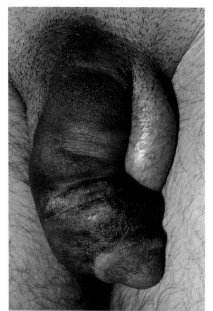

**Fig. 8.3
Hematoma.**
Penis. (Courtesy
of Dr Jeremy
Gilkes, London,
UK.)

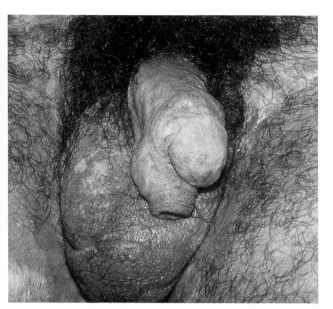

Fig. 8.1 Dorsal perforation of the prepuce. Severe
hidradenitis suppurativa, groins. Note: the penile head has
perforated dorsally through the prepuce, now lying
ventrally. (Courtesy of Prof. Bhushan Kumar, Chandigarh,
India.)

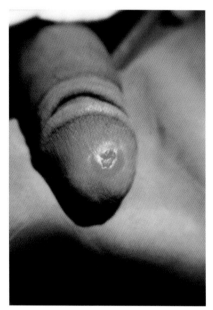

**Fig. 8.4 Human
bite.** Glans penis.
Traumatic ulcer.
(Courtesy of
Dr P Sugathan,
Kerala, India.)

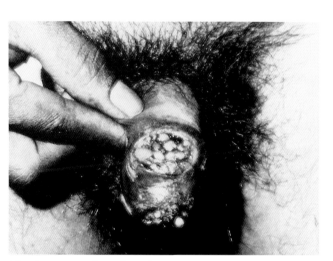

Fig. 8.2 Dorsal perforation of the prepuce. Penis.
(Courtesy of Prof. Bhushan Kumar, Chandigarh, India.)

Dorsal perforation of the prepuce (**Figs 8.1, 8.2**) is a
recently highlighted complication of several ulcerative
penile diseases, sexually and non-sexually acquired, as
listed in **Table 8.5** (Gupta & Kumar 2000, 2001).
Penile necrosis is a rare but devastating presentation
with an important differential diagnosis (**Table 8.6**).

TRAUMA

The genitals may be traumatized by sexual activity. The
penis is very vascular and hematoma formation (**Fig.
8.3**) is not uncommon; 'fracture' (penile rupture) however, is more rare (see page 223). Sometimes the penis
gets bitten by another person (**Figs 8.4, 8.5**). The effects

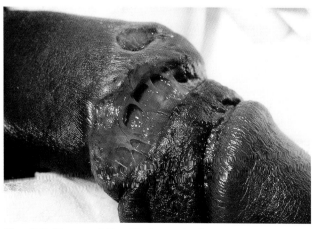

Fig. 8.5 Human bite. Shaft, penis. (Courtesy of
Dr Nicholas Soter, New York, NY, USA.)

137

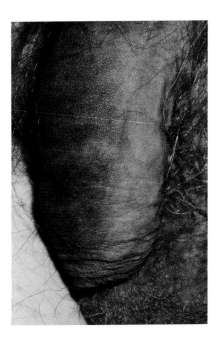

Fig. 8.6 Hematoma. Penis. Post-injection: self-medication for erectile impotence.

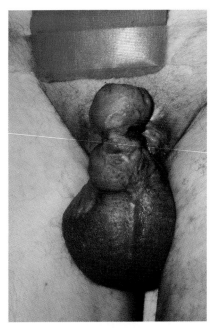

Fig. 8.8 Genital self-mutilation. Penis, scrotum, groins. Lacerations both groins, distal shaft strangulation, suprapubic catheter.

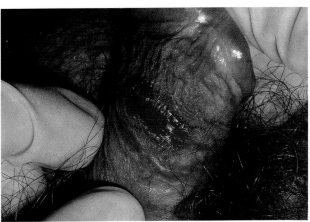

Fig. 8.7 Trapped hair. Ventral shaft, penis. Erosion.

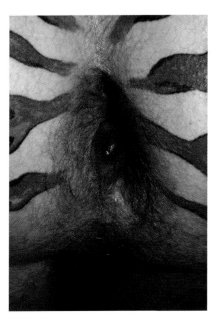

Fig. 8.9 Perianal hematoma. Anus.

of animal bites to the genitals have been reviewed by Gomes et al (2000). Degloving injuries can occur in accidents with industrial or agricultural equipment (Serrano Ortega et al 1980; Rutkow 1997; Hrbaty & Molitor 2001). Electric burns are rare (Xu et al 1999).

Sex aids can result in abrasions, eczema and ulceration. Injection of agents such as alprostadil prescribed for erectile dysfunction can be complicated by hematoma (**Fig. 8.6**). The penis may be incarcerated by ring devices (Wasadikar 1997), including vacuum erection equipment (Ganem et al 1998), rubber bands or hair (Haddad 1982; Pohlman 2000), and erosion (**Fig. 8.7**), ulceration and strangulation, necrosis and auto-amputation can supervene – the tourniquet syndrome. A retained, buried, condom ring following a tear during intercourse can cause an urethrocutaneous fistula (Tash & Eid 2000). The penis may be traumatized by external urinary devices employed to counter urinary incontinence (Fauer & Morrow 1978).

Seriously mentally ill patients have been known to mutilate their genitalia, as have transvestites (Greilsheimer & Groves 1979), but non-psychotic genital self-mutilation can also occur (**Fig. 8.8**). Australian aborigines slit the penis – opening the urethra ventrally, creating hypospadias – and this is called subincision. It has been mimicked pathologically (Pounder 1983). Ritual female circumcision in Islamic culture and male circumcision in Jewish culture, Islam and Western society may be perceived as similar tendencies.

Foreign body, lipogranuloma and silicon granuloma are discussed on pages 175 and 176.

Anal trauma is not uncommon. The two most common causes of acute, painful anal ulceration in homosexual men are trauma and herpes simplex. Primary syphilis, followed by chancroid, lymphogranuloma venereum, granuloma inguinale and amoebiasis are much less common (McMillan & Smith 1984). Post-traumatic hematoma can be seen (**Fig. 8.9**).

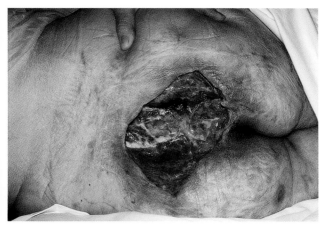

Fig. 8.10 Pressure sore. Lumbosacral area. (Courtesy of Dr Ron Zeegen, London, UK).

Table 8.8 Anogenital mimics of child abuse
Nappy rash
Innocent skin tags and fissures
Threadworms
Eczema
Phytophotodermatitis
Lichen sclerosus
Henoch-Schönlein purpura
Acute hemorrhagic edema of childhood
Anogenital streptococcal dermatitis
Causes of diarrhea 　Hemolytic uremic syndrome 　Crohn's disease
Causes of constipation 　Hirschsprung's disease

PRESSURE SORE

Pressure sores/decubitus ulcers in the sacral area (**Fig. 8.10**) are common despite measures taken to prevent this complication in the immobile or bed-ridden patient. The other common site is the heel. Ischemic compression or shearing forces over a bony prominence are the main nosogenic factors but sensory disturbance and debility also contribute (Kennedy 1998). Squamous carcinoma may eventuate as with all chronic ulceration.

CHILD ABUSE

The disquieting topic of physical and sexual child abuse is beyond the scope of this book but it should be suspected in the differential diagnosis of erosions and ulcers, vesicles and blisters of the anogenital area of children. The perianal signs of childhood sexual abuse in children generally have been described by Clayden (1987) and in girls by McCann and Voris (1993). Anal signs should be interpreted with caution (Clayden 1987; Hobbs & Wynne 1997; Priestley 1997) (**Table 8.7**). Re-examination should be avoided (Wynne & Hobbs 2000).

Child abuse may be erroneously suspected in the presentation of several diseases (**Table 8.8**). The bloody diarrheal prodrome of hemolytic uremic syndrome leading to perianal redness, anal dilatation and alternating

contraction and relaxation of the anal sphincter led to such suspicions in two girls (Vickers et al 1988).

The significance of anogenital warts in pointing to the possibility of child sexual abuse is controversial (Yun & Joblin 1993; Gibbs 1998). Hicks (1993) reported perianal warts in a three-year-old boy abused by his uncle. However, early recognition as a marker for child sexual abuse is in the child's long-term best interest (Hobbs & Wynne 1999).

EXTRUSION OF TESTICULAR PROSTHESIS

This has been reported to cause scrotal ulceration due to the presence of a sinus tract (Gordon & Schwartz 1979).

EMBOLIZATION

Localized gangrene of the scrotum and penis due to arterial embolization with particulate matter complicating accidental femoral self-injection of heroin in an addict has been reported (Somers & Lowe 1986).

DERMATITIS ARTEFACTA

Dermatitis artefacta focalized to the anogenital area is sometimes encountered (**Figs 8.11 8.13**). Dermatitis artefacta is recognized by dermatologists as unexplained erosions or ulcers that fail to heal or inexplicably break down despite treatment. The lesions are often geometrical, angulated and rectilinear. Sometimes they are induced by needles, knives, instruments, cigarette burns and extraneous foreign material may be introduced into the skin

Table 8.7 Anogenital signs of child abuse
Overall context 　Emotional disturbance 　Passivity on anogenital examination
Anal relaxation/dilatation
Purpura, bruising, tearing
Signs of sexually transmitted disease

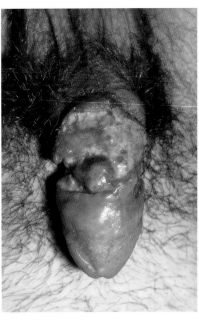

Fig. 8.11 Dermatitis artefacta. Penis.

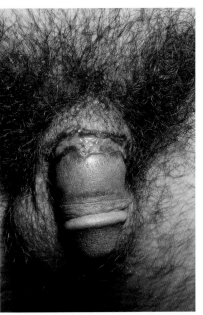

Fig. 8.12 Dermatitis artefacta. Penis. (Reproduced with permission from Bunker CB and Mallon E, Management of penile erosions and ulcers, Postgraduate Doctor Middle East, 1998; 21: 163–168. Copyright © Professional Managerial and Healthcare Publications Limited.)

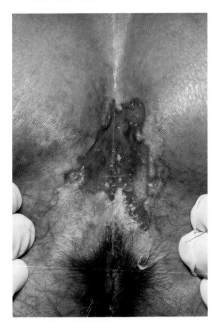

Fig. 8.13 Dermatitis artefacta. Natal cleft. Central ulceration and surrounding lichenification.

(lipogranuloma and silicon granuloma are discussed on page 176). The psychological ambience is characteristic. A belle indifference may be prevalent. There may be depression but rarely is a major psychiatric diagnosis sustainable. Confronting the patient with the suspected diagnosis is widely regarded as dangerous with an attendant risk of suicide. Alternatively, the injuries may be sustained in the course of sadomasochistic sexual gratification (Sonderbo & Nyfors 1986) due to algolagnia (love of pain).

Histology is usually obtained to exclude penile cancer but it is also important to consider pyoderma gangrenosum, which is rare but frequently omitted from the differential diagnosis of penile ulceration by non-dermatologists.

Management must be medically (infection treated and the lesions dressed and nursed) and psychologically supportive. Sometimes patients may be induced to take antipsychotic medication usually on a pretext. Pimozide has the reputation of being the drug of choice. Rarely will patients acquiesce to psychiatric evaluation and it may not be useful.

APHTHAE

Aphthous ulceration of the penis and scrotum does occur but this is not an acceptable diagnosis in the perianal skin or genitalia without overt exclusion of sexually transmitted diseases and other causes of genital ulceration, especially Behçet's syndrome. This is a different scenario from oral ulceration where to make a clinical diagnosis is reasonable practice. The causes of aphthae are obscure. The histology of idiopathic aphthous ulceration is non-specific.

The impression is that aphthae and idiopathic orogenital ulceration are more common in HIV infection and worse, symptomatically and morphologically. Giant lesions may occur (**Fig. 8.14**). Idiopathic perianal ulcer-

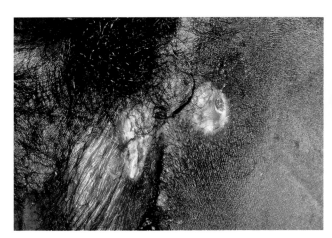

Fig. 8.14 Major aphthae/HIV. Scrotum and groin. Biopsy non-specific and culture negative.

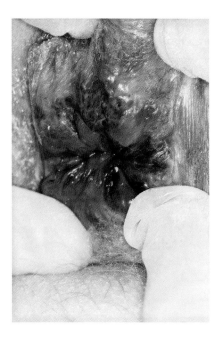

**Fig. 8.15
Idiopathic
ulceration/HIV.**
Perianal
ulceration.
(Courtesy of Prof.
Tim Allen-Mersh,
London, UK.)

ation is recognized (**Fig. 8.15**). In HIV all mucocutaneous ulcers must be biopsied and cultured; several pathologies may coexist. Treatment of simple aphthae is with topical corticosteroid/antibiotic/anti-candidal combinations. In HIV, thalidomide may be efficacious (Bunker & Staughton 2002).

PENILE NECROSIS

This serious situation has a number of causes and a wide differential diagnosis. Many of the causes are discussed in this or other chapters, for example decubitus ulcer (see page 139), the strangulation and tourniquet syndromes and other auto-erotic misadventures and causes of artefact (see page 175), priapism (see page 225), pyoderma gangrenosum (see page 154), infections such as herpes simplex (see page 163), ecthyma gangrenosum (see page 156) and Fournier's gangrene (see page 158) or complicating serious illness, such as mucormycosis in acute myeloblastic leukemia (Grossklaus et al 1999).

Necrosis can be the result of diabetic small vessel *and* end-stage renal disease (Bour & Steinhardt 1984; Frydenberg 1988) and chronic renal failure with secondary hyperparathyroidism and calciphylaxis (Lowe & Brendler 1984) can complicate polycythemia, thrombocytopenia and leukemia, cryoglobulinemia and vasculitis.

Inferior vena caval thrombosis as part of disseminated intravascular coagulation can lead to necrosis and gangrene of the penis (Sodal et al 1978). Heparin necrosis is a coagulopathy due to heparin-induced thrombocytopenia. Warfarin necrosis is a state of acquired protein C dysfunction (Harmanyeri et al 1998; Piette 2003).

SPONTANEOUS SCROTAL ULCERATION

Five cases of spontaneous scrotal ulceration in young, previously fit men have been described by Pinol Aguade et al (1974). Histology showed non-specific vasculitis and spontaneous resolution occurred. This entity may be related to idiopathic scrotal panniculitis and fat necrosis. Idiopathic scrotal necrosis in a two-month-old boy has been documented by Sarihan (1994): trauma, extreme cold and Fournier's gangrene were excluded.

PILONIDAL SINUS

Pilonidal sinus probably derives from the perineal pilosebaceous unit (Millar 1970). Precursor pits (not the common congenital sacral pits, see Fig. 1.53) associated with trapped hairs (**Fig. 8.16**) are thought to be important (Allen-Mersh 1990). Clinically pilonidal sinus is considered by dermatologists to constitute part of the 'follicular-occlusion tetrad' alongside hidradenitis suppurativa, acne conglobata, and dissecting cellulitis of the scalp. The pattern of cytokeratin expression supports this (Kurokawa et al 2002).

Presentations include itch, pain, recurrent abscess (**Fig. 8.17**), purulent discharge and persistent nodule (**Fig. 8.18**). Pilonidal sinus occurs in the midline and although the sacrococcygeal location is the most common site they have been reported to occur on the pubis, anterior perineum and very rarely the penis (usually in the coronal sulcus). Some of the penis cases have been complicated by actinomycosis (Rashid et al 1992; Val-Bernal et al 1999) and another has been

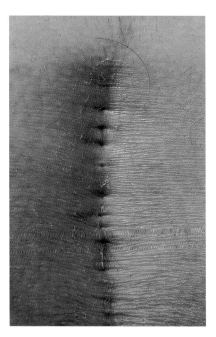

**Fig. 8.16
Pilonidal sinus.**
Natal cleft.
Precursor pits.
(Courtesy of Prof.
Tim Allen-Mersh,
London, UK.)

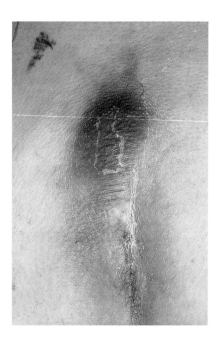

Fig. 8.17 Pilonidal abscess. Natal cleft. (Courtesy of Prof. Tim Allen-Mersh, London, UK.)

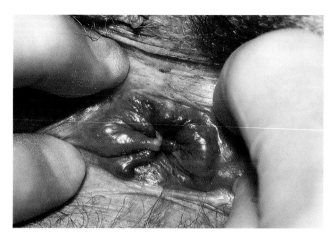

Fig. 8.19 Anal fissure. (Courtesy of Prof. Tim Allen-Mersh, London, UK.)

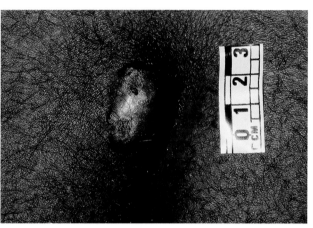

Fig. 8.18 Pilonidal granuloma. Natal cleft. (Courtesy of Prof. Tim Allen-Mersh, London, UK.)

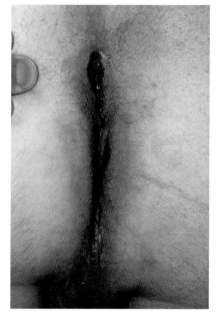

Fig. 8.20 Crohn's disease. Buttocks. Large fleshy perianal skin tag and fissure.

associated with a dermoid cyst (never previously reported on the penis but possibly missed or obliterated by granulomatous inflammation and fibrosis complicating pilonidal sinus, Tomasini et al 1997).

Treatment is surgical (Allen-Mersh 1990). Squamous carcinoma can supervene (Sagi et al 1984).

ANAL FISSURE

An anal fissure (**Fig. 8.19**) is a linear midline perianal ulcer: 90% posteriorly, 10% anteriorly. Many are idiopathic: the cause is probably related to defecation of a hard stool causing pressure trauma and necrosis. Other causes include sexually transmitted diseases, Crohn's disease (**Fig. 8.20**) and post-operative complication. Pain, bleeding, mucous discharge and constipation constitute the symptomatology. On examination there may be a 'sentinel pile' at the anal pole of the ulcer. Proctoscopy is mandatory. Management is surgical.

ANAL FISTULA

A perianal fistula is a communication between the anal canal and the perianal skin (see Fig. 3.6). Low-level fistulae open into the anal canal below the anorectal ring and high-level fistulae above it. Sixty percent are found in the midline posteriorly (there may be several perianal openings) and 20% anteriorly. Most first originate from infection and abscesses within the anal glands, although the anal opening may disappear. Most perianal fistulae are idiopathic but Crohn's disease, foreign body and tuberculosis are classical causes; an important differential diagnosis is hidradenitis suppurativa. Cancer is a rare complication. Fourteen percent of HIV-positive patients were found to have a fistula (Yuhan et al 1998).

The presentation is usually related to seropurulent discharge inducing pruritus ani but there may be pain of abscess formation. Surrounding skin may be indurated.

The management is the preserve of the colorectal surgeon.

ERYTHEMA MULTIFORME/STEVENS-JOHNSON SYNDROME

Erythema multiforme is a widespread symmetrical but centrifugal (i.e. concentrated on acral parts such as hands and feet) eruption of erythematous papules and plaques that grow to develop target or iris lesions (**Fig. 8.21**). Mucosal involvement of the mouth (**Fig. 8.22**) and the genitals (**Figs 8.23, 8.24**) occurs frequently. It is a common reaction pattern triggered by some infections such as herpes simplex, mycoplasma and orf and drugs, although many cases may be idiopathic. Severe disease with systemic upset, fever and florid mucocutaneous manifestations is called the Stevens-Johnson syndrome, which in itself is part of a spectrum of serious cutaneous reaction pattern of which toxic epidermal necrolysis is the most severe (with an appreciable mortality).

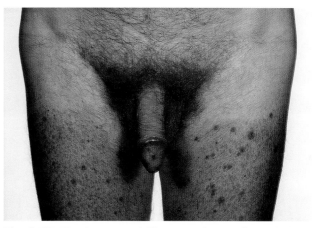

Fig. 8.23 Erythema multiforme. Pelvic girdle and glans penis. Target lesions.

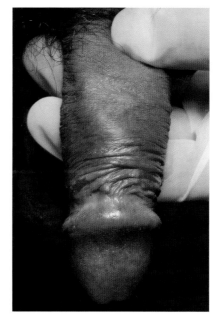

Fig. 8.24 Erythema multiforme. Prepuce, penis. Erythema and erosion.

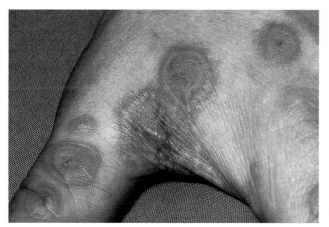

Fig. 8.21 Erythema multiforme. Hand. Target lesions.

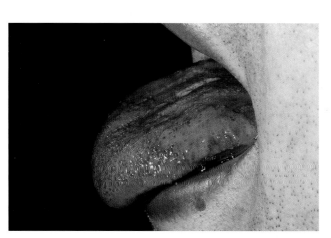

Fig. 8.22 Erythema multiforme. Lateral border of tongue. Erythematous erosions and ulcers.

PENILE ACNE

This is not an entity that appears in the literature but it is occasionally encountered in clinical practice. Young men complain of spots or boils or blackheads and on examination have comedones, papules, pustules and inflammatory nodules of the proximal penile shaft (**Figs 8.25, 8.26**). An important differential diagnosis of acneiform disease presenting at any site is chloracne, due to occlusion of the skin with machine oil. Conventional treatment for acne is prescribed in a hierarchical manner; topical keratolytics, antibiotics and retinoids, oral antibiotics; even isotretinoin may be justified.

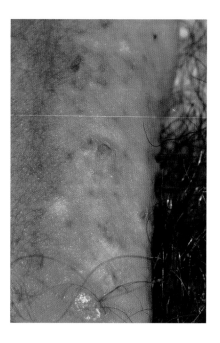

Fig. 8.25 Penile acne. Proximal shaft, penis. Comedones, cysts and healing inflamed lesions.

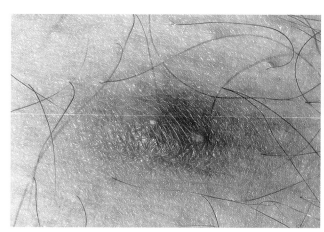

Fig. 8.27 Pili incarnati. Groin. Inflamed follicular lesion. Patient within hidradenitis suppurativa spectrum. Same case as Figs 5.1 and 5.2.

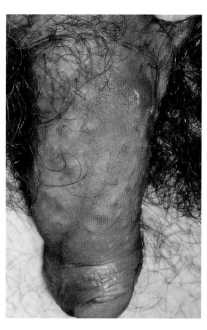

Fig. 8.26 Penile acne. Proximal shaft, penis. Comedones, papules, nodules.

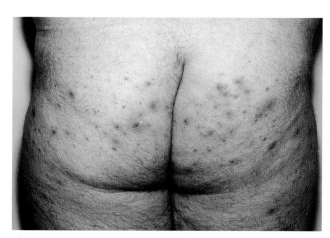

Fig. 8.28 Hidradenitis suppurativa. Buttocks. Borderline disease. Folliculitis, furunculosis, abscesses and nodules.

HIDRADENITIS SUPPURATIVA

Hidradenitis suppurativa (termed chronic perianal pyoderma in Japan) can be a painful disease. There is a clinical spectrum overlapping with chronic folliculitis, e.g. of the buttocks and 'penile acne'. Pili incarnati (ingrowing hairs) and secondary folliculitis are a common problem in the 'bikini' area in women but are rarely encountered in men (Fig. 8.27, see also Figs 5.1, 5.2).

In full-blown hidradenitis bridged comedones, folliculitis and furunculosis (Figs 8.28, 8.29), deep discharging sinuses, nodules, cysts, and scars in the groins (Fig. 8.30) and axillae (Fig. 8.31), the natal cleft and buttocks (Coda & Ferri 1991) may all be present and

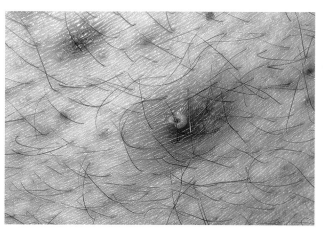

Fig. 8.29 Furunculosis/hidradenitis suppurativa. Buttocks. Same case as Fig. 8.28.

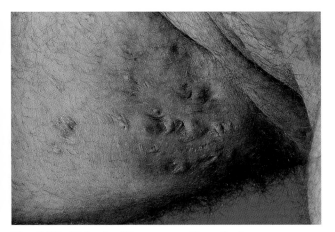

Fig. 8.30 Hidradenitis suppurativa. Groin.

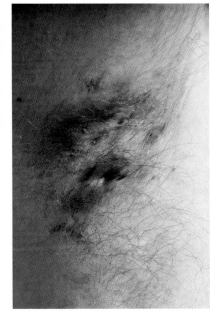

Fig. 8.31 Hidradenitis suppurativa. Axilla.

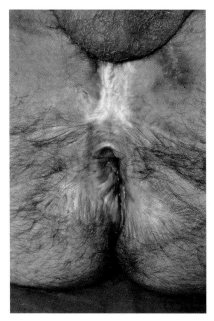

Fig. 8.32 Hidradenitis suppurativa. Perineum. Scars from disease and surgical treatment. (Courtesy of Prof. Tim Allen-Mersh, London, UK).

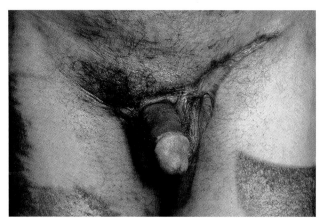

Fig. 8.33 Hidradenitis suppurativa. Groins. Note graft sites.

then the clinical picture is near-pathognomic. It is more common in black individuals and affects the axillae preferentially in women and the perineum in men. A urethral cutaneous fistula and phimosis has been reported (Chaikin et al 1994). It is a cause of dorsal perforation of the penis (Gupta & Kumar 2000, 2001, see also Fig 8.1). Some patients may also have severe conglobate acne. Scarring from the disease and its treatment can be extensive (**Figs 8.32, 8.33**). The morbidity of hidradenitis may be appalling, interfering with sitting, sleeping, walking, defecation and sexual activity. It is not surprising that depression is common.

Hidradenitis suppurativa is considered to be analogous to acne (a disorder of the pilosebaceous unit) affecting the apocrine sweat gland. Indeed, patients sometimes also have cystic or conglobate acne. The role of endocrine factors is unknown. Occlusion leads to comedone formation and purulent infection due to secondary infec-

tion with Gram-negative and Gram-positive organisms. *Staphylococcus aureus, Streptococcus milleri, Bacteroides* sp. (Highet et al 1988) and more recently *Chlamydia trachomatis* (Bendahan et al 1992) have been implicated in the pathogenesis.

Chronicity and tissue destruction lead to the classical physical signs. Disease that has persisted for more than 20 years carries a significant risk of progression to squamous cell carcinoma (Black & Woods 1982; Shukla & Hughes 1995; Ishizawa et al 2000) and rarely verrucous carcinoma (Cosman et al 2000).

Hidradenitis is usually a clinical diagnosis. Swabs should be taken for bacteriological evaluation and to guide therapy, but the patient should be fully evaluated (with appropriate specimens collected) for sexually transmitted diseases should the presentation be in any way suspicious. Chloracne has been mentioned above.

Rarely a biopsy may be necessary to exclude carcinoma or Crohn's disease. Perineal Crohn's disease

145

mimics hidradenitis with its granulomatous inflammation ulceration and fistula formation but it is less painful. Also, the disease is absent from the axillae and it is rare for patients to be free of overt gastrointestinal symptoms. Very florid perianal disease can be seen in myeloma and leukemia (Alexander-Williams & Buchmann 1980), in homosexual men and AIDS (Carr et al 1989).

Treatment is with oral antibiotics (erythromycin 250mg qds or 500mg–1g bd, flucloxacillin 250mg tds, ciprofloxacin 250–500mg bd, metronidazole 200–400mg bd) and topical antiseptics offering the lynch-pin of medical management. Hormonal manipulation with antiandrogens such as cyproterone acetate is an option in women. Oral prednisolone can be used alongside antibiotics to control intercurrent exacerbations. Oral isotretinoin (1mg/kg) for six to eight months helps some but not, disappointingly, all patients.

Surgical resection and reconstruction must be considered for extensive, recalcitrant disease (Slauf et al 1993). Local excision is also a good treatment for localized disease, as is sometimes encountered.

CROHN'S DISEASE

Crohn's disease can affect any part of the gut and its cutaneous borders from the mouth (**Fig. 8.34**) to the anus. Perianal disease may occur in as many as 75–90% of patients (Fielding 1972; Gruwez et al 1983). Crohn's disease may have other cutaneous manifestations (**Table 8.9**).

Anogenital features of Crohn's disease (**Table 8.10**) (McCallum & Kinmont 1968; Boggs 1970; Lockhart-Mummery 1972; Rankin 1979; Alexander-Williams & Buchmann 1980; Palder et al 1991) include those common to most chronic diarrheal illnesses such as pruritus ani, skin maceration and erosions with secondary infection.

Table 8.9 Other cutaneous features of Crohn's disease
Granulomatous cheilitis (Melkersson-Rosenthal syndrome)
Chronic vulval edema
Metastatic granuloma
Erythema nodosum
Granulomatous vasculitis
Acrodermatitis enteropathica (zinc malabsorption)
Epidermolysis bullosa acquisita

Iatrogenic
  acne
  warts
  mollusca

Table 8.10 Anogenital features of Crohn's disease
Pruritus ani
Maceration
Erosion
Secondary infection
Skin tags
Fissures
Anal stenosis
Fistula in ano
Abscess
'Metastatic' granulomatous plaques
Balanoposthitis and phimosis
Anogenital granulomatosis/granulomatous lymphangitis

Skin tags, larger, thicker and harder than are normally encountered, are common (**Fig. 8.35**). Deep, undermined, angulated fissures (**Fig. 8.36**, see also Fig. 8.20), with cyanotic edges to adjoining skin that may fuse to form 'flying buttress' skin bridges, are characterized by relative lack of pain. Anal stenosis is present when the anal canal will not admit one let alone two (as is normal) examining fingers. Fistulae in ano are less common than fissures. They are typified by an indurated orifice in the skin that exudes pus and a palpable track running towards the anus and are often asymptomatic even when multiple. Pain usually means that an abscess has formed due to blockage of a fistula. Multiple external openings can be encountered all over the buttock (**Fig. 8.37**), on the scrotum and on the thigh. Again, a distinctive sign is the cyanotic hue of the indurated skin.

Fecal incontinence is the most serious complication of perianal Crohn's disease. Carcinoma can complicate

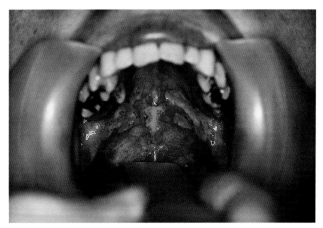

Fig. 8.34 Crohn's disease. Palate. Oral ulceration. (Courtesy of Dr Ron Zeegen, London, UK.)

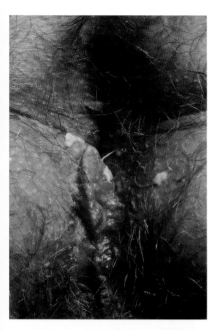

**Fig. 8.35
Crohn's disease.**
Perianal skin.
Large, thick, hard
tag.

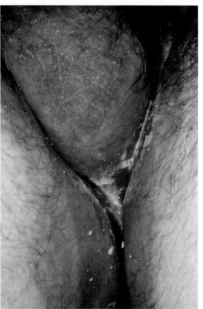

**Fig. 8.36
Crohn's disease.**
Groins and
scrotum. Erosions
and fissures. Note
cyanotic hue.

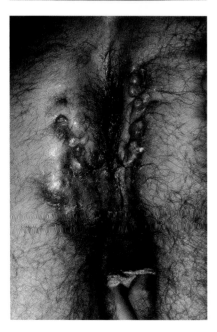

Fig. 8.37 Crohn's
disease. Buttocks
and perianal area.
(Courtesy of
Dr Ron Zeegen,
London, UK.)

any site of chronic inflammation and Crohn's is no exception (Slater et al 1984).

Crohn's disease of the penis and scrotum is rare but metastatic erythematous granulomatous plaques and ulceration have been encountered (Goh et al 1998; Corazza et al 1999; Lehrnbecher et al 1999; Acker et al 2000) as has metastatic cutaneous ulceration of the penile shaft, multiple scrotal urinary fistulae and destruction of the proximal urethra (Slaney et al 1986). Balanoposthitis and phimosis have been reported (Phillips et al 1997).

The etiology of Crohn's disease is not known. It is an idiopathic disorder of granulomatous inflammation of the gastrointestinal tract. Fistulae are thought to arise from infection of an anal gland or from more proximal intestinal Crohn's ulcers. The pathological process is granulomatous inflammation. It has been suggested that some perianal lesions may be analogous to intestinal 'skip' lesions and be due to retrograde lymphatic flow (Fielding 1972).

Clinical diagnosis may be achieved in the context of symptoms, signs and investigation results (e.g. radiography and gut biopsy) consistent with Crohn's disease. Any anal lesion in a patient who is known to be suffering from Crohn's disease is likely to have perianal Crohn's (Alexander-Williams & Buchmann 1980). The difficulty comes when the anogenital disease just happens to be the first manifestation of the Crohn's disease. Histologically positive perianal disease of all clinical types may predate frank gastrointestinal Crohn's disease by several years (Baker & Milton-Thompson 1971), including in children (Palder et al 1991). The relative lack of pain, the multiplicity of lesions, the edema of skin tags and the eccentricity of fissures are important pointers (Alexander-Williams & Buchmann 1980). Biopsy is helpful and sigmoidoscopy and biopsy of intestinal mucosal lesions is mandatory.

Occasionally perineal biopsy may be necessary in the face of cryptic lesions (e.g. a solitary papule or nodule on the penis). Swabs should be taken and the patient fully evaluated (with appropriate specimens collected) for sexually transmitted diseases should the presentation be in any way atypical.

The differential diagnosis encompasses the causes of pruritus ani and includes simple non-specific anal fissures and fistulae. Hidradenitis suppurativa presents with nodules, sinuses and purulence but is more painful: other sites may be involved and severe acne is often present. Similarly, florid perianal disease can be seen in myeloma and leukemia (Alexander-Williams & Buchmann 1980). Proctitis, perianal ulceration, abscess, fissure and fistula are prevalent in homosexual men and HIV infection (Carr et al 1989; Denis et al 1992). Perineal pyoderma gangrenosum has been misdiagnosed as Crohn's disease. A solitary granulomatous nodule with or without ulceration poses a differential diagnosis including sarcoid, schistosomiasis, leishmaniasis, tuberculosis, atypical mycobacterial infection, deep fungal infection, granuloma inguinale, lymphogranuloma venereum, chancroid and syphilis and mucocutaneous malignancy (squamous cell carcinoma, basal cell carcinoma, Kaposi's sarcoma and amelanotic malignant melanoma). Crohn's disease should be excluded in patients with chronic penile edema.

As a generalization the treatment of the skin manifestations of Crohn's disease depends to some extent on treatment of active intestinal disease. Local measures include soaks with potassium permanganate and aluminum acetate, potent or very potent topical corticosteroid/antibiotic combinations and oral antibiotics (as for hidradenitis). A special place has been claimed for long-term, oral metronidazole (20mg/kg per day in divided doses (Bernstein et al 1980; Brandt et al 1982). Although extensively used for the management of the enteric disease, rarely are systemic corticosteroids indicated for cutaneous disease alone but in this exiguous circumstance the morbidity can be profound (as it can be for hidradenitis) and so justify such treatment with its attendant side effects and risks. Perianal abscess may respond to sulphasalazine and anal fissure to prednisolone and azathioprine (Rankin 1979).

Management of anal stenosis, fissures, and fistulae should involve a surgeon. The general approach is conservative although stenosis may require dilatation and abscesses, decompression. Proctectomy is rarely indicated (Lockhart-Mummery 1972; Buchmann et al 1980; Hibbiss & Scofield 1982). Particular conservatism is advocated in the management of the perianal complications of pediatric and adolescent Crohn's disease (Palder et al 1991).

BEHÇET'S DISEASE

Dr Hulusi Behçet (a Turkish dermatologist) described a syndrome of recurrent orogenital ulceration and inflammatory eye disease in 1937 (Behçet 1937). Dr Benediktos Adamantiades, a Greek ophthalmologist, described a probable case in 1930 but other likely cases can be found in the earlier literature; Behçet's disease was probably first described by Hippocrates of Kos (460–377 BC) (Zoubolis & Keitel 2002). Essentially, Behçet's disease is a systemic vasculitis that may have involved many organs so that protean presentations and complications are possible (Shelley & Shelley 1992; Pickering & Haskard 2000).

The diagnostic criteria of The International Study Group for Behçet's Disease (Lancet 1990) are given below (**Table 8.11**). In other words: oral ulceration must be present, then patients must also either manifest genital ulceration and ophthalmic involvement *or* genital ulceration and skin signs (or a positive pathergy test); if patients do not have genital ulceration then they must have ophthalmic and dermatological involvement *or* a positive pathergy test.

In practice there are many patients who have an incomplete syndrome. Despite not satisfying these rigid

Table 8.11 Diagnostic criteria for diagnosis of Behçet's disease

Recurrent oral ulceration	Minor aphthous, major aphthous or herpetiform ulceration observed by the physician or patient, which have recurred at least three times in one 12-month period
Plus two of:	
Recurrent genital ulceration	Aphthous ulceration or scarring observed by the physician or the patient
Eye lesions	Anterior uveitis, posterior uveitis, or cells in the vitreous on slit-lamp examination; or retinal vasculitis observed by the ophthalmologist
Skin lesions	Erythema nodosum observed by the physician or the patient. Pseudofolliculitis or papulopustular lesions; or acneiform nodules observed by the physician in adult patients off steroid treatment (i.e. not acne)
Positive pathergy test	Read by physician at 24–48h

diagnostic criteria, 'possible' or 'probable' Behçet's disease is an acceptable label for everyday practical purposes.

Other clinical manifestations include malaise, fever, arthralgia, myalgia thrombophlebitis (Haim et al 1974), epidermitis and urethritis (Kirkali et al 1991), spontaneous hematocele (from venous rupture due to lymphocytic venulitis; Orhan et al 1999), erectile dysfunction (Aksu et al 2000) and cardiac, renal, neurological and rheumatological effects (**Table 8.12**).

The classical oral ulceration of Behçet's disease consists of painful lesions anywhere in the oral cavity (lips, buccal mucosa (**Fig. 8.38**), gingiva, tongue (**Fig. 8.39**), palate (**Fig. 8.40**) and pharynx contributing to a focal or generalized stomatitis. Single or multiple, local or multifocal, they start as papules which ulcerate within 48 hours, achieving a size anywhere between 2mm and 1cm. The central base is sometimes yellow and there is an erythematous rim. Healing can occur without scarring but it may be protracted (several weeks) and scars are commonplace (especially if lesions recur at the same site).

The genital ulcers in men (**Figs 8.41–8.44**) are painful (can be very painful and this distinction can be helpful)

Table 8.12 Clinical manifestations of Behçet's disease

Malaise

Fever

Headache

Facial and retrosternal pain

Arthralgia

Myalgia

Sore throat and tonsillitis

Abdominal pain

Melena

Epididymitis

Urethritis

Neurovasculitis including venous thrombosis

Psychiatric syndromes

Aneurysms

Thrombophlebitis

Skin pathergy

Proteinuria, nephrotic syndrome and amyloidosis

Erectile dysfunction

Spontaneous hematocele

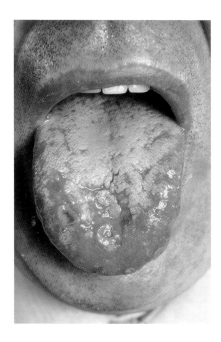

Fig. 8.39 Behçet's disease. Tongue. Painful ulceration. Same case as Fig. 8.38.

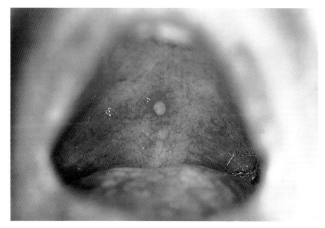

Fig. 8.40 Behçet's disease. Hard palate. Painful ulceration. Same case as Fig. 8.38.

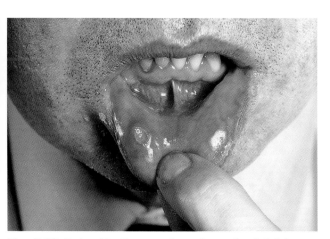

Fig. 8.38 Behçet's disease. Inner lower lip. Painful ulceration.

and occur anywhere on the genitalia including the scrotum and perianal skin. As a generalization they are bigger and deeper than in the mouth. It is also said that they are fewer and less recurrent.

Other cutaneous complications are listed in Tables 8.11 and 8.12 and include a sterile non follicular acneiform pustulosis (Fig. 8.45)

Patients with relapsing polychondritis (sore, red, swollen, ulcerative lesions of the helix; saddle nose deformity) and Behçet's disease have been reported and the acronym MAGIC (mouth and genital ulcers with

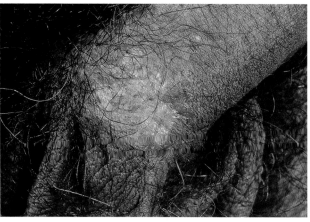

Fig. 8.41 Behçet's disease. Ulcer, penis root.

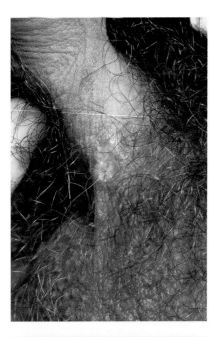

Fig. 8.42 Behçet's disease. Root of penis. Painful ulcer. Same case as Fig. 8.38.

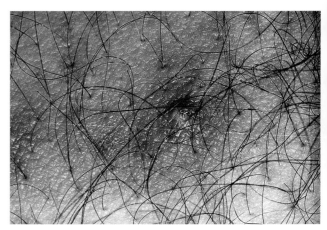

Fig. 8.45 Behçet's disease. Back. Non-follicular sterile pustulosis. Same case as Fig. 8.38.

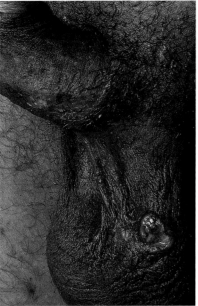

Fig. 8.43 Behçet's disease. Scrotum. Ulcer. (Courtesy of Dr Brian Gibberd, London, UK).

Table 8.13 Differential diagnosis of the systemic features of Behçet's disease

Systemic lupus erythematosus

Relapsing polychondritis (MAGIC syndrome)

Familial Mediterranean fever

Reiter's syndrome

inflamed cartilage) syndrome proposed (Firestein et al 1985; Orme 1990).

The cause of Behçet's disease is not known. A viral etiology is possible and it may be a post-streptococcal syndrome. Childhood infection has been invoked (Cooper et al 1989). Some foods have been implicated. Familial cases have been reported (Dundar et al 1985; Woodrow et al 1990) and there is an association with the HLA class I antigen B 51 (Pickering & Haskard 2000).

Histology is usually non-specific and does not distinguish idiopathic aphthae although sometimes necrotizing vasculitis can be discovered.

No particular blood test is diagnostic. Patients under investigation should be screened for systemic disease (Tables 8.12, 8.13) and sexually transmitted diseases. It is possible that asymptomatic organ involvement (e.g. of the central nervous system and of fibrinolysis) may not be detectable by routine tests (Markus et al 1992).

The pathergy test is the development of a sterile pustule or a tuberculin-like reaction 24–48 hours after the intradermal injection of 0.2ml normal saline. Pathergy refers to the development of a skin reaction at the site of any invasive trauma.

Topical treatment with corticosteroid/antimicrobial combinations may suffice. However, some patients will require systemic modalities including colchicine (Vordermark & Hudson 1984), prednisolone, azathioprine and cyclosporin (Suss et al 1993). Thalidomide has been used to treat the mucocutaneous lesions (Hamuryudan et al 1998) and associated pyoderma gangrenosum

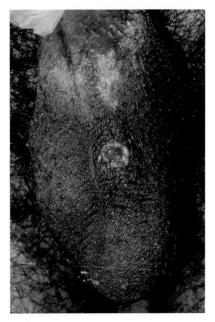

Fig. 8.44 Behçet's disease. Scrotum. Ulcer.

(Munro & Cox 1988; Rustin et al 1990; Stirling 1998). Many things have been tried and new approaches are under evaluation (Russell et al 2001).

AUTOIMMUNE BULLOUS DISEASES

Pemphigus

Pemphigus is a group of rare immunobullous disorders where loss of epidermal cohesion causes blistering and erosion of mucocutaneous sites (**Figs 8.46, 8.47**). Therefore the penis is often involved but possibly never in isolation. Sami & Ahmed (2001) have described the clinical features of twelve patients in none of whom was the penis the only site of the disease. The glans penis is the site of predilection.

Histology shows acantholysis, direct immunofluorescence; intercellular epidermal IgG and C3 and indirect immunofluorescence; a titre of circulating IgG intercellular antibody proportionate to the severity of the disease. Treatment requires high-dose systemic corticosteroids and often other immunosuppressant medication. Despite this the mortality is still high.

Pemphigus vegetans

Pemphigus vegetans is a rare variant where moist and verrucous plaques occur in intertriginous areas at the site of blister and erosion formation. A case (Castle et al 1987) presenting as four years of indolent tender balanitis has been described where the glans penis was involved with a moist, vegetative plaque with beefy, red erosions separating irregular hyperkeratotic mounds. Other sites were uninvolved. Histology showed acanthosis, papillomatosis, suprabasalar clefting, acantholysis and an eosinophil-rich inflammatory infiltrate. Immunofluorescence (direct and indirect) was positive. Treatment was with oral and topical corticosteroids and dressings.

Bullous pemphigoid

Bullous pemphigoid is common in elderly folk. It is thought to be due to autoimmune damage to the hemidesmosome of the cutaneous basement membrane, but the initiating factors are not known.

The primary lesions are often not blisters, the patient first developing erythematous urticated and eczematous areas on the trunk and limbs, often around the pelvic girdle (**Fig. 8.48**). Tense blisters then appear in these sites and are sometimes mistaken for bullous impetigo

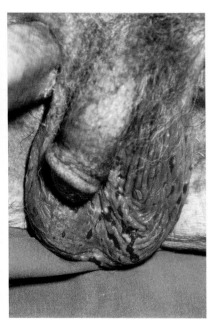

Fig. 8.46 Pemphigus. Scrotum. Erythema and erosions. (Courtesy of the late Dr Gerald Levene, London, UK.)

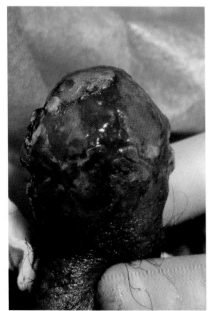

Fig. 8.47 Pemphigus. Ventral glans and distal shaft, penis. Severe erosion.

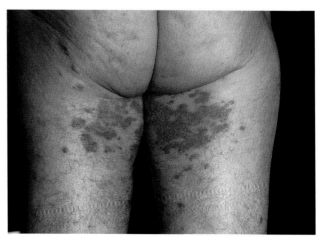

Fig. 8.48 Bullous pemphigoid, prodrome. Buttocks and upper thighs. Urticated plaques. (Courtesy of Prof. Richard Groves, London, UK.)

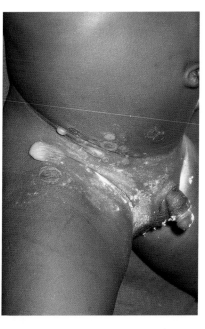

Fig. 8.49 Bullous impetigo. Right pelvic girdle. Blisters and erosions. (Courtesy of Dr Peter Copeman, London, UK.)

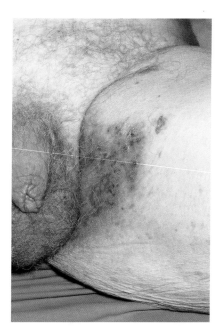

Fig. 8.51 Bullous pemphigoid. Right groin. Hemorrhagic (frictional) bullae and erosions. This patient was discovered to have an underlying lung cancer.

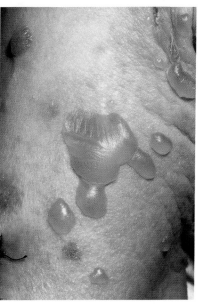

Fig. 8.50 Bullous pemphigoid. Right groin. Tense blisters.

(**Fig. 8.49**). Pelvic girdle lesions are often seen but rarely in isolation (**Figs 8.50, 8.51**). Mucosal lesions are uncommon: their presence suggests another diagnosis or underlying neoplasm.

The diagnosis of bullous pemphigoid is confirmed by histological evidence of a subepidermal blister with positive direct immunofluorescence of perilesional skin, where IgG and C3 are demonstrated at the basement membrane zone. Circulating antibodies to the basement membrane zone (indirect immunofluorescence) are often but not always found in the serum. Seronegative disease may be a harbinger of internal malignancy.

Most patients respond well to prednisolone 40–60mg daily, which is given until the blisters begin to heal and no new blisters are appearing. The dose is reduced over a few weeks and many patients remain free of lesions after treatment is stopped. Azathioprine is often introduced (50–150mg daily) as a corticosteroid-sparing agent.

Cicatricial pemphigoid

Cicatricial (cicatrizing) pemphigoid or (benign) mucous membrane pemphigoid is a rare variant of bullous pemphigoid. Blisters affect the skin and the mucous membranes. Skin lesions are usually less widespread than in bullous pemphigoid and may heal with scarring. Oral lesions predominantly involve the palate and gingivae, but there may be esophageal involvement with dysphagia and conjunctival disease with the formation of symblepharon can lead to blindness. Involvement of the penis may be with blisters, erosions, ulcers, transcoronal adhesions, scarring and phimosis (Kirtschig et al 1998; Ramlogan et al 2000, Fueston et al 2002) (see Figs 2.24, 2.29).

Although direct immunofluorescence is usually positive (see above), circulating antibodies (indirect immunofluorescence) to the basement membrane zone are rarely found.

Patients often respond poorly to oral steroids but dapsone or other sulpha-drugs such as sulphamethoxy-pyradazine can be strikingly effective (Kirtschig et al 2003). Regular hematology screening is mandatory with dapsone because agranulocytosis has been reported. Most patients develop a degree of hemolytic anemia that is tolerated in view of the benefit obtained.

Dermatitis herpetiformis

This very rare disease occurs in young adults with a second peak of incidence in old age. Intensely itchy groups of small blisters on an urticarial base occur over the elbows, knees, buttocks (**Figs 8.52, 8.53**) or face; often only excoriations may be seen.

An association with HLA B8, DR3 and DQw2 suggests an autoimmune basis but circulating antibodies

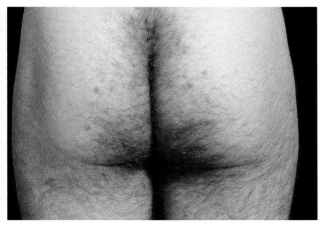

Fig. 8.52 Dermatitis herpetiformis. Buttocks. Impetiginized excoriations.

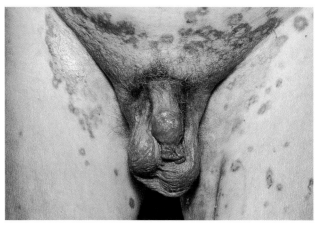

Fig. 8.54 Linear IgA disease. Pubis, upper thighs and genitalia. Antibiotic induced.

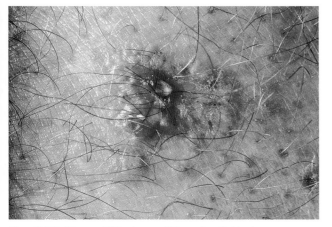

Fig. 8.53 Dermatitis herpetiformis. Buttocks. Herpetiform vesicles Same case as Fig. 8.52.

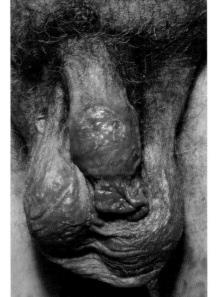

Fig. 8.55 Linear IgA disease. Penis and scrotum. Same case as Fig. 8.54.

are not found. However, histology reveals subepidermal blisters and microabscesses in the dermal papillae and direct immunofluorescence shows IgA in the papillary tips. Endoscopy and biopsy may be necessary because patients often have a gluten-sensitive enteropathy, which may be clinically silent and inapparent on simple screening (e.g. FBC, serum iron, and folate and red cell folate) and because there is the risk of gastrointestinal lymphoma. The itch and rash responds to dapsone within a few days. A strictly controlled gluten-free diet may mean that dapsone can be avoided.

Linear IgA disease

Linear IgA disease is an uncommon bullous eruption that presents acutely with widespread tense blisters of the skin and erosions and ulcers of the mucosae. Many cases are attributed to drugs, especially antibiotics (Figs 8.54–8.56). The name is derived from the characteristic deposition of IgA in a linear band at the dermo-epidermal junction on direct immunofluorescence. Management is broadly as for bullous pemphigoid.

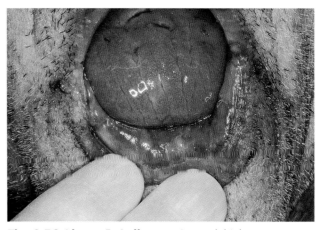

Fig. 8.56 Linear IgA disease. Lower labial mucosa. Same case as Fig. 8.54.

153

NECROBIOSIS

Two cases have been reported of erythematous ulcerated lesions of the glans penis due to necrobiosis. One patient was diabetic and had lesions on the legs – the classical and common presentation of this common dermatosis (Lecroq et al 1984) – the other had penile lesions only and was cured with oral pentoxifylline (Espana et al 1994).

PYODERMA GANGRENOSUM

There are a handful of case reports of pyoderma gangrenosum involving the penis in adults (**Figs 8.57, 8.58**). It has also occurred on the scrotum (Bigler et al 1995) manifesting in one case as the vegetative variant, superficial granulomatous pyoderma (Calikoglu 2000).

It may occur as a Koebner phenomenon following local trauma such as urological surgery (Farrell et al 1998). One of the penis cases was associated with ulcerative colitis (Sanusi et al 1982) and another with chronic lymphocytic leukemia (Wahba & Cohen 1979), where the role of herpes simplex (HSV 2) isolated from the multifocal ulceration was questionable, but the others occurred without any associated disease (Harto et al 1985; Sanchez et al 1997; Gungör et al 1999; Park et al 2000). One case was initially misdiagnosed as Fournier's gangrene (Baskin et al 1990).

Pyoderma gangrenosum is also rare in pediatric practice but a predilection for the anogenital region (**Figs 8.59, 8.60**), as well as the head and face, in children has been proposed (Graham et al 1994).

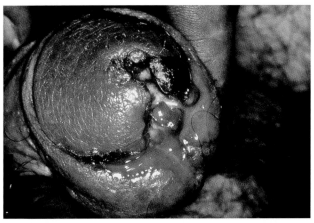

Fig. 8.57 Pyoderma gangrenosum. Penis. (Courtesy of Dr Martin Black, London, UK. Reproduced by kind permission of Blackwell Science Ltd from Farrell AM et al. Pyoderma gangrenosum of the penis. Br J Dermatol. 1998; 138(2): 337–40.)

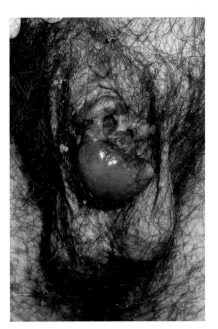

Fig. 8.58 Pyoderma gangrenosum. Penis. Despite healing following aggressive medical treatment, patient lost all ability to achieve an erection. (Reproduced by kind permission of Blackwell Science Ltd from Farrell AM et al. Pyoderma gangrenosum of the penis. Br J Dermatol. 1998; 138(2): 337–40.)

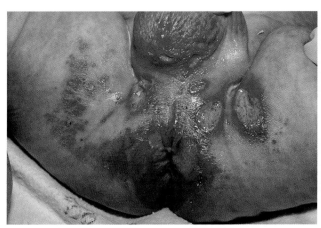

Fig. 8.59 Pyoderma gangrenosum. Anus, perineum, thighs, scrotum. Three weeks old. (Courtesy of Dr Nancy B Esterly, Milwaukee, Wisconsin, USA. Reprinted by permission of Blackwell Science Inc from Graham JA et al. Pyoderma gangrenosum in infants and children. Pediatr Dermatol. 1994; 11(1): 10–7.)

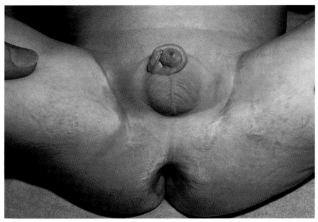

Fig. 8.60 Pyoderma gangrenosum. Anus, perineum, thighs, scrotum. 17 months old. Fully healed following treatment with intralesional steroid and oral prednisolone (four weeks). (Courtesy of Dr Nancy B Esterly, Milwaukee, Wisconsin, USA. Reprinted by permission of Blackwell Science Inc from Graham JA et al, Pyoderma gangrenosum in infants and children. Pediatr Dermatol. 1994; 11(1): 10–7.)

Pyoderma gangrenosum is a diagnosis made when other causes of purulent ulceration such as infection (sexually acquired and exotic), malignancy and artefact have been excluded.

Aggressive therapeutic measures are often required including high-dose oral corticosteroids or intravenous methylprednisolone. Cyclophosphamide has been reported to be effective in some cases (Crawford et al 1967; Baskin et al 1990). Minocycline (Berth-Jones et al 1989) and thalidomide (Venecie 1982; Munro & Cox 1988; Rustin et al 1990; Stirling 1998) may be beneficial in pyoderma gangrenosum unresponsive to corticosteroids and in pyoderma gangrenosum associated with Behçet's disease.

NECROTIZING VASCULITIS

Penoscrotal ulceration due to necrotizing vasculitis in association with Wegener's granulomatosus (Osada et al 1974; Matsuda et al 1976), systemic lupus erythematosus (Tripp et al 1995), systemic vasculitis (Koga et al 1996), polyarteritis nodosa (Downing & Black 1985, **Fig. 8.61**) and hereditary spherocytosis with recurrent vascular necrosis (Horner et al 1991) has been reported. Rubio et al (1999) describe a case of isolated penile ulceration due to a necrotizing vasculitis, with no evidence of systemic vasculitis, that responded to systemic steroids. Fournier's gangrene may show histological evidence of necrotizing vasculitis (Schultz et al 1995) and priapism (see page 225) has been documented as a manifestation of isolated genital vasculitis (Lakhanpal et al 1991).

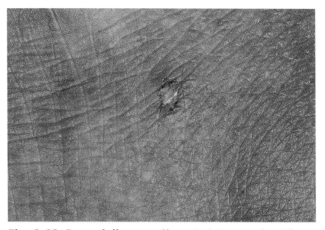

Fig. 8.62 Degos' disease. Characteristic macule with erythematous halo and porcelain-white central scar.

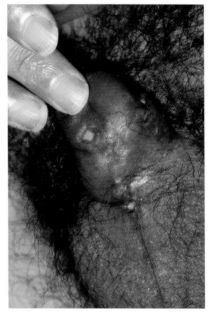

Fig. 8.63 Degos' disease. Ventral shaft, penis. Ulceration. (Courtesy of Dr Allan Highet, York, UK.)

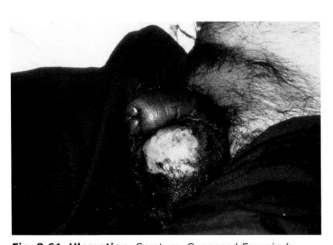

Fig. 8.61 Ulceration. Scrotum. Supposed Fournier's gangrene caused by polyarteritis nodosa. (Courtesy of Mr Richard Downing, Worcester, UK. Reproduced by kind permission of Blackwell Science Ltd from Downing R, Black J. Polyarteritis nodosa: an unrecognised cause of Fournier's gangrene. Br J Urol. 1985; 57(3): 355–6.)

DEGOS' MALIGNANT ATROPHIC PAPULOSIS

Degos' disease is a very rare lymphocyte-mediated obliterative vasculopathy with the potential for devastating multisystem involvement. Characteristic skin lesions occur (**Fig. 8.62**). Thomson & Highet (2000) describe a case of a 47-year-old man who presented to a genitourinary department with penile ulceration (**Fig. 8.63**). This preceded the observation of the rash and eventual fatal involvement of other organs, despite aggressive treatment.

CALCIPHYLAXIS

Calciphylaxis is a rare but serious complication of chronic renal failure (Hafner et al 1998). Extending ischemic gangrenous necrosis affects acral tissues, fingers and toes, and sometimes the thighs and buttocks.

There may be extensive metastatic calcification of soft tissues. The pathogenesis is ill understood but histology shows subcutaneous arteriolar medial calcification and intimal hyperplasia and patients often have an elevated calcium-phosphate product and parathormone level. The genitals can be the seat of involvement (Ivker et al 1995; Siami & Siami 1999; Boccaletti et al 2000).

HYPEREOSINOPHILIC SYNDROME

The hypereosinophilic syndrome (Morgan et al 1994) encompasses a wide spectrum of acute, chronic, benign and fatal conditions characterized by persistent blood eosinophilia of more than $1.5 \times 10^9/l$ with infiltration of the heart, lymph nodes, bone marrow and, in up to 50% cases, the skin (orogenital ulceration, erythroderma and urticaria. It may occur in HIV infection.

BULLOUS IMPETIGO

Bullous impetigo is a manifestation of streptococcal (sometimes staphylococcal) cutaneous infection and is common in children. The disease may be localized to the face (sometimes the genitocrural area). Blisters, erosions (**Fig. 8.49**), and golden-yellow crusts and swabs are seen. Oral and topical antibiotics are prescribed.

ECTHYMA GANGRENOSUM

This is usually due to pseudomonas septicemia (Bodey et al 1983; Greene et al 1984). A red macule rapidly progressing to a blue bulla will rupture to form a necrotic ulcer with a central erythematous halo or painful, tense grouped vesicles, which rapidly become necrotic and form ulcers with black necrotic eschars, are the clinical characteristics of ecthyma gangrenosum. It occurs in immunosuppressed, ill patients including children with leukemia, cancer or AIDS (Greene et al 1984; Smith et al 1995) and has a predilection for the acral and anogenital extremities and may affect the penis in isolation leading to gangrene (Rabinowitz & Lewin 1980). The prognosis is poor. A case affecting the penis has been reported (**Fig. 8.64**) that was probably caused by direct arterial septic embolization from femoral heroin injection (Cunningham & Persky 1989). In the acute presentation herpes simplex was misdiagnosed.

Patients with hematological malignancy may develop the disease without evidence of pseudomonas septicemia and in these cases the prognosis is better (Huminer et al 1987; Wolf et al 1989). Perianal infiltration, ulceration or abscess occurs in 5% of hematological malignancy and rarely may be the presenting feature (Vanheuverzwyn et al 1980).

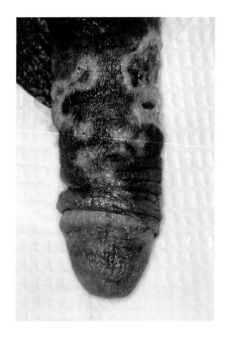

Fig. 8.64 Ecthyma gangrenosum. Penis. Pseudomonas. Due to embolic dissemination following femoral heroin injection. (Courtesy of Dr David Cunningham, Ocala, Florida, USA and reprinted with permission from Cunningham DL, Persky L. Penile ecthyma gangrenosum. Complication of drug addiction. Urology. 1989; 34(2): 109–10. Elsevier Science Inc.)

Sick patients with leukemia may develop a necrotizing anorectal ulcer due to pseudomonas. The presentation is with severe anal pain, anorectal ulceration, local pseudomonas infection, pseudomonas septicemia (including other cutaneous manifestations such as ecthyma gangrenosum), with a very high mortality. Anorectal ulceration may be the portal of entry of the pseudomonas infection or a consequence of it (Givler 1969).

CHANCROID

This sexually transmitted disease begins as a red vesicle or papule (about 3–6 days after inoculation) on the external genitalia (especially where traumatized frictionally during sex) but this rapidly ulcerates with pain. There may be several lesions that become confluent to form serpiginous and herpetiform patterns. After about a week the inguinal glands enlarge painfully (buboes) and they may fistulate (**Fig. 8.65**).

The causative organism is *Haemophilus ducreyi*. However, the bubo, once developed progresses despite the administration of effective anti-*H. ducreyi* drugs: it is possible that other bacteria, e.g. the anaerobes *B. melaninogenicus* and *fragilis*, are involved (Kumar et al 1991). Chancroid is rare but resurgent in the developed world. In warmer Third World areas where hygiene is poor and sexually transmitted diseases are not well controlled it is the most prevalent cause of genital ulceration. Like all forms of genital ulceration it is a risk factor for the transmission of HIV.

Diagnosis is confirmed by smear and staining of a swab from the primary ulcer or discharging bubo. Treat-

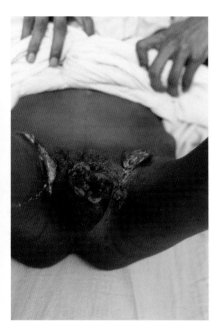

Fig. 8.65 Chancroid. Groins and penis. Confluent phagedenic penile ulceration and inguinal lymphadenopathic fistulation. (Courtesy of Prof. Bhushan Kumar, Chandigarh, India.)

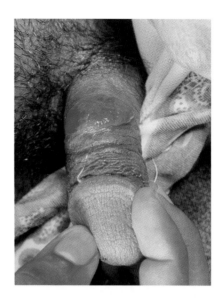

Fig. 8.66 Granuloma inguinale. Dorsal shaft, penis. Painless large, well-demarcated ulcer. (Courtesy of Dr Paramoo Sugathan, Kerala, India.)

ment is currently with azithromycin ceftriaxone, ciprofloxacin or erythromycin. Antibiotic resistance has been a problem in the past. Suppurative nodes should be incised, circumcision may be necessary. Relapse (probably due to reinjection) occurs in 5% (Lautenschlager & Eichmann 2003).

DONOVANOSIS (GRANULOMA INGUINALE)

Granuloma inguinale is probably a sexually transmitted disease. It begins (about 2–4 weeks after exposure) as a painless button-like papule, which ulcerates over a few days to give a large, well-demarcated, painless ulcer of the distal penis (**Figs 8.66, 8.67**). Spread of the ulcer occurs chronically, often centrifugally (ulcerovegative variant). Centripetal nodular (subcutaneous) extension also occurs into the inguinal and perineal region (nodular variant) with eventual ulceration. In the groins this may be mistaken for lymphadenopathy (pseudo bubo). Primary perianal disease may occur in the ano-receptive homosexual (Goldberg & Bernstein 1964).

Although lymph gland enlargement is rare lymphatic obstruction occurs in chronic cases causing lymph-oedema (even elephantiasis of the penis and scrotum). Other clinical forms of chronic disease include grossly vegetating or verrucous masses (hypertrophic form) and slowly spreading irregular scarring (cicatricial form). The clinical manifestations of granuloma inguinale are given in Table 8.14.

The differential diagnosis of lymphoedema and of diffuse indurated inflammatory nodules in the ano-genital region is given in **Tables 9.5–9.9** in Chapter 9 and **Table 10.1** in Chapter 10, respectively.

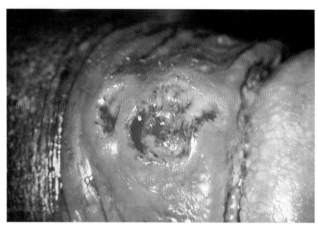

Fig. 8.67 Granuloma inguinale. Sub-coronal lateral penile shaft. Ulcer. (Courtesy of Dr Peter Copeman, London, UK.)

Table 8.14 Clinical forms of granuloma inguinale

Button nodule

Primary ulcer

Ulcerovegative (spreading ulcers)

Nodular (spreading infiltrated subcutaneous disease)

Cicatricial

Hypertrophic (vegetative masses)

Lymphoedema/elephantiasis

Donovanosis is thus a slowly progressive infiltrative and ulcerative disease of the anogenitalia and the important differential diagnosis includes cancer and pyoderma gangrenosum (as well as other sexually transmitted diseases) but may include the causes of swelling (idiopathic penile edema, filariasis), diffuse infiltrated nodular disease (hidradenitis, cutaneous tuberculosis, actinomycosis) and verrucous masses (verrucous carcinoma, Buschke-Lowenstein tumor).

Calymmatobacterium granulomatis is the pathogenic micro-organism. It is prevalent in tropical and subtropical areas and infection is a risk factor for HIV dissemination. The diagnosis is made by staining a smear from the active edge of an ulcer to demonstrate the pathogen.

Management depends upon effective systemic antibiotic treatment, e.g. azithromycin or ciprofloxacin (Richens 1999).

LYMPHOGRANULOMA VENEREUM

This sexually transmitted disease may present as a painless papule or ulcer, sometimes unnoticed, anywhere on the anogenitalia about 1–2 weeks after exposure. This lesion usually heals spontaneously but may be herpetiform.

The more common presentation is of unilateral or bilateral painful inguinal lymphadenopathy about three or four weeks later. A palpable groove in the inguinal adenopathic mass is described due to separation of confluent matted nodes by the inguinal ligament. The lymphadenitis can also cause a palpable cord-like lesion on the penis, proctitis, wart-like lymphatic hyperplasia (lymphorrhoids) of the perineum. The lymphatics may ulcerate at any site and there can be anogenital abscesses and fistulae and gross penile scarring. Sometimes these syndrome complexes are called the inguinal or anogenitorectal syndromes and have as their causes any chronic infection or infiltration of the pelvic nodes. Lymphatic obstruction can cause genital elephantiasis (**Fig. 8.68**).

Lymphogranuloma venereum is caused by *Chlamydia trachomatis* (of which there are several serotypes). It is endemic in tropical and subtropical areas. Diagnosis is achieved by demonstrating intracellular inclusions in stained lesional smears or transfected cells in tissue culture.

Treatment is with anti-chlamydial antibiotics such as a tetracycline or a macrolide.

FOURNIER'S GANGRENE

In 1883 the Parisian dermatologist Alfred Fournier described five cases of spontaneous genital gangrene and ulceration but Baurienne (1764) probably reported this condition first. Since then several hundred other case reports have appeared in the literature with the elucidation of the principal predisposing factors and the identification of the clostridial (gas gangrene) and non-clostridial causative micro-organisms important in the pathogenesis (Rosenberg et al 1978; Biswas et al 1979; Bubrick & Hitchcock 1979; Jones et al 1979; Nickel & Morales 1983; Spirnak et al 1984; Enriquez et al 1987; Smith et al 1998).

Patients present with systemic upset, painful erythematous swelling of the genital, perianal or lower abdominal skin and may be in urinary retention. An 'ominous' black spot may appear on the scrotum (Bubrick & Hitchcock 1979). Rapid necrosis of skin and deeper tissues supervenes (**Figs 8.69–8.71**) and death ensues (the mortality may be higher than 50%) unless diagnosis is prompt and radical management instituted. There is gross systemic toxicity and no suppuration. In its clinical picture it overlaps with necrotizing fasciitis and Meleney's gangrene (Meleney 1924) of other sites. In children there may not be systemic toxicity (Adams et al 1990).

Risk factors (Flanigan et al 1978; Hughes-Davies et al 1991) are debilitation, alcoholism, diabetes, colorectal

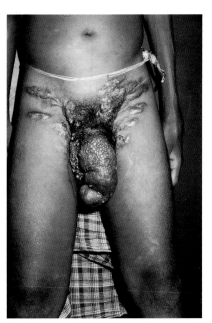

Fig. 8.68 Lymphogranuloma venereum. Groins and penis. Destroyed lymph glands and penile elephantiasis – saxophone penis.(Courtesy of Prof. Bhushan Kumar, Chandigarh, India.)

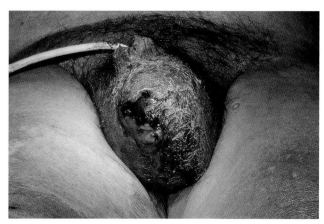

Fig. 8.69 Fournier's gangrene. Scrotum. Diffuse hemorrhagic necrotizing ulceration. Note gross preputial edema.

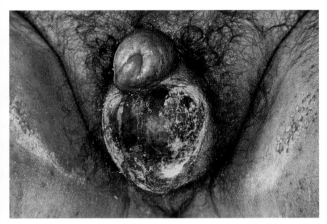

Fig. 8.70 Fournier's gangrene. Scrotum. (Courtesy of Dr Erwin Schultz, Erlangen, Germany and reproduced by kind permission of Blackwell Science Ltd from Schultz ES et al. Systemic corticosteroids are important in the treatment of Fournier's gangrene: a case report. Br J Dermatol. 1995; 133(4): 633–5.)

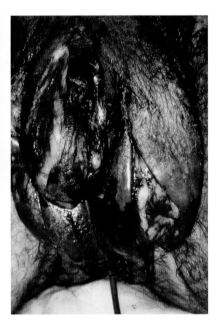

Fig. 8.71 Fournier's gangrene. Penis and scrotum. Severe necrosis and ulceration. (Courtesy of Prof. Jan der Meer, Leeuwarden, Netherlands.)

Table 8.15 Risk factors for Fournier's gangrene
Diabetes mellitus
Alcoholism
Anogenital infection
Chemotherapy
HIV
Post-instrumentation
Post-operative (urological and colorectal)
Heroin addiction
Trauma
Unconventional sexual practices

Table 8.16 Differential diagnosis of Fournier's gangrene
Trauma
Herpes simplex
Cellulitis (streptococcal, staphylococcal)
Streptococcal necrotizing fasciitis
Gonococcal balanitis and edema
Ecthyma gangrenosum
Allergic vasculitis
Polyarteritis nodosa
Migratory necrolytic erythema
Vascular occlusion syndromes
Warfarin necrosis

disease and surgery, anogenital infection, chemotherapy, granulocytopenia, HIV (Murphy et al 1991), urological disease, instrumentation and surgery; including vasectomy (Chantarasak & Basu 1988) and especially in 'at risk' patients (e.g. the immunocompromised, such as post-transplant patients, Walther et al 1987), heroin addiction, trauma and sexual perversion (Table 8.15).

The process probably begins with appendageal or urethral infection and polybacterial infection develops. Most of the organisms isolated from cases prove to be resident urethral or lower gastrointestinal flora and most patients have mixed infections. What then follows is a necrotizing vasculitis (see page 155), perhaps exotoxin-mediated, affecting skin, subcutis, fascia and muscle – the human counterpart of the local Shwartzman phenomenon (van der Meer et al 1990; van der Meer & de Jong 1992; Schultz 1995). In children the most com-

monly isolated pathogens are staphylococci and streptococci (Adams et al 1990). Radiological studies may show soft tissue gas (Fisher et al 1979).

The differential diagnosis (Table 8.16) includes: cellulitis (streptococcal, staphlyococcal), acute herpes simplex, streptococcal necrotizing fasciitis, gonococcal balanitis and edema, ecthyma, allergic vasculitis, migratory necrolytic erythema (see Fig. 6.203), diabetic small vessel disease (Frydenburg 1988), secondary hyperparathyroidism in chronic renal failure (Lowe & Brendler 1984), vascular occlusion syndromes and warfarin necrosis.

A general approach to the management of genital skin loss has been articulated by Wessells (1999) who acknowledged that Fournier's gangrene is the most common and morbid cause. If the clinical diagnosis of Fournier's gangrene is entertained then drastic emergency management is required. Surgical, microbiological and intensivist assistance are required.

Radical surgical debridement of all affected tissue is undertaken and broad therapy systemic antibiotic therapy initiated. One paper has advocated limited debridement with radical drainage (Kearney & Carling 1983). If the patient survives then plastic surgical repair can be undertaken. Hyperbaric oxygen treatment has been advocated (Schweigel et al 1973; Bubrick & Hitchcock 1979; Radaelli et al 1987; Chantarasak & Basu 1988), as has high-dose systemic corticosteroid treatment (van der Meer 1990; Schultz et al 1995). Children can be treated with more conservative surgery and the mortality rate is lower (Sussman et al 1978; Adams et al 1990).

In adults the mortality is around 25% and is highest in disease of anorectal rather than urogenital origin reflecting a less typical presentation and longer delay in diagnosis (Enriquez et al 1987).

TUBERCULOSIS

Penile tuberculosis is extremely rare (Minkin et al 1972). Fournier described the first case in 1878. Primary penile ulceration (solitary and multiple) with or without inguinal lymphadenopathy due to sexual infection or contact with infected clothing may occur (Schnitzler 1972; Agarwalla et al 1980; Jaisankar et al 1994; Martinez et al 1994; Rossi et al 1999), or the ulceration (**Figs 8.72, 8.73**) may be secondary to tuberculosis elsewhere, for example, the lung (Burns & Sarkany 1976). A cold abscess of the corpus cavernosum presenting as erectile failure has been reported (Murali & Raja 1998).

Perianal tuberculosis (which is more common) presents as a large, painful ulcer. Sinus and fistula formation may

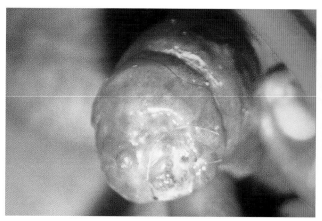

Fig. 8.73 Tuberculosis. Glans penis. Ulceration (Courtesy of Prof. Bhushan Kumar, Chandigarh, India.)

occur. Tuberculosis cutis orificialis is thought to arise from auto-inoculation of organisms contained in swallowed sputum from pulmonary lesions. It may occur in the immunocompromised and has been reported alongside Evans' syndrome – autoimmune hemolytic anemia and immune thrombocytopenia (Kim et al 1995).

Perineal scrofuloderma (secondary skin involvement from underlying lymph node disease) may cause diagnostic confusion (Polakova 1993).

Tuberculides are eruptions that are thought to result from hematogenous dissemination of relatively small numbers of organisms, the signs being due to local granulomatous hypersensitivity to the bacilli, which cannot usually be cultured. The clinical manifestations include superficial ulcers and/or crops of chronic or recurrent, discrete, dusky red, lichenoid or granulomatous papules with crusting, ulceration and scarring of elbows, knees, legs, hands and feet, face and ears, and buttocks and penis (**Figs 8.74, 8.75**). Cases where the penis alone was

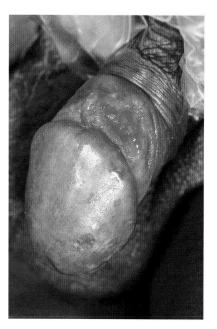

Fig. 8.72 Tuberculous ulceration. Penis distal, lateral shaft. British Indian immigrant. (Courtesy of Dr Tony Burns, Leicester, UK, and Dr Imrich Sarkany, London, UK, and reprinted by kind permission of the Royal Society of Medicine Press Ltd from Burns DA, Sarkany I. Tuberculous ulceration of the penis. Proc R Soc Med. 1976; 69(12): 883–4.)

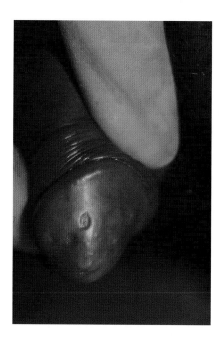

Fig. 8.74 Papulonecrotic tuberculide. Glans penis (Courtesy of Prof. Bhushan Kumar, Chandigarh, India.)

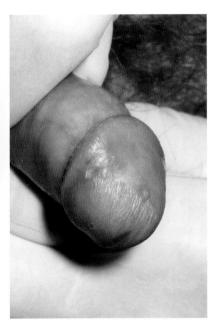

Fig. 8.75 Papulonecrotic tuberculide. Glans penis. Ulceration. Part of a generalized eruption in a patient with HIV.

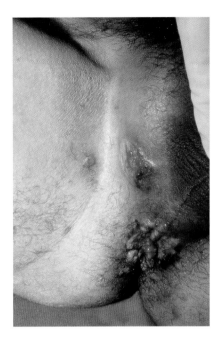

Fig. 8.76 Syphilis. Groins and anus. Primary inguinal chancre and perianal condyloma lata (Courtesy of Prof. Bhushan Kumar, Chandigarh, India.)

affected have been published (Nishigori et al 1986; Jeyakumar et al 1988; Kashima et al 1999).

Diagnosis is made on the basis of culture and histopathology. Pyoderma gangrenosum, Crohn's disease, hidradenitis, neoplasia, artefact, sexually transmitted diseases, amoebiasis and deep mucoses appear in the differential diagnosis (Betlloch et al 1994).

Treatment is by suitable combination chemotherapy. There may be a place for concomitant surgery for large ulcerative lesions (Kaufman & Silver 1954).

SYPHILIS

Syphilis was the name of a fabled shepherd, the subject of a 16th century Italian poem, who died of a disease new to Europe at that time. The causative organism is the spirochete *Treponema pallidum*. All types of syphilis can affect the external genitalia and anal region. If there is a primary presentation in syphilis (it is such an important disease because of the serious sequelae and the fact that the primary disease and secondary disease may go unnoticed and hence untreated) then the most common lesion is a genital chancre (**Fig. 8.76**).

The chancre can occur at any mucocutaneous site including the anorectum (Samenius 1966; Gluckman et al 1974; Drusin et al 1976) and mouth. Before the ulcer of the chancre develops, about 2–4 weeks after infection, a dusky red macule gives way to a button-like, firm dermal papule or nodule (of variable size) that then erodes after a few days. Neither morphological form is in itself painful. The norm is for there to be a solitary lesion but 'kiss' appearances are well recognized.

Slightly tender inguinal lymphadenopathy may appear after a week or two. A primary syphilitic balanitis – of Follmann (Lejman & Starzycki 1975) – is

probably more common than is appreciated. Rectal pain (due to secondary infection), discharge and bleeding, fissures (especially laterally) and fistulae should arouse suspicion of anorectal primary syphilis (Gluckman et al 1974; Bassi et al 1991). Syphilitic proctitis without detectable anal lesions does occur (Akdamar et al 1977). Without treatment a classical chancre will heal after one or two months without scarring.

If there is a secondary presentation of syphilis (again, the signs may go unremarked by the patient) then possibilities include (**Table 8.17**) a widespread rash (syphilide, see below), mucous patches or ulcers, condylomata lata, alopecia, lymphadenopathy or, very unusually, systemic symptoms, occurring 6–8 weeks

Table 8.17 Manifestations of secondary syphilis

Primary chancre still visible

Syphilides
    several morphological forms
    post-inflammatory hypopigmentation

Mucous patches

Mucous snail track ulcers

Diffuse alopecia

Condylomata lata

Lymphadenopathy

Constitutional symptoms due to systemic disease
    hepatitis
    arthritis
    bone pain
    deafness
    hoarseness

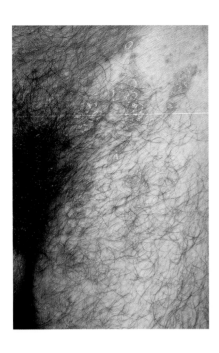

Fig. 8.77 Secondary syphilis. Groin. Part of a widespread papulosquamous eruption.

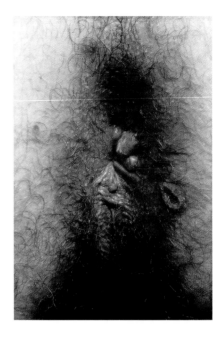

Fig. 8.78 Anus and perineum. Condyloma lata of secondary syphilis.

(sometimes much longer, even a year) after infection and due to bacteremic dissemination of the causative organism.

The syphilides are classified according to their morphology (hence roseolar, macular, papulosquamous (slightly scaly), pustular, ulceronecrotic (malignant) syphilides. They are all broadly characterized by being symmetrical (with a predilection for the palms and soles, Fig. 2.1o, see page 25) and widespread and having a coppery hue to their erythema (**Fig. 8.77**).

Mucous patches are well-defined, red, not particularly scaly lesions (although some will have a superficial, diphtheria-like gray surface membrane). Around the genitalia they may manifest as punched out, rather herpetiform lesions and in and around the mouth as snail track ulcers, so from a pedantic dermatological point of view 'patch' is not an ideal term for them.

Condylomata lata are moist, flesh-colored or brown, flat-topped, monomorphic papules that coalesce into verrucous clumps in the intertriginous sites so perianal and inguinal involvement is what is seen in the male (**Figs 8.76, 8.78**).

All of these secondary expressions of syphilis are infectious especially those that affect the mucosa and intertriginous sites (mucous patches and condylomata lata). They will heal spontaneously without scarring but there may be some post-inflammatory hyperpigmentation evident after a syphilide.

Latent syphilis may persist in an asymptomatic manner and some patients will die from other causes. This is probably much more common than it once was because now it is almost impossible to live anywhere on the planet without being treated at some stage, if not frequently, with antibiotics for some other bacterial infection. A large number of antibacterial agents have antiluetic potency.

The granulomatous gumma is the lesion of tertiary syphilis. It may affect the anogenital area as an ulcer, a white plaque or as an atrophic scar. Pseudo-chancre redux is rare but describes gummatous (tertiary stage) recurrence at the site of the primary chancre (Evans & Summerly 1964). A presentation as a red plaque on the penis has been described where the clinical differential diagnosis was considered to be fixed drug eruption, granuloma annulare, lichen planus and lymphocytoma cutis. Other cardiovascular, neurological and skeletal consequences are beyond the scope of this book.

Syphilis is endemic throughout the world. Although now much less common now than it was, even in homosexual men, from the point of view of the dermatologist, it should never be allowed to slip from the memory as a possible cause of oro-ano-genital ulceration, red scaly rashes, anogenital warts, hair loss, lymphadenopathy, leg ulcers, trophic foot ulcers and cryptic systemic disease.

Diagnosis is by dark-field examination of a smear from the chancre or secondary syphilitic lesion for the spirochete. Occasionally dermatologists will biopsy a cryptic rash and suspect syphilis if the inflammatory infiltrate is plasma cell rich. Histology is even more helpful in the rare circumstances where gummatous tertiary syphilis is on the cards and the inflammatory picture here is granulomatous.

Serological testing of blood (and sometimes cerebrospinal fluid) is crucial in most instances. It is as well to get expert assistance in interpretation if in doubt. Only about 60% of patients will have positive serology at the time of presentation with primary syphilis but nearly all should be positive when secondary syphilis occurs. The presentation of syphilis, hence its clinical diagnosis and the interpretation of serological testing, can be problematic in HIV infection (Gregory et al 1990).

The treponeme responds to penicillin but the evaluation and treatment should be discussed with an experienced specialist. As with other sexually transmitted diseases, the patient and partner(s) should be screened for concomitant venereal pathology.

NON-SYPHILITIC SPIROCHAETAL ULCERATIVE BALANOPOSTHITIS

This condition is recognized in the tropics and South Africa presenting as large, serpiginous, foul-smelling ulcers in uncircumcised men, associated in some with non-tender inguinal lymphadenopathy. Treatment is with penicillin or metronidazole (Piot et al 1986).

YAWS

Yaws is a treponemal disease of the rural tropics. It is a non-venereally transmitted, potentially crippling contagion caused by *Treponema pallidum* subspecies *pertenue*. There is an early stage, characterized by infectious skin lesions and a late stage, of which the hallmark is destructive involvement of skin, bone and joints.

After the primary cutaneous lesion of yaws, the mother yaw (2–6 months), heals or prior to healing, daughter yaws appear, initially as papules but rapidly becoming ulcerated, crusted plaques. These have a predilection for periorificial sites on the face and around the perineum (as well as the palms and soles).

An ulcerated, crusted and papillomatous lesion has been reported on the prepuce (**Fig. 8.79**) of a young Indonesian boy (Engelkens et al 1990) as part of dis-

seminated early yaws with other skin lesions elsewhere. The lower limb is the common portal of entry for this tropical treponemal infection and the mother remembered a leg lesion three months previously. The genital lesion probably arose from autoinoculation. Diagnosis was achieved by dark-field demonstration of motile treponemes and positive serology. He was treated with a single dose of intramuscular penicillin. He was living in an endemic area and several family members were also infected.

HERPES SIMPLEX

Herpes simplex (Oates 1983) is an acute, sexually acquired anogenital affliction presenting with clusters of painful vesicles on an erythematous base within a week of exposure. There may be prodromal constitutional and local symptoms. The ulcers rapidly break down to leave erosions or ulcers (**Figs 8.80–8.83**, see also Fig. 2.11) and secondary infection occurs readily, sometimes

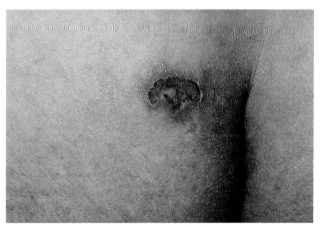

Fig. 8.80 Herpes simplex. Buttock.

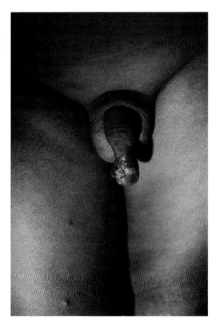

Fig. 8.79 Disseminated early yaws. Prepuce, Indonesian boy aged 3 years. Presented with this and similar disseminated skin lesions. (Courtesy of Dr Herman Jan Engelkens, Rotterdam, Holland. Reprinted by permission of Blackwell Science Inc from Engelkens HJ et al. Disseminated early yaws: report of a child with a remarkable genital lesion mimicking venereal syphilis. Pediatr Dermatol. 1990; 7: 60–2.)

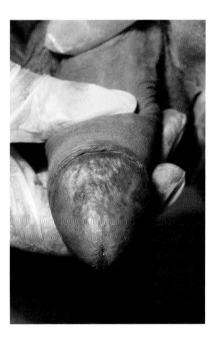

Fig. 8.81 Herpes simplex. Glans penis.

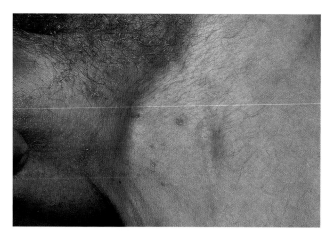

Fig. 8.82 **Herpes simplex.** Groin.

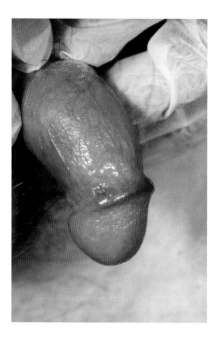

Fig. 8.83
Herpes simplex.
Coronal sulcus.

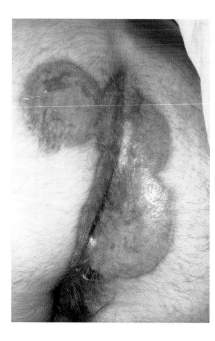

Fig. 8.84
**Chronic herpes
simplex.**
Buttocks and
perianal skin. HIV
pre-HAART era.

In HIV the problem can be particularly serious and chronic, especially in the perianal area (**Fig. 8.84**, Denis et al 1992; Bunker 1996; Yuhan et al 1998; Bunker & Staughton 2002). This was a big management challenge before the advent of antiviral therapy with AZT and its eventual successor drugs.

More recently, a phenomenon of chronic recrudescence, erosive and verrucous herpes (**Figs 8.85–8.87**) in patients with HIV, who were otherwise relatively successfully treated by highly active antiretroviral treatment with significant immuno-reconstitution, has been described (HAART) by my colleagues and me (Fox et al 1999). Treatment is difficult but the stratagem of circumcision, topical cidofovir and oral prednisolone proves successful in most cases (**Fig. 8.88**). Others have used topical imiquimod (Gilbert et al 2001).

HSV 2 causes most anogenital infections due to herpes simplex. Diagnosis is made by electron microscopy, cytology (Naib 1981), culture or viral antigen detection.

causing cellulitis. Dysuria, urinary retention (Oates & Greenhouse 1978) and lymphadenopathy may be found. Acute anal pain and ulceration may be the symptoms and signs in homosexuals (McMillan & Smith 1984).

Healing occurs spontaneously in about 5–10 days. Scarring and post-inflammatory hyperpigmentation are possibilities. Occasionally genital herpes may be acquired non-sexually, e.g. during contact sports like rugby football (Esteve et al 1998).

Recurrent disease affects many patients. Systemic prodromal symptoms or local paresthesia herald an attack, often following trauma, sex, or stress. The clinical features are as for the primary attack and often at the same site. The tendency is for the frequency and severity of recrudescences to become attenuated with time but many patients with recurrent herpes simplex have considerable physical and psychological morbidity. Herpes simplex, acute or recurrent, is a common cause of erythema multiforme.

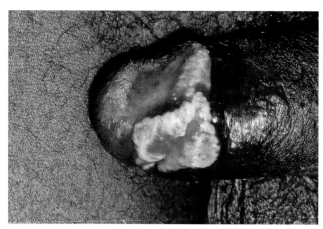

Fig. 8.85 **Chronic verrucous and erosive herpes simplex in HIV.** Glans penis.

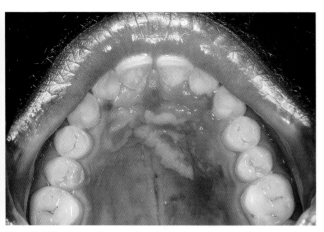

Fig. 8.86 Chronic erosive herpes simplex in HIV. Palate. Same case as Fig. 8.85.

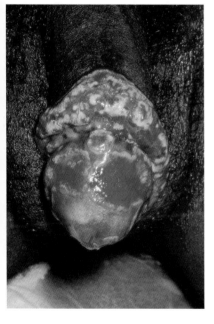

Fig. 8.87 Chronic verrucous and erosive herpes simplex in HIV. Glans penis.

Treatment consists of local toilet (potassium permanganate soaks), topical corticosteroid/antibiotic combination, systemic antibiotics and systemic antivirals. Aciclovir 200mg, five times daily for five days has been used for some years. Topical aciclovir is of limited clinical usefulness and confers no additional benefit when used concomitantly with oral acyclovir (Kinghorn et al 1986). Newer agents exist now and different drugs and regimens are under evaluation.

Recurrent attacks can be managed by early initiation of antiviral therapy at the first intimation of local or systemic prodromal symptoms or, if this does not improve the quality of life, long-term prophylactic antiviral treatment (Douglas et al 1986; Mindel et al 1984; Strauss et al 1984), for example, acyclovir 400mg bd. A role for oral isotretinoin in some recalcitrant cases has been proposed (Kanzler & Rasmussen 1988).

In HIV and AIDS aciclovir resistance (due to strains of the virus negative for thymidine kinase-required for acyclovir activation) may be overcome by treatment with intravenous trisodium phosphonoformate – foscarnet (Erlich et al 1989).

HERPES ZOSTER/SHINGLES

Sacral herpes zoster is relatively rare but can be associated with severe morbidity due to urinary symptoms (nocturia, dysuria, hesitancy), acute retention and constipation and fecal retention. Painful, grouped, crusting vesicopustular lesions may be found on the buttock (**Fig. 8.89**), in the perineum, on the scrotum and penis (**Fig. 8.90**), in the groins and on the upper thigh. Hospitalization, urological assessment, observation and possibly catheterization and sigmoidoscopy, and assisted fecal extraction are indicated (Fungelso et al 1973; Waugh 1974). Treatment should be with intravenous acyclovir.

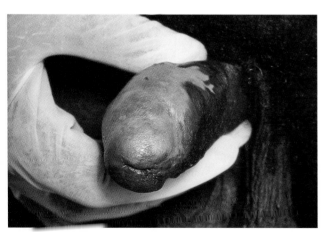

Fig. 8.88 Healed chronic herpes simplex. Glans and shaft penis. Post-inflammatory hypopigmentation. Same case as Fig. 8.85.

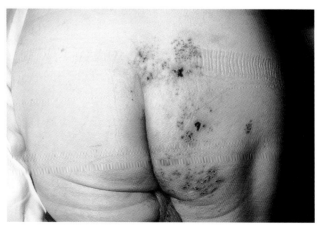

Fig. 8.89 Herpes zoster (shingles). Buttocks.

165

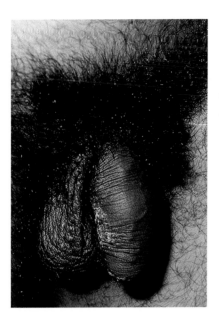

**Fig. 8.90
Herpes zoster.**
Shaft of penis
(Courtesy of Prof.
Bhushan Kumar,
Chandigarh,
India.)

Table 8.18 Causes of penile and scrotal ulcers in HIV infection

Aphthae

Pseudomonas

Syphilis

Chancroid

Herpes simplex

Penicilliosis

Amoebiasis

Fournier's gangrene

Squamous carcinoma

Kaposi's sarcoma

Drugs, e.g. foscarnet

HUMAN IMMUNODEFICIENCY VIRUS (HIV) INFECTION

Ulcerative anogenital disease is a risk factor for acquiring HIV (Stamm et al 1988) but anogenital ulceration may also be a consequence of HIV infection (Copé & Debou 1995; Yuhan et al 1998). **Tables 8.18** and **8.19** list the main causes. Infectious causes must always be considered, for example, due to pseudomonas (Berger et al 1995), Fournier's gangrene (Murphy et al 1991), syphilis, tuberculosis (see page 160) and atypical mycobacteria, herpes simplex (see page 163) and CMV (see page 165) and fungi (see page 168), e.g. penicilliosis (Chiewchanvit et al 1991; Wortman 1996). Intraepithelial and frank invasive squamous carcinoma should always enter the differential diagnosis, as should Kaposi's sarcoma and lymphoma (Puy-Montbrun et al 1992; Yuhan et al 1998). Therefore biopsy with special stains and culture is mandatory.

Other anogenital problems in HIV such as psoriasis, warts, herpes simplex, intraepithelial neoplasia, squamous carcinoma and Kaposi's sarcoma are discussed elsewhere.

Genital ulcers can occur in acute primary HIV infection (Hulsebosch et al 1990; Lapins et al 1996). Acute, erosive genitocrural intertrigo has been reported (Calikoglu et al 2001). It is believed that the majority of infections with HIV are clinically silent. However, received wisdom and experience suggests that 25–75% of patients may develop symptoms 2–6 weeks after exposure, accompanying seroconversion. Symptoms are often those of a non-specific viral infection, such as infectious mononucleosis (Gaines et al 1990).

Skin involvement occurs in up to 75% of those who manifest symptomatic seroconversion (Kinloch de Loes et al 1993). A symmetrical maculopapular erythematous exanthem, notably of face, palms and soles occurs. Pale pink macules and perifollicular erythematous papules

Table 8.19 Causes of anal ulceration in HIV

Idiopathic

Hemorrhoids

Fissures

Sepsis

Syphilis (chancre)

Herpes simplex

Cytomegalovirus

Kaposi's sarcoma

Non-Hodgkin's lymphoma

Squamous carcinoma

have been described (Alessi & Cusini 1995). Occasionally there may be vesicles, urticaria and alopecia. One-quarter of these patients will have painful oral ulceration and a few will develop genital ulceration (Kinloch de Loes et al 1993). Stevens-Johnson syndrome has been described (Mortier et al 1994). It has been suggested that the exanthem represents infection of cutaneous Langerhans cells and that the orogenital erosions or ulcers appear at sites of viral inoculation (Porras-Luque et al 1998).

Although idiopathic anogenital aphthous ulceration may occur in established HIV (Figs 8.14 & 8.15) and may be the most common cause of perianal ulceration (Yuhan et al 1998) this should be a diagnosis of exclusion: all HIV-associated anogenital ulcers should be biopsied and cultured to exclude infection and cancer (Denis et al 1992). Thalidomide can be useful, as in the treatment of oral ulceration (Stirling 1998; Bunker & Staughton 2002).

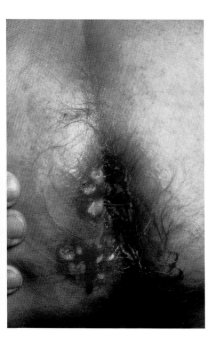

Fig. 8.91 Cytomegalovirus in HIV. Anus. Severe perianal ulceration. (Courtesy of Dr Nick Soter, New York, NY, USA.)

Foscarnet is a *cause* of genital ulceration in HIV (Evans & Grossman 1992; Gross & Dretler 1993).

Cytomegalovirus is a major cause of disease in AIDS and an independent predictor of death (Gallant et al 1992). Reactivation of CMV in HIV occurs with a CD4 count <50×10⁶/l. Despite the frequency of systemic disease, skin involvement with CMV is relatively uncommon in HIV but when CMV affects the skin the mortality is about 85% in six months (Lee 1989). Purpura, papules, nodules, verrucous plaques and ulcers, and nodular prurigo have been described (Chiewchanvit et al 1993). A CMV epididymitis has been reported (Randazzo et al 1986). The differential diagnosis of these clinical possibilities is broad. Herpes simplex and CMV skin involvement may be seen concurrently (Smith et al 1991) and concomitant CMV, M. tuberculosis and M. avium-intracellulare have been documented (Nunez et al 1997). Perianal ulceration can be severely disabling (**Fig. 8.91**) and recalcitrant to treatment and its diagnosis is not always straightforward (Yuhan et al 1998). Biopsy, with special stains for organisms and immunochemistry for viruses and with separate material sent for culture, is crucial (Cohen et al 1994; Nico et al 2000). CMV infection should be suspected histologically if dermal capillary neoangiogenesis, fibrinoid thrombi, necrotic endothelial cells, epidermal hyperplasia, acantholysis, and keratinocyte degeneration are seen. Keratinocytes and endothelial cells contain characteristic cytomegaloviral inclusions. Syringosquamous metaplasia has been observed (Chetty et al 1999; Dauden et al 2000). Immunohistochemistry, in situ hybridization and electron microscopy may be employed. Skin biopsy material can be cultured with human fibroblasts to demonstrate the cytopathic effect; the demonstration of a CMV viremia can be similarly achieved by the co-culturing of a patient's leucocytes (Toome et al 1991). Serological testing may be difficult

to interpret. Argument continues about true infection and latent infection. The differential diagnosis of perianal ulceration in HIV is as given above (Yuhan et al 1998), including chronic ulceration with herpes simplex (Fig. 8.84, page 164), with which CMV can co-occur.

Treatment and prophylaxis centers on immuno-reconstitution with HAART but a severe cutaneous ulcerative eruption has been reported after the initiation of HAART and possibly representing IRD (Qazi et al 2002). Intravenous foscarnet, ganciclovir and cidofovir are specific treatments (Charthaigh et al 1993; Moyle & Gazzard 2002). Mutations in the viral kinase allow the development of drug resistance. Other drugs are under evaluation.

LEISHMANIASIS

Cutaneous leishmaniasis can assault the genitalia (Cain et al 1994; Schubach et al 1998). As at other sites of bites by infected sand flies, painless papules or pustules progress to chronic ulceration (**Fig. 8.92**) of the penis or scrotum (Cabello et al 2002) without regional lymphadenopathy. An erythematous scaly plaque on the glans has been reported (Crunwald et al 1998).

The disease is due to one of several protozoal organisms and is endemic in the Middle East, Asia and South America. Disseminated leishmaniasis in HIV infection can involve the skin and genitalia, presenting with ulcers (Agostini et al 1998). Diagnosis depends on biopsy where there is granulomatous inflammation and necrosis and the 1–3μm Leishman-Donovan bodies can be found within macrophages and giant cells stained with hematoxylin and eosin (or Giemsa).

Treatment is controversial but the antimony derivative sodium stibogluconate intravenously is usually recommended. Oral ketoconazole or itraconazole is promising. Some lesions may heal spontaneously but with scarring.

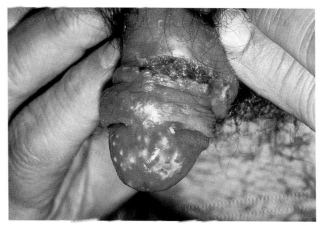

Fig. 8.92 Leishmaniasis. Glans penis and prepuce (Courtesy of Dr Mary Stone, Iowa City, IA, USA and reproduced from Cain C et al. Nonhealing genital ulcers. Cutaneous leishmaniasis. Arch Dermatol. 1994; 130: 1315–6.)

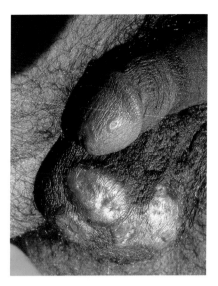

Fig. 8.93 Post-kala-azar dermal leishmaniasis. Scrotum and glans penis (Courtesy of Prof. Bhushan Kumar, Chandigarh, India.)

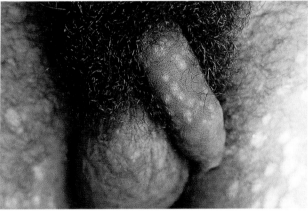

Fig. 8.94 Post-kala-azar dermal leishmaniasis. Thighs, scrotum and shaft of penis (Courtesy of Prof. Bhushan Kumar, Chandigarh, India.)

Post-kala-azar dermal leishmaniasis of the penis and scrotum is illustrated in **Figs 8.93, 8.94**.

DEEP FUNGAL INFECTIONS

Although histoplasmosis is a common cause of disseminated fungal infection in the United States, urological, cutaneous and genital infection is rare. Palmer et al (1942) published the first account of mucocutaneous (including anogenital ulceration) manifestations in the United States. Curtis & Cawley (1947) describe genital ulceration and inguinal adenopathy in association with disseminated extragenital lesions. Penile ulceration and abdominal pain are reported by Jayalakshmi et al (1990). Preminger et al (1993) document orogenital ulceration, inguinal and umbilical intertrigo and hepatosplenomegaly. All these patients were ill. Mankodi et al (1970) saw an otherwise well man with a small warty nodule on the glans penis. One ill patient with a penile ulcer transmitted the disease venereally to his wife (Sills et al 1973).

In blastomycosis the genitourinary tract is involved in 20–30% of cases (prostate and epididymis, Craig et al 1970). Involvement of the genital skin is rare but lesions of the prepuce and perianal skin have been recorded (Eickenberg et al 1975; English et al 1997). Paracoccidioidomycosis (South American blastomycosis) can be the cause of scrotal swelling and warty genital papules and nodules and erosions (Hay 1996; Severo et al 2000).

Actinomycosis can be responsible for multifocal perineal and buttock ulceration in G6PD deficiency (Millet et al 1982).

AMEBIASIS

Cooke & Rodriguez (1964) describe cases of amoebiasis presenting as balanitis. Painful swelling and ulceration are the principal clinical features but frequency, dysuria and retention may be complications. This must be one of the rarest manifestations of *Entamoeba histolytica* infection, so most case reports have come from tropical countries, particularly Papua New Guinea. Contamination from an amoebic bowel infection is thought to be the route of infection either by self-inoculation, or by heterosexual intercourse where the female partner has amoebic vaginitis, or by sodomy, which seems the most likely mechanism in Papua New Guinea. Diagnosis is by demonstration of the *E. histolytica* trophozoites in the mucopurulent discharge or in a biopsy or the circumcised prepuce, circumcision being necessary as part of the treatment.

Amoebiasis can be a cause of genital ulceration in which case underlying HIV infection should be suspected (Gbery et al 1999). It can be very destructive (Wynne 1980) and perianal and buttock ulceration may simulate malignancy (Venkataramaiah et al 1982).

Treatment is by debridement, circumcision and oral metronidazole.

LYMPHOMA AND LEUKEMIA

Ulceration of the penis due to leukemic infiltration secondary to chronic lymphocytic leukemia has been reported (Knight et al 1979; Gatto-Weis et al 2000). Scrotal ulceration (**Fig. 8.95**) due to leukemia cutis in acute myelogenous leukemia has also occurred (Zax et al 1989). Lymphoma may present with perianal ulceration abscess and suppuration (Steele et al 1985). Indeed, perianal infiltration, ulceration or abscess occurs in 5% of hematological malignancy (Vanheuverzwyn et al 1980). Pseudomonas infection and Fournier's gangrene are discussed on pages 156 and 158 respectively.

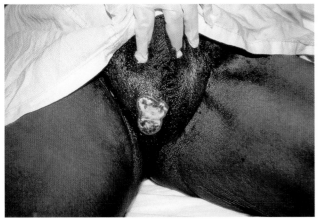

Fig. 8.95 Leukemia cutis. Scrotum. Ulceration. Acute myelogenous leukaemia. (Courtesy of Dr Jeffrey Callen, Louisville, KY, USA. Reprinted with permission from Zax RH et al. Leukemia cutis presenting as a scrotal ulcer. J Am Acad Dermatol. 1989; 21: 410–3.)

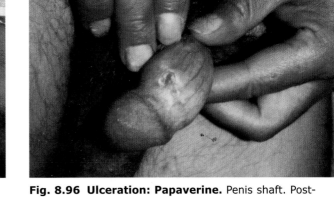

Fig. 8.96 Ulceration: Papaverine. Penis shaft. Post-self-administration for erectile impotence (Courtesy of Dr Eric Borgstrom, Stockholm, Sweden. Reprinted with permission from Borgstrom E. Penile ulcer as complication in self-induced papaverine erections. Urology. 1988; 32: 416–7. Elsevier Science Inc.)

Pyoderma gangrenosum can be associated with leukemia (see page 154).

DRUG REACTIONS

Fixed drug eruptions can ulcerate and are discussed on page 123. Ulceration has been reported due to papaverine (**Fig. 8.96**) when inadvertently injected subcutaneously for the treatment of erectile impotence (Borgstrom 1988).

Dequalinium is a topical antibacterial that was developed for the treatment of impetigo and moniliasis fifty years ago. It caused a necrotizing balanitis with ulceration when used for the treatment of balanitis in uncircumcised men (Coles & Wilkinson 1965).

Heparin and warfarin induced skin necrosis of the genitalia (Harmanyeri 1998) are discussed on page 141.

All-*trans*-retinoic acid has been reported to induce scrotal ulceration in a patient with acute promyelocytic leukemia (Esser et al 2000).

Foscarnet is a recognized cause of genital ulceration in HIV-infected patients (Evans & Grossman 1992; Gross & Dretler 1993; Moyle et al 1993).

Lisinopril has been reported to cause genital angio-edema (Henson et al 1999).

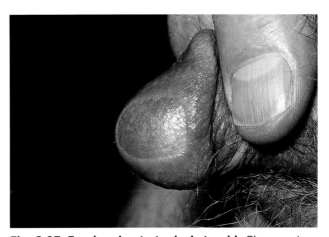

Fig. 8.97 Erosion due to topical steroid. Glans penis (Courtesy of Dr Peter Copeman, London, UK.)

The cutaneous side effects of topical steroids are well known. Striae are illustrated in Figs 4.9 and 4.10. Atrophy, erythema, telangiectasia and modification of cutaneous, bacterial, viral and fungal (Figs 6.21, 6.22) infections occur commonly. Erosion has been seen (**Fig. 8.97**).

Drugs can also cause pruritus and urticaria (see pages 38 and 41).

Palpable lesions–lumps and bumps

Inflamed as well as neoplastic tissue can present as *palpable lesions* (lumps and bumps) so in this chapter are considered the presentation of benign and malignant tumors of the anogenital area as well as papular, pustular, nodular, plaque and cystic inflammatory disease (**Tables 9.1–9.9**).

Papules (arbitrarily <1cm) are smaller than *nodules* (>1cm); *micropapules* (1–2mm) are smaller still. *Pustules* are papules containing pus. *Plaques* are large

---

Table 9.1 Causes of anogenital flesh-colored micropapules

Acrochordons (skin tags)

Angiofibroma (pearly penile papules)

Fordyce's (ectopic sebaceous glands) spots

Scrotal calcinosis

Lichen nitidus

Viral warts

Mollusca

Genital smooth muscle hamartoma

Table 9.2 Causes of anogenital red micropapules

Angioma

Angiokeratoma

Lichen nitidus

Inflamed viral warts

Inflamed mollusca

Angiokeratoma corporis diffusum

Carcinoma erysipeloides

Table 9.3 Causes of anogenital pustules

Behçet's disease

Folliculitis
    Staphylococcal/streptococcal
    Gonorrhea
    Tuberculide (acne scrofulosorum)
    Steroid acne
    Occlusional

Candidosis

Herpes simplex

Herpes zoster

---

and thick and flat topped: they may represent a confluence of papules (e.g. lichen planus, acanthosis nigricans; **Fig. 9.1**) or a single lesion (epidermal nevus (**Fig. 9.2**). *Cysts* are nodules with a central space containing fluid (e.g. pus) or tissue (e.g. keratin). Aggressive inflammation or malignant neoplasia leads to rupture of cysts and ulceration of nodules and plaques.

Lymphadenopathy is a cause of nodular subdermal swelling and inguinal lymphadenopathy has an important differential diagnosis (**Table 9.10**). Other causes of swelling in the groin are listed in **Table 9.11**.

MEDIAN RAPHE CYSTS

Cystic median raphe anomalies may remain clinically indistinct and asymptomatic or present as quiet, cystic or nodular and linear swellings of the ventral penis (**Fig. 9.3**), commonly near the glans, until adulthood when they are more likely to become traumatized or infected (e.g. with staphylococci, gonorrhea or trichomonas) and present as tender, erythematous, purulent nodules (**Fig. 9.4**; Neff 1936; Duperrat et al 1969; Sowmini et al 1972; Asarch et al 1979; Civatte et al 1982; Dupré et al 1982; Claudy et al 1991; Nagore et al 1998).

Table 9.4 Causes of anogenital flesh-colored papules

Common causes	Rare causes
Pearly penile papules (angiofibromas)	Median raphe cyst
Sebaceous hyperplasia	Mucoid cyst
Acrochordons (skin tags)	Tick bite/tick in situ
Scrotal calcinosis	Sclerosing lymphangitis
Viral warts	Lichen nitidus/lichen planus
Mollusca	Amyloid
Basal cell papilloma	Mucinous syringometaplasia
Epidermoid cyst	Demodicidosis
	Squamous hyperplasia
	Syringoma
	Leiomyoma
	Genital smooth muscle hamartoma
	Neurofibroma
	Lymphangioma circumscriptum
	Malignant melanoma
	Malignant schwannoma
	Lipoid proteinosis

Table 9.5 Causes of anogenital red papules

Common causes	Rare causes
Melanocytic nevus	Angioma
Angiokeratoma	Tick bite/tick in situ
Lichen planus	Insect bites
Inflamed viral warts	Granuloma annulare
Inflamed mollusca	Sarcoid
Scabies	Amyloid
Venous varicosities	Primary granuloma inguinale (Donovanosis)
Hemorrhoids	Primary lymphogranuloma venereum
Bowenoid papulosis	Tuberculide (lichen scrofulosorum)
	Leprosy
	Early chancre of primary syphilis
	Schistosomiasis
	Inflamed epidermoid cyst
	Syringoma
	Dermatofibroma
	Juvenile xanthogranuloma
	Pseudo Kaposi's sarcoma
	Kaposi's sarcoma
	Langerhans cell histiocytosis

Table 9.6 Causes of anogenital pigmented papules

Common causes	Rare causes
Melanocytic nevi	Angioma
Angiokeratoma	Tick bite/tick in situ
Skin tags (acrochordons)	Amyloid
Lichen planus	Superficial phaeohyphomycosis
Viral warts	Acanthosis nigricans
Basal cell papilloma	Nevus comedonicus
Venous varicosities	Syringomas
Bowenoid papulosis	Dermatofibroma
	Malignant melanoma
	Langerhans cell histiocytosis
	Xanthoma disseminatum
	Metastases

Table 9.7 Causes of anogenital plaques

Leprosy

Epidermal nevus

Basal cell papilloma

Verruciform xanthoma

Squamous hyperplasia

Squamous carcinoma

Buschke-Lowenstein tumor

Extramammary Paget's tumor/verrucous carcinoma

Table 9.8 Causes of exudative and verrucous anogenital plaques

Lichen sclerosus

Granuloma inguinale

Atypical mycobacterial infection

Secondary syphilis

Yaws

Confluent condylomata

Herpes simplex

Candidosis

Deep mycoses, e.g. blastomycosis

Halogenoderma

Bowenoid papulosis

Buschke-Lowenstein tumor/verrucous carcinoma

Xanthoma disseminatum

Table 9.9 Causes of anogenital cysts or nodules

Common causes	Rare causes	Rare causes (Cont'd)
Median raphe cysts	Segmental urethral hypospadias	Fibrous hamartoma of infancy
Scrotal calcinosis	Urethral/mucoid cysts	Leiomyoma
Sclerosing lymphangitis	Hernias and herniation	Neurofibroma
Hidradenitis suppurativa	Foreign body	Hemangioma
Crohn's disease	Lipogranuloma	Masson's tumor
Scabies	Keloid	Epithelioid hemangioma
Epidermoid cyst	Scrotal fat necrosis	Angiolymphoid hyperplasia with eosinophilia/Kimura's disease
Pilar cyst	Sarcoid	Lymphangioma circumscriptum
Squamous carcinoma	Amyloid	Solitary reticulohistiocytic granuloma
	Granuloma inguinale (Donovanosis)	Penile horn
	Bacillary angiomatosis	Keratoacanthoma
	Leprosy	Basal cell carcinoma
	Giant condyloma	Extramucosal anorectal carcinoma
	Histoplasmosis	Malignant melanoma
	Paracoccidioidomycosis (South American blastomycosis)	Merkel cell carcinoma
	Schistosomiasis	Malignant eccrine poroma
	Onchocerciasis	Sarcoma
	Benign appendageal tumors	Malignant schwannoma
	Myxoma	Kaposi's sarcoma
	Dermoid cyst	Chronic lymphocytic leukemia
	Granular cell tumor	Langerhans cell histiocytosis
	Giant cell fibroblastoma	Metastases
	Connective tissue nevus	

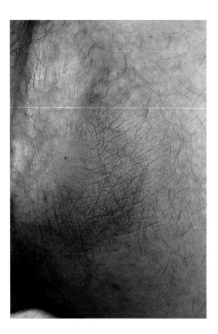

Fig. 9.1 Pseudo-acanthosis nigricans. Left groin. Brown, velvety, warty plaque. Associated with obesity and insulin resistance.

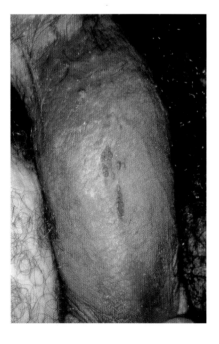

Fig. 9.2 Epidermal nevus. Dorsal shaft, penis. (Courtesy of Dr Nicholas Soter, New York, NY.)

Table 9.10 Causes of inguinal lymphadenopathy

Localized
  Infection
    Sexually transmitted diseases
      Chancroid
      Lymphogranuloma venereum
      Syphilis
      Herpes simplex
    Plague
    Tularemia
    Tuberculosis
  Angiolymphoid hyperplasia with eosinophilia/Kimura's disease
  Carcinoma
    Penis
    Scrotum
    Anus
    Rectum
    Lower limb
  Teratoma
  Seminoma
  Melanoma
    Anogenital
    Lower limb
  Lymphoma, e.g. Hodgkin's disease

Generalized
  Sarcoidosis
  Infection: tuberculosis, glandular fever, HIV, toxoplasmosis, brucellosis
  Carcinomatosis and melanomatosis
  Lymphoma
  Chronic lymphatic leukemia

Table 9.11 Causes of inguinal masses

Lymphadenopathy

Hernia-inguinal
  Femoral

Hydrocele

Spermatocele

Incompletely descended testis

Femoral aneurysm

Tumor (benign, malignant)

Oshin & Bowles (1962) speculate that congenital cysts of the scrotal and perineal raphe arise from rests formed during invagination and closure of the genital folds. Alternatively, they may represent outgrowths of epithelium split off from the raphe after closure of the genital folds. They are either dermoid or mucoid depending on their epithelial lining. Very rarely the basal epithelial lining of the cysts may contain melanocytes and endow the lesion with brown/black pigment (median raphe cysts with melanosis, Urahashi et al 2000). Serotonin containing cells have been found in several morphological types of median raphe cysts of the penis arguing for an endodermal urethral origin for these lesions (Fetissof et al 1985).

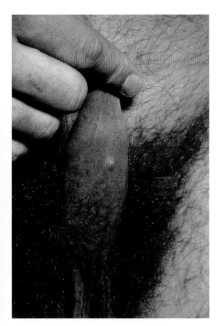

Fig. 9.3 Median raphe cyst.
Ventral mid-shaft penis.
Histologically the cyst was lined by pseudo-stratified columnar epithelium.

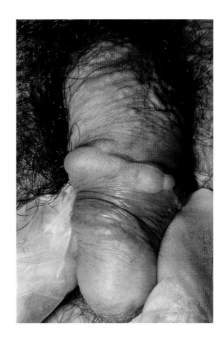

Fig. 9.5 Cyst.
Dorsal shaft penis. Precise nature of cyst not established as patient lost to follow-up.

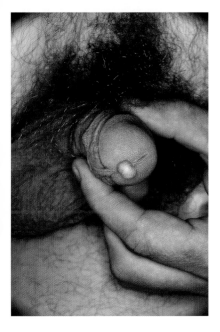

Fig. 9.4 Median raphe cyst.
Glans penis. Translucent cystic swelling.
(Courtesy of Dr Richard Asarch, Grand Rapids, MI, USA.)

urethral meatus to the anus and present at any age in life. The assessment of such cysts should involve the exclusion of secondary infection, for example gonorrhea. They are treated by surgical excision.

FOREIGN BODY

The circumstances surrounding self-instrumentation of the external genitalia may be categorized as autoerotic, psychiatric, therapeutic (relief of itch (Franzblau 1973; Al-Durazi et al 1992), aiding voiding, cleaning) or accidental (Aliabadi et al 1985). Complications include frequency, hematuria, abscess, retention, fistulae and calculi.

The diagnosis is made by palpation and radiography. Endoscopic removal is usually possible for foreign bodies below the urogenital diaphragm.

Foreign bodies are occasionally introduced into the rectum (**Fig. 9.6**).

Glass beads, pieces of plastic or small, smooth stones may be introduced into the skin of the penis for erotic reasons. However, this can cause clinical and radiographic confusion. If oil, petroleum jelly or silicon (**Fig. 9.7**) are used they can elicit a paraffinoma, silicone granuloma or (sclerosing) lipogranuloma (see below).

In the Philipines the practice is called 'bulleetus', in Sumatra 'persimbraon' and in Korea 'chagan ball'. In Thailand it is called 'mukhsa' or 'tancho' (after a Japanese hair pomade the glass container of which is melted down and fashioned into glass balls that are then inserted subcutaneously in the penile shaft). The insertion of real pearls – 'papular pearly penile pearls' – has been reported (**Fig. 9.8**) (George 1989). These practices are believed to have started in the Far East after the Second World War.

MUCOID CYSTS

These are rare lesions that present as small flesh-colored, mobile papules (2mm) to nodules (25mm), usually easily determined to be cystic on clinical grounds (**Fig. 9.5**, see also Figs 1.61, 2.14). They do not have a punctum. Either they are asymptomatic or they become infected or interfere with coitus. They have usually been present from birth or childhood and are found on the glans or foreskin. The histological features suggest that they arise from ectopic urethral tissue during embryological development (Cole & Helwig 1976).

The occurrence of a ventral cystic, often translucent, lesion of the penis should arouse the suspicion of this diagnosis (Asarch et al 1979). They are common near the glans penis but may occur anywhere from the

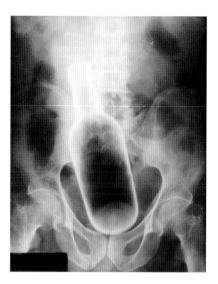

Fig. 9.6 Foreign body, rectum. Plain abdominal radiogram. (Courtesy of Prof. Bhushan Kumar, Chandigarh, India.)

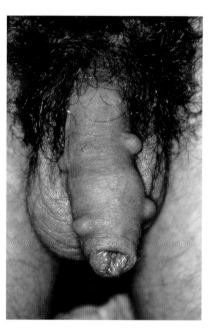

Fig. 9.7 Artificial penile nodules. Penis shaft. This patient also had secondary syphilis. (Courtesy of Dr Peter Wolf, Graz, Austria.)

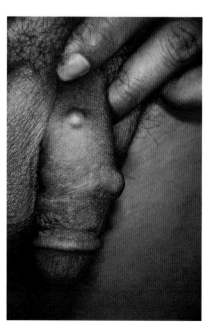

Fig. 9.8 Papular pearly penile pearls, 'mukhsa'. Dorsal shaft penis. Thai adult. Real pearls implanted. (Courtesy of Dr William M George, Doha, Qatar. Reproduced with permission from George WM. Papular pearly penile pearls. J Am Acad Dermatol. 1989; 20: 852.)

LIPOGRANULOMA

Mineral oil, petroleum jelly and silicon introduced into the genital skin can elicit lipogranuloma (Datta & Kern 1973; Sundaravej & Suchato 1974; Nitidanhaprabhas 1975; Stewart et al 1979; Cohen & Kim 1982; Gilmore et al 1983; Du 1984; Lim et al 1986; Sugathan 1987; Coldiron & Jacobson 1988; Wolf & Kerl 1991; Santucci et al 2000).

One patient presented with a nodule at the base of the penis, which rapidly became more generally uncomfortable and swollen (**Fig. 9.9**). Two months previously he said he had dressed a laceration of the penis with Johnson's Baby Oil ®. Surgical extirpation of the sclerosising lipogranuloma (**Figs 9.10, 9.11**) and plastic repair was necessary. The presence of a paraffin hydrocarbon in the tissue identical to a constituent of the oil was confirmed (Armstrong & Hackett 1981). A

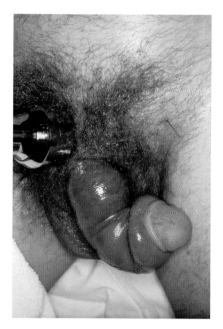

Fig. 9.9 Lipogranuloma. Penis. (Courtesy of Dr Lance Armstrong, Rotorua, New Zealand.)

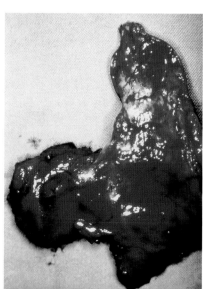

Fig. 9.10 Lipogranuloma. Penis. Surgical specimen. (Courtesy of Dr Lance Armstrong, Rotorua, New Zealand.)

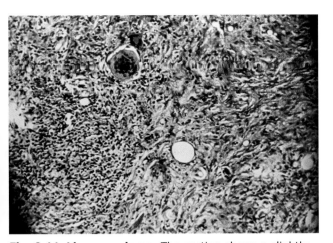

Fig. 9.11 Lipogranuloma. The section shows a slightly fibrotic lesion in which there is dense chronic inflammation, occasional multinucleated giant cells (of foreign body and of Touton type) and in the center of the picture some lipid type vacuoles. (Courtesy of Dr Lance Armstrong, Rotorua, New Zealand.)

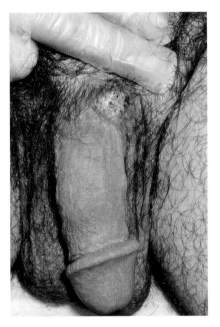

Fig. 9.12 Foreign body granuloma. Base of penis. Granulomatous nodule and ulceration. The patient had ground up acyclovir tablets, dissolved them in hydrogen peroxide solution and injected the solution to try to cure chronic recurrent genital herpes simplex (Courtesy of Dr Richard Staughton, London, UK.)

similar case due to topical vitamin E application has been reported (Foucar et al 1983). The patient illustrated in **Fig. 9.12** prepared a solution of acyclovir from grinding up the tablets he had been prescribed for chronic recurrent genital herpes simplex and dissolving them in hydrogen peroxide solution which he then injected into the root of his penis (Porter et al 1999).

Other cases of genital lipogranuloma have been described and it is likely that most are self-induced, either to create testicular prostheses or to increase penile size, enhance sexual pleasure, mutilate or malinger (Oertel & Johnson 1977; Coldiron & Jacobson 1988), although some may be accidental. One patient injected his penis with an industrial high-pressure pneumatic grease gun (Kalsi et al 2002).

Endogenous fat liberation is a possible mechanism (Carlson 1968) and idiopathic cases have been published (Foucar et al 1983; Golomb et al 1992) including predominantly from Japan (Tomioka et al 1987; Yoshida et al 1987; Iwakawa & Hammo 1989). Matsuda et al (1988) reported four cases of characteristic painless 'Y'-shaped swelling of the scrotum embracing the penile root. These patients had sclerosing eosinophilic lipogranuloma on histology and electron microscopy and blood eosinophilia (one patient had arthralgia), but no exogenous lipids were found. Spontaneous resolution occurred.

TICK BITE

Sometimes if the vascular penis attracts a blood sucking insect like a tick and the tick attaches asymptomatically to an oblivious host it can grow rapidly into a papule or nodule that is flesh, red or darkly colored (**Figs 9.13, 9.14**) and the differential diagnosis of melanoma is sometimes alarmingly considered.

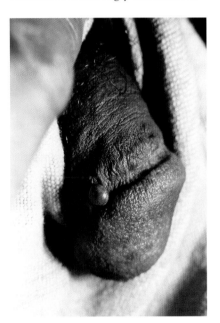

Fig. 9.13 Tick bite. Lateral coronal sulcus, penis. Tick in situ. (Courtesy of Dr Paramoo Sugathan, Kerala, India.)

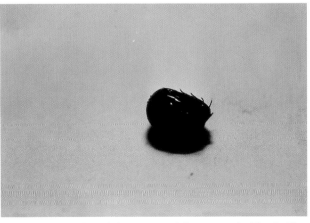

Fig. 9.14 Ixodes tick. Extracted from case in Fig. 9.13. (Courtesy of Dr Paramoo Sugathan, Kerala, India.)

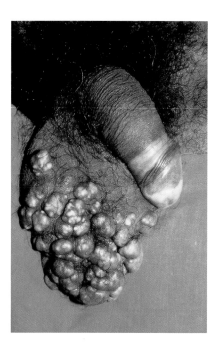

**Fig. 9.15
Scrotal
calcinosis.**
(Courtesy of Prof.
Bhushan Kumar,
Chandigarh,
India.)

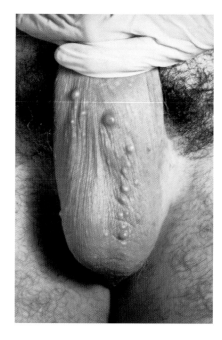

**Fig. 9.16
Scrotal
calcinosis.**
Multiple rock-hard
nodules.

SCROTAL CALCINOSIS

Scrotal calcinosis is a relatively common, benign idiopathic disorder presenting as rock hard, smooth white papules or nodules on the scrotum, multiple (**Figs 9.15–9.17**) or solitary (**Fig. 9.18**, see also Fig. 2.8) Interestingly, these lesions are much rarer on the vulva (Jamaleddine et al 1988). Occasionally they may become secondarily inflamed or infected following trauma. Rarely a lesion or lesions occur on the penis (Lucke et al 1997; Cecchi & Giomi 1999). The differential diagnosis includes epidermoid cyst (**Fig. 9.19**).

The occurrence of calcified nodules within the scrotum was first described by Hutchinson (1888). Shapiro et al (1970) reported 13 cases and reviewed nine in the literature and ascribed the term 'idiopathic scrotal calcinosis'. The few reports (e.g. Fisher & Dvorettzky 1978) contributed since then have debated whether they are indeed idiopathic or whether they arise from epidermoid cysts (Shapiro et al 1970), eccrine duct milia (Dare & Axelsen 1988), eccrine epithelial cysts (Ito et al 2001) or dystrophy of the dartos muscle (King et al 1979).

A number of other etiologies for scrotal calcinosis have been previously proposed. Trauma (Veress & Malik 1975) and the presence of foreign bodies (e.g. thorn or even oncherciasis, Browne 1962) have been suggested as contributing to the formation of calcified scrotal cysts. Swinehart and Golitz (1982) pointed out that calcification of the scrotum may occur with increased frequency in a variety of conditions including meconium peritonitis with leakage of meconium through the processus vaginalis and in testicular tumors such as teratomas, gonadoblastoma and Leydig-cell tumors, although there was no clinical evidence of such problems in any of our

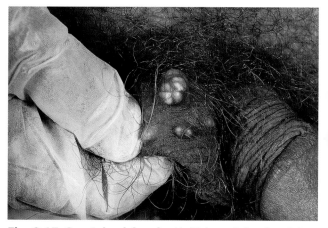

Fig. 9.17 Scrotal calcinosis. Multiple rock-hard nodules.

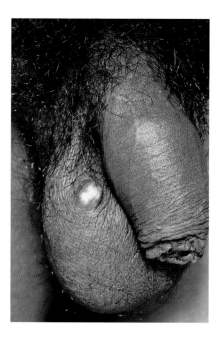

**Fig. 9.18
Scrotal
calcinosis.**
Scrotum. Solitary,
rock-hard lesion.

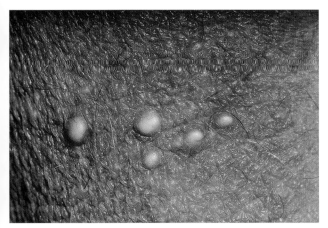

Fig. 9.19 Epidermoid cysts. Scrotum. These firm papules were diagnosed clinically as scrotal calcinosis but the histology was of epidermoid cysts.

cases. King et al (1979) proposed that they arose due to dystrophic calcification within the dartos muscle but they found no evidence of dartos muscle within the calcified mass. My colleagues and I (Farrell et al 1996) did not observe staining with smooth actin antibodies within the calcified nodules themselves to support such a theory.

Dare and Axelson (1988) reported that in three out of four subjects studied there was evidence on light microscopy of communication of the cysts with eccrine ducts and staining with CEA, an immunohistochemical marker for eccrine duct derivatives. However, we did not reproduce these findings in any of our 15 calcified nodules.

Several studies have furnished histological evidence of preceding epidermoid cysts (Swinehart & Golitz 1982; Sarma & Weilbaecher 1984; Song et al 1988) although others were unable to detect any trace of epithelium around these nodules (Fisher & Dvoretzzky 1978; Takayama et al 1982). None of the 15 classical calcified cysts examined by us (Farrell et al 1996) demonstrated a lining of keratinizing stratified squamous epithelium. Furthermore, none of the 15 calcified nodules stained with the antibody to pancytokeratin. This result is consistent with the other previous immunohisto-chemical study using the anti-keratin monoclonal anti-bodies LP34 and PKK1 where no staining was observed around 63 nodules (Wright et al 1991).

It is still possible that the calcified nodules that we studied did originally arise from epidermoid cysts (or even eccrine glands) but were examined at a stage when the structures of origin had been lost by either degeneration or destruction by inflammatory cells. Indeed Song et al 1988 studied 51 nodules which had appeared over two years in one patient and noted that keratinizing stratified squamous epithelium was present in 37 nodules, absent in 13 and partially destroyed in one. None of the cysts with intact walls had a significant surrounding inflammatory reaction, but of the 13 that lacked a stratified squamous epithelium, 10 had a significant inflammatory infiltrate. The one structure with a partially destroyed squamous epithelium was also surrounded by an inflammatory infiltrate. The authors suggested that this inflammatory response resulted in destruction of this epithelial lining and since only one of the 51 nodules showed both inflammation and remnants of a cysts wall, resorption of the cysts wall appeared to be a relatively rapid process.

Again, of the lesions we examined, the seven that were histologically epidermoid cysts had very little calcification within them, and if calcified scrotal nodules did indeed derive from epidermal cysts, the fact that we did not find intermediate structures with features of both, suggests that such calcification would have to be a relatively rapid process. Biopsies of many early nodules may be required to establish the etiology of calcified scrotal nodules but it may be that subjects do not present at an early enough stage for such informative histology to be obtained.

Why scrotal skin should be particularly prone to develop calcification is uncertain. Contributing factors may be the lower temperature compared to other parts of the body, the presence of layers of several organized cell types including muscle fibers in close apposition and trauma. The facial skin shares these features and is also a site where calcification can occur in the form of sub-epidermal, calcified nodules. Interestingly, one of the cysts in our series had the histological features of a subepidermal, calcified nodule.

I treat these unsightly and embarrassing lesions by incision and eventration under local anesthesia in several sessions of 12 or so at a time. The scrotum heals with minimal visible scarring because of its innate rugosity.

In endemic areas of onchocerciasis (e.g. West Africa) calcified scrotal cysts may be due to the living or dead nematodes of *O. volvulus* but patients will invariably have evidence of the disease elsewhere (Browne 1962; Akogun et al 1992). Onchocercal nodules are more common on the iliac crests and the rib cage (see page 185).

KELOID

Denis Browne asserted that the skin of the penis 'never' forms keloid (Browne 1949) but it has occurred following circumcision in a 10-year-old West African boy (**Fig 9.20**) as documented by Warwick & Dickson (1993) and others maintain that this complication of circumcision is more common than suspected (Gurunluoglu et al 1999). Keloid has also been reported following the surgical removal of a post-traumatic cyst in an 8-year-old black boy (Parsons 1966) and after a laceration and a burn in an adult Caucasian (Kormoczy 1978).

Keloid has been simulated on the dorsum of the penis (**Figs 9.21** and **10.5**) by chronic edema caused by a condom catheter (Bang 1994).

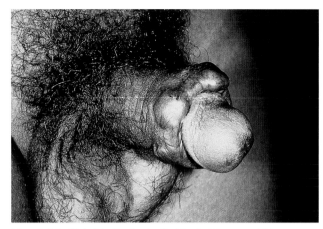

Fig. 9.20 Keloid. Penis shaft. Black 10-year-old boy. Post-circumcision. (Courtesy of Mr William Dickson, Swansea, UK. Reproduced from Warwick DJ, Dickson WA. Keloid of the penis after circumcision. Postgrad Med J. 1993; 69: 236–7.)

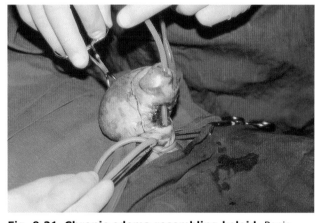

Fig. 9.21 Chronic edema resembling keloid. Penis. Note: dorsal proximal swelling and ventral urethral fistula. (Courtesy of Dr Rameshwar Bang, Safat, Kuwait. Reproduced by kind permission of Scandinavian University Press from Bang RL. Penile oedema induced by continuous condom catheter use and mimicking keloid scar. Scand J Urol Nephrol. 1994; 28: 333–5.)

SCLEROSING LYMPHANGITIS

Non-venereal sclerosing lymphangitis/penile venereal edema/Mondor's phlebitis/localized penile (venereal) lymphedema/penile lymphocele is increasingly recognized and probably went previously unrecorded (Helm & Hodge 1958; El-Hoshy & Mizguchi 1998). Patients present with a serpiginous mass in the coronal sulcus, spreading sometimes on to the dorsal penis (**Fig 9.22**). The lesion may appear for the first time or become tender and enlarge after prolonged or frequent sexual intercourse with a passive 'hardened and sexually non-participating partner'. In circumcised men the circum-

ferential scar may be a predisposing factor. A chlamydial etiology has been posited (Kristensen & Scheibel 1981). The problem may resolve spontaneously or require surgical excision (Harrow & Sloane 1963; Canby et al 1973; Hutchins et al 1977; Broaddus & Leadbetter 1982; Kraus et al 2000).

It is probably erroneous to describe this entity as a lymphangitis. The lymphatics of the skin of the penis form a superficial network with fine dorsal drainage; larger vessels have not been described. Whereas the veins (Stieve 1930) '… comprise emissary channels from the erectile tissue which perforate the tunica albuginea and join a series of circumflex vessels curving around the penis shaft to the deep dorsal vein. They have many valves, a fibrous coat, some elastica and a variable amount of muscle. The most distal circumflex set, lying deep to the preputial attachment behind the corona glandis, is usually plexiform (the retroglanular plexus) and is the set subject to particular stretching and torsion when congested …' (Findlay & Whiting 1977). These authors argue that histological evidence points to post-traumatic thrombosis of the superficial venous plexus as the cause of the phlebitis; affected cutaneous vessels stain with factor VIII-related antigen (Tanii et al 1984). McMillan (1976) proposed that localized penile lymphedema or lymphocele were better descriptive terms for this condition.

Phlebitis of scrotal veins has been reported in three patients. One had been injured by a golf ball but the others developed idiopathically (Harrow & Sloane 1963).

Thrombophlebitis of superficial penile and scrotal veins is analogous to Mondor's phlebitis of the chest wall (Harrow & Sloane 1963). But HSV, polyarteritis nodosa and thromboangiitis obliterans may initiate it (Coldiron & Jacobson 1988). Penile thrombophlebitis

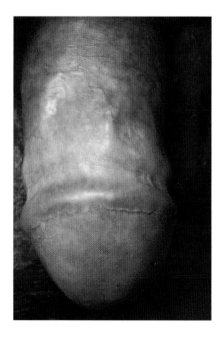

Fig. 9.22 Sclerosing lymphangitis. Dorsal distal penis. Firm cord-like inverted 'Y' in coronal sulcus.

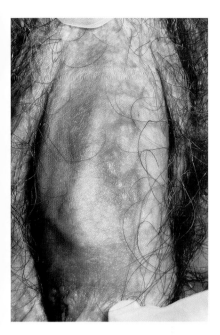

Fig. 9.23
Granuloma annulare. Shaft, penis.

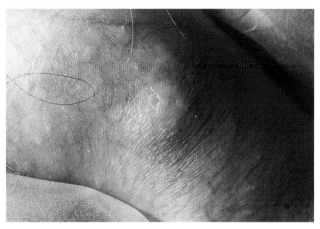

Fig. 9.25 Granuloma annulare. Shaft, penis.

uncircumcised (**Figs 9.23–9.25**). Only one of my cases had granuloma annulare elsewhere.

SARCOID

Sarcoid is an idiopathic non-caseating, granulomatous, multisystem disease. There are very few reports of genital cutaneous sarcoid (**Figs 9.26, 9.27**) in the literature. Occasionally patients with generalized cutaneous disease will present with genital lesions (Wei et al 2000). Tender erythematous induration of the distal shaft of the penis and several yellowish subcutaneous nodules on the glans have been described where biopsy showed non-caseating granulomas and the patient's past and subsequent medical history was compatible with sarcoidosis (Rubinstein et al 1986). Topical corticosteroids were effective treatment in this case. A case presenting with penile ulceration has been documented by Mahmood et al (1997).

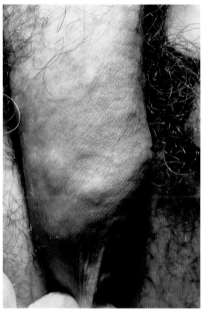

Fig. 9.24
Granuloma annulare. Proximal prepuce, penis.

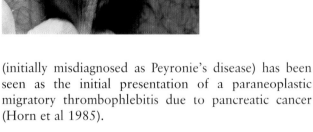

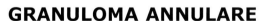

(initially misdiagnosed as Peyronie's disease) has been seen as the initial presentation of a paraneoplastic migratory thrombophlebitis due to pancreatic cancer (Horn et al 1985).

GRANULOMA ANNULARE

A few cases of granuloma annulare affecting the penis have been reported. In its localized form it usually affects the hands and feet, perhaps associated with trauma. In its generalized form it may be associated with diabetes mellitus. Erythematous smooth, round and linear nodules are described (Kossard et al 1990; Hillman et al 1992; Laird 1992; Trap & Wiebe 1993; Narouz et al 1999). All the five cases I have seen have been

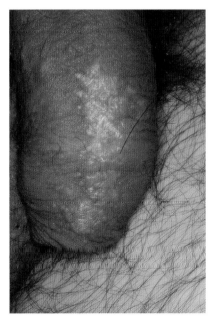

Fig. 9.26
Sarcoid. Penis, dorsal shaft. Confluent plaque of granulomatous papules. (Courtesy of Dr Howard Stevens, Barnet, UK.)

181

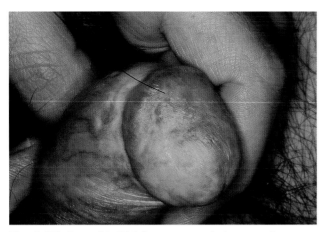

Fig. 9.27 Sarcoid. Distal prepuce and glans, penis. Granulomatous papules. Same case as Fig. 9.26. (Courtesy of Dr Howard Stevens, Barnet, UK.)

Patients presenting with anogenital swelling and chronic penile edema may need a biopsy to exclude anogenital granulomatosis which may be idiopathic or associated with sarcoid, Crohn's disease or Behçet's disease (van de Scheur et al 2003).

Testicular malignancy can be simulated by gross testicular and epididymal involvement with sarcoid. Although rare, it is an important cause of a testicular mass and hilar lymphadenopathy in a young black man – tuberculosis, syphilis and mycosis must also be considered in the differential diagnosis (Turk et al 1986; Sieber & Duggan 1988; Gross et al 1992).

AMYLOID

Although very rare, the non-tender, smooth, yellowish, waxy (occasionally hemorrhagic) papules that constitute the most common cutaneous lesion of primary systemic amyloidosis have a predilection for the anogenital region, particularly the sacrum (Yanagihira 1981; Mukai et al 1986) and the face (especially the eyelids), scalp and neck (Brownstein & Helwig 1970). A soft tissue mass in the penis has been reported unassociated with systemic amyloid (Leal et al 1988).

Primary amyloid of the urethra is very rare indeed, but accurate diagnosis is essential, as it presents like carcinoma, with dysuria, bloody discharge and tender induration of the penis (Provet et al 1989), or as an obstructive voiding syndrome with tender periurethral masses and irregular urethral strictures (Noone & Clark 1997).

BENIGN MUCINOUS METAPLASIA

One case only of this benign reactive process has been described affecting the prepuce: a 6mm lesion consisting of acid mucin-containing cells replacing the superficial epidermis (Val-Bernal & Hernandez-Nieto 2000).

MUCINOUS SYRINGOMETAPLASIA

This is an extremely rare, benign disorder of acrosyringial tissue. A case of an ulcerated papule on the shaft of the penis has been published (Kappel & Abenoza 1993).

FOLLICULITIS AND FURUNCULOSIS

Hirsute humankind is prone to infection of the hair follicles and the anogenital area is particularly susceptible, mainly the buttocks and thighs of men. *Staphylococcus aureus* is the most common organism. Severe involvement with furunculosis and abscesses suggests overlap with hidradenitis. Nasal carriage, diabetes and immunodeficiency (**Fig. 9.28**) should be excluded.

BACILLARY ANGIOMATOSIS

This is an important entity in the differential diagnosis of AIDS-related KS, discussed on page 119. A case where the presenting tender, red nodules affected the scrotum and groins has been published (Fagan et al 1995). It is due to the cat-scratch organism (*Rochalimaea* or *Bartonella henselae* or *quintana*) and responds readily to erythromycin or doxycycline, hence the desirability of prompt diagnosis.

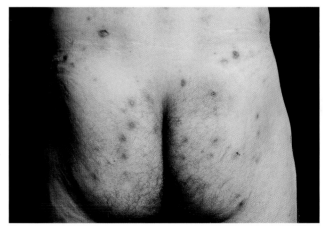

Fig. 9.28 Common variable immunodeficiency. Buttocks. Chronic folliculitis and furunculosis.

LEPROSY

About two million people worldwide have leprosy (Noordeen & Pannikar 1997). Nasal or cutaneous dissemination and infection by *Mycobacterium leprae* result in transmission but the manifestations of infection are determined by host genetic and immunological features. Variable degrees of inflammation in skin and nerves account for three classical clinical forms: lepromatous, tuberculoid and borderline (dimorphous).

Lepromatous lesions (LL-multibacillary form in patients with poor immunity) present initially as multiple non-pruritic, non-anesthetic macules, red in pale skins and coppery in dark skins with a hypopigmented rim found anywhere on the skin including the buttocks but *unusually* distributed in the groins and perineum and on the external genitalia. With advancing disease papules, nodules and ulcers form and there may be hair loss including of the brows and lashes. Neural involvement leads to sensory and motor dysfunction and palpable peripheral nerves at classical sites, but skin lesions are not anesthetic unless in a region affected by sensory neuropathy.

Tuberculoid (TT-paucibacillary form in patients with good immunity) leprosy skin lesions or nerve is asymmetrically localized to one or a few areas. Skin lesions are macules or plaques and are anesthetic and anhidrotic. Macules are red in white skins and hypopigmented in dark skins whereas plaques are annular, erythematous, red or brown, pebbly with central flattening and healing and peripheral well-marginated indurated edges. Buttock lesions are common but genital involvement is not. Peripheral neuropathy may result in trophic ulceration of skin, deformities and palpable nerves.

Borderline leprosy presents with erythematous or hypopigmented (depending on skin type) anesthetic macules or infiltrated, purple-brown, smooth, shiny, annular, nodular or linear anesthetic plaques with sloping (down away from the surface to the edge) surfaces and well-defined central areas and poorly defined peripheral margins (BL or BT). Apart from the buttocks anogenital skin is rarely affected. Nerve involvement manifests as paraesthesia and hyperalgesia, asymmetrical neuropathy and palpable nerves.

Diagnosis relies on clinical grounds (principally classical skin lesions, thickened nerves, anesthesia and demonstration of the organism in skin, the nasal mucosa or biopsy). Treatment is a specialist area: rifampicin, dapsone and clofazimine are the main drugs.

A review by Kumar et al (2001) elegantly describes and illustrates the nuances of involvement of the male genitalia with leprosy. Genital lesions were seen in 6.6% of their male patients; 25% of patients with lepromatous leprosy, 13.3% of patients with borderline lepromatous leprosy and 1.4% of patients with borderline tuberculoid leprosy had penile or scrotal involvement (**Figs 9.29–9.34**).

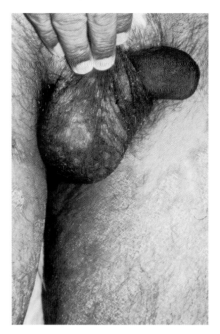

Fig. 9.29 Leprosy. Scrotum. BL in reversal. Subsiding reaction on thighs (Courtesy of Prof. Bhushan Kumar, Chandigarh, India. Reproduced with kind permission from LEPRA.)

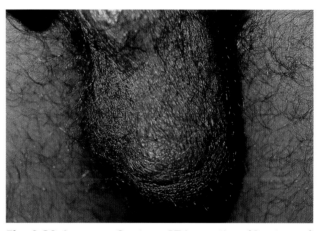

Fig. 9.30 Leprosy. Scrotum. BT in reaction. (Courtesy of Prof. Bhushan Kumar, Chandigarh, India. Reproduced with kind permission from LEPRA.)

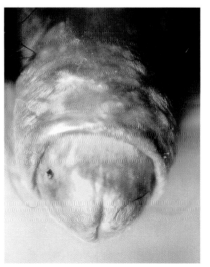

Fig. 9.31 Leprosy. Glans penis and foreskin. Multiple necrotic lesions of ENL on glans penis and prepuce. LL/erythema nodosum leprosum. (Courtesy of Prof. Bhushan Kumar, Chandigarh, India. Reproduced with kind permission from LEPRA.)

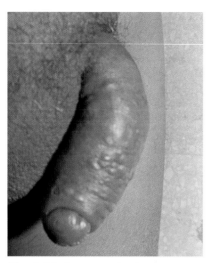

Fig. 9.32 Leprosy. Penis. BL disease with histoid lesions. (Courtesy of Prof. Bhushan Kumar, Chandigarh, India. Reproduced with kind permission from LEPRA.)

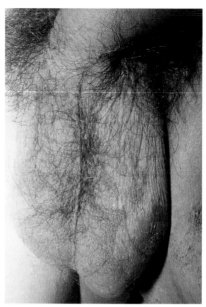

Fig. 9.33 Leprosy. Scrotum. Infiltrated plaque. LL disease. (Courtesy of Prof. Bhushan Kumar, Chandigarh, India. Reproduced with kind permission from LEPRA.)

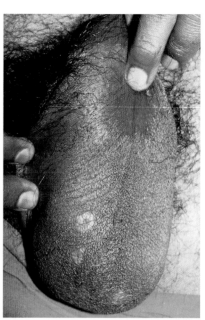

Fig. 9.34 Leprosy. Scrotum. Infiltrated papules. BL disease. (Courtesy of Prof. Bhushan Kumar, Chandigarh, India. Reproduced with kind permission from LEPRA.)

SUPERFICIAL PHEOHYPHOMYCOSIS

A unique case of multiple, 1–3mm, pigmented papules, resembling seborrheic keratoses, on the scrotum of an HIV-positive patient appears in the literature. A potassium hydroxide preparation showed a mass of mycelia and two organisms were cultured: *Bipolaris* and *Curvularia*, both dematiaceous fungi (Duvic & Lowe 1987).

SCHISTOSOMIASIS

Perineal granulomatous lesions are a rare manifestation of schistosomiasis (*Schistosomia haematobium*), which is endemic in many parts of the world and is contracted by swimming in water harboring infected freshwater snails. It may present with skin symptoms and signs at the time of infection or later with hematuria. Rarely genital skin lesions may lead to the diagnosis.

Cercariae are disseminated throughout the tissues but mature into adult worms in the liver. They then migrate to the pelvic plexus of veins where natural egg production takes place. Cutaneous schistosomiasis (which is unusual) is thought to occur because ova are deposited in skin by female worms that have migrated from the pelvic venous plexuses to the superficial veins through anastomoses. The rare occurrence of genital lesions is

due to ova shed by worms that have entered the perineal vessels (Adeyemi-Doro et al 1979).

Cutaneous manifestations of schistosomiasis include swimmers itch (due to invasion of the skin by infective cercariae), urticaria, edema, fever, pruritus, hypersensitivity reactions to infection and granulomatous papules and nodules (due to ectopic deposition of ova).

The papules and nodules may be skin-colored, pink or brown, scattered or grouped, affecting the penis scrotum (and vulva). They can spread onto the perineum and around the anus and may develop into soft warty vegetating lesions, but remain relatively asymptomatic. Ulceration is rare. But, even more rarely, concomitant carcinoma has been reported (El-Zawahry 1965).

Diagnosis is by biopsy, which shows eosinophilic infiltration (there may be a blood eosinophilia) or frank giant cell granuloma formation around viable and calcified *S. haematobium* ova with a characteristic terminal spine. Other granulomatous conditions, especially tuberculosis, may be suspected. Ova may be recovered from urine or stool.

ONCHOCERCIASIS

Onchocerciasis (river blindness) is caused by infection with the helminth *Onchocerca volvulus* transmitted by the *Simulium* blackfly. About 18 million people in Africa and South America are infected. The *dermatological* consequences are pruritus, 'leopard skin' hypo-pigmentation (shins and scrotum), nodules (ileal crests, rib-cage, scrotum), dermatitis including 'lizard skin' lichenification, 'hanging groin' and scrotal enlargement (Akogun et al 1992; McMahon & Simonsen 1996). The differential diagnosis of the scrotal enlargement includes bancroftian filiariasis (Akogun et al 1992).

The diagnosis is made by demonstrating microfilariae in skin snips.

VIRAL WARTS

Warts and verrucae are extremely common human afflictions due to human papillomaviruses (HPV: Majewski & Jablonska 1997). HPV can be found in normal skin of immunocompetent hosts (Astori et al 1998). Genital warts (condyloma acuminata) have been recognized since ancient times and were first wrongly attributed to syphilis and then gonorrhea (Oriel 1971; van Krogh 1992). The estimated lifetime risk of acquiring HPV sexually is near 80% (van Krogh 1992). Incidence rates are rising (Anon 2000) including in children (Allen & Siegfried 1998). Circumcised men are more likely to have genital warts than those who are uncircumcised yet warts in the latter group tend to affect the distal portion of the organ (Cook et al 1993). Consistent condom use significantly reduces the risk of acquiring genital warts (Wen et al 1999). Congenital and acquired immunosuppression increases susceptibility to HPV infection or recrudescence, including of the ano-genital region, and progression to dysplasia and worse (Daneshpouy et al 2001).

Lesions are papillomatous, plane or papular, filiform or verrucous, essentially flesh-colored, sometimes inflamed (**Fig. 9.35**), sometimes pigmented, epidermal lesions (**Figs 9.36–9.47**, see also Fig. 2.6). Clinically

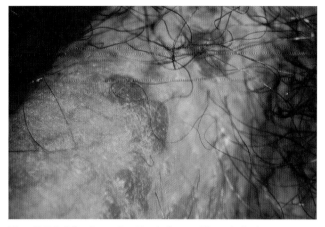

Fig. 9.36 Viral warts. Penis base. Chronic lesions. Alcoholic. Clinically suspected to be Bowenoid papulosis but histology showed no dysplasia.

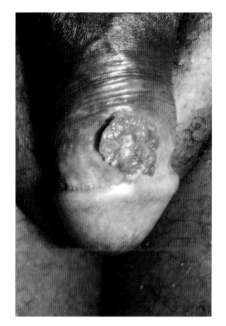

Fig. 9.37 Viral wart. Doral distal shaft, penis.

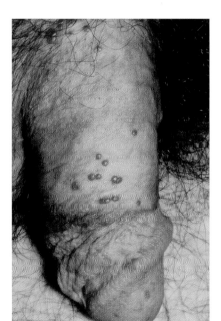

Fig. 9.35 Viral warts. Shaft penis. Red papules. This patient had previously been treated for biopsy-proven lichen nitidus of the penis with a potent topical steroid.

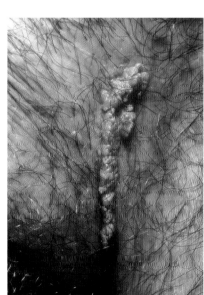

Fig. 9.38 Viral warts. Groin. Florid linear exophytic plaque.

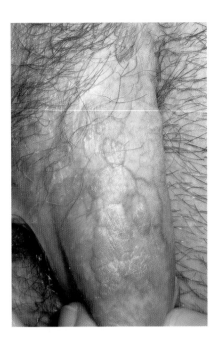

Fig. 9.39 Viral warts. Dorsal shaft, penis. Flesh-colored planar plaques.

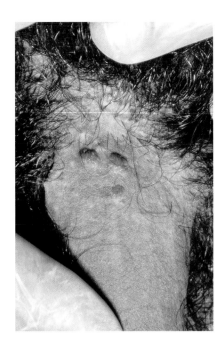

Fig. 9.42 Viral warts. Dorsal root, penis. Pigmented papules.

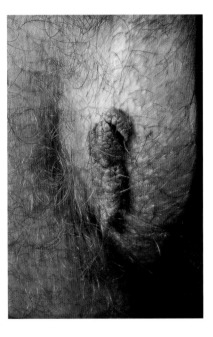

Fig. 9.40 Viral wart. Scrotum. Pigmented cxophytic plaque.

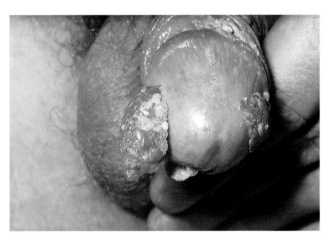

Fig. 9.43 Viral warts. Glans penis. Florid exophytic lesions. (Courtesy of Dr Richard Staughton, London, UK.)

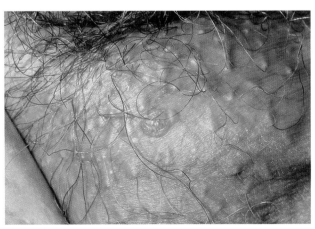

Fig. 9.41 Viral wart. Scrotum and ventrolateral root, penis. Solitary flesh-colored papule.

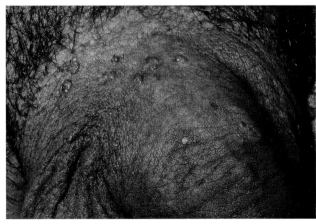

Fig. 9.44 Viral warts. Dorsal proximal shaft, penis. Multiple flesh-colored papules. (Courtesy of Dr Peter Copeman, London, UK.)

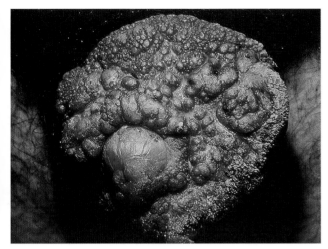

Fig. 9.45 Viral warts. Penis. Florid confluent exophytic lesions.

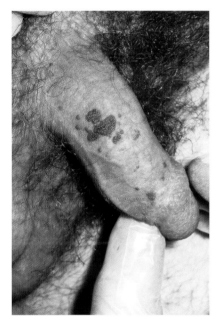

Fig. 9.46 Viral warts. Penis, lateral penile shaft. Exuberant pigmented lesions.

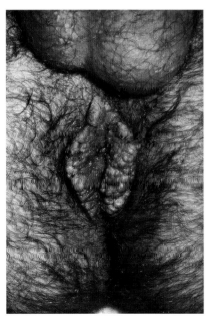

Fig. 9.47 Viral warts. Perianal skin. Florid exophytic condylomata. (Courtesy of Prof. Tim Allen-Mersh, London, UK.)

inapparent disease may present as balanoposthitis (Lowhagen et al 1993; Wikström et al 1994). It is held that 5% acetic acid can aid the visualization of HPV infection, e.g. macular lesions and areas of dysplasia (Aynaud et al 1992; Steinberg et al 1993) but biopsy and HPV PCR screening suggests that the acetowhite test is not very specific (Mazzatenta et al 1993; Wikström et al 1992; Voog et al 1997). The visible urethra should be examined (Yamamoto et al 1993) and the otoscope has been proposed as the instrument of choice (O'Brien & Luzzi 1995). Some clinicians extol examination under magnification using a colposcope-peniscopy (Boon et al 1988; Aynaud et al 1992; Costa et al 1992).

Anogenital warts are due to multicentric (Hillman et al 1993b) infection (usually, but not exclusively, sexually acquired) with several subtypes of the human papilloma virus (HPV), especially HPV 6 and 11 (von Krogh 1991; Handley et al 1992; Hillman et al 1993c; Wen-yuan et al 1993; Lambropoulou et al 1994). High-risk HPV types (16, 18, 31, 33, 35) may be found in papular and macular lesions (Lowhage et al 1993) but in general there is a poor correlation between clinical morphology and HPV type (Rock et al 1992). In benign lesions the HPV DNA exists in circular form separate from the host genome but in malign lesions it is usually integrated (Durst et al 1985)

There is evidence that male urethral HPV infection is prevalent in the presence or absence of genital warts (Green et al 1991; Wikström et al 1991; Hillman et al 1993a) and that female consorts of men with genital condyloma are infected in the absence of clinical evidence of genital warts (Kiss et al 1993) and vice versa (Scneider et al 1988). Subclinical or latent genital HPV infection may be 100 times more common than classical condyloma (van Krogh 1992). Immunocompromise is a predisposing factor; so may be drug abuse, especially cannabis (Gross et al 1991).

Although it is assumed that some cases of anal warts may be due to anal intercourse in homosexuals there is neither evidence that this is the case in heterosexuals, nor that anal warts are related to receptive anodigital insertion (Sonnex et al 1991). Voltz et al (1999) found anogenital warts in 165 of all HIV-positive males nearly half of whom showed histological signs of intraepithelial neoplasia. In children anogenital warts may be due to HPV infection acquired by vertical infection from the maternal birth canal, sexual abuse (Hicks 1993), sexual precociousness or of unknown source (Handley et al 1993; Yun & Joblin 1993).

Anogenital HPV infection is a risk factor for anogenital cancer particularly of the anus (and cervix) yet it is rare for condylomata to contain HPV 16, which has a well-documented association with anal carcinoma. Homosexual men have a higher incidence of both perianal warts and anal carcinoma both in situ and invasive. HIV infection may alter and worsen the expression and consequences of anogenital HPV infection (Arany et al 1998); for example an HIV-positive

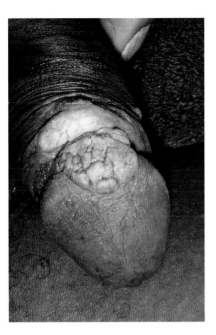

Fig. 9.48 Giant condyloma. Glans penis. Patient on prednisolone for chronic asthma. Histology showed HPV changes and mild dysplasia.

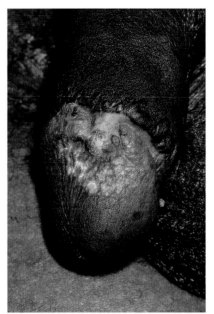

Fig. 9.49 Giant condyloma. Glans penis. Recurrence. Same patient as Fig. 9.48. Post-surgical treatment including circumcision. Further curettage showed identical histology.

man with HPV 16-positive anal warts has been reported to develop carcinoma in situ (Bradshaw et al 1992), high-grade dysplasia associated with high-risk HPV types have been found in genital warts from HIV-positive individuals (Bryan et al 1998) and high-grade squamous intraepithelial lesions manifest significantly different tissue gene-expression patterns (IL-6, TNF α, HPV E7) compared with low-grade lesions and condyloma (Arany et al 2001). However, overall, the risk of progression of anal intraepithelial neoplasia (AIN) associated with anal HPV wart infection to invasive squamous carcinoma is low (Morgan et al 1994).

HPV infection can usually be diagnosed with clinical certainty but condylomata lata (secondary syphilis) and lichen planus enter the differential diagnosis, as do mollusca and Bowenoid papulosis. Pearly penile papules may be confusing to the tyro but classically affect the coronal rim in rows; if they occur on the shaft then they may confuse the expert (O'Neil & Hansen 1995). Solitary lesions have a wider differential diagnosis including many of the other conditions discussed in this chapter. Squamous carcinoma is the most important condition not to miss. Large lesions/giant condyloma (**Figs 9.48, 9.49**) may be part of the Buschke-Lowenstein verrucous carcinoma spectrum (see page 214). Transitional cell carcinoma of the distal urethra has presented as a warty lesion at the urethral meatus (Langlois et al 1992).

Biopsy should be performed if there is any diagnostic uncertainty (**Fig. 9.50**) or if dysplasia is suspected. Histologically, HPV infection is characterized by papillomatous and acanthotic epithelial hypertrophy with confluence and rounding of the rete pegs. No nuclear atypia of keratinocytes is seen but there may be koilocytes in the subcorneal layers (**Fig. 9.51**). Immuno-histochemistry, in situ demonstration of HPV DNA or HPV PCR can be informative (Law et al 1991; Tsutumi et al 1991; Lassus et al 1992).

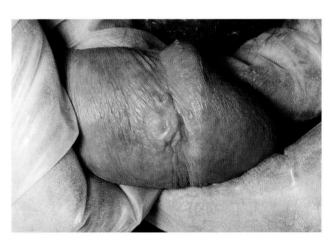

Fig. 9.50 Viral wart. Lateral coronal sulcus. Atypical, irregular keratotic nodule. Biopsy necessary. Benign histology.

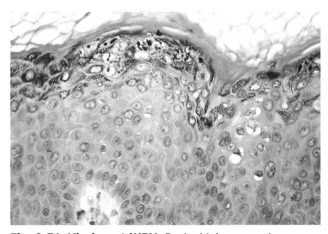

Fig. 9.51 Viral wart/HPV. Penis, high-power view. Increased keratohyaline granules; some perinuclear vacuolation; no dysplasia. (Courtesy of Dr Nick Francis, London, UK.)

Table 9.12 Treatments for anogenital warts

Surgery	Curettage (with electro- or chemocautery)
	Scissor amputation (supplemented by electro- or chemocautery)
	Circumcision
	Penile resurfacing with split-skin grafting
Cryosurgery	Liquid nitrogen
	Nitrous oxide
Electrosurgery*‡	Electrocautery
	Hyfrecation
	Direct electrical current
Laser surgery	CO_2 laser*#
	Circumcision
Topical	Podophyllin and podophyllotoxin
	Trichloroacetic acid
	5-fluorouracil
	Interferon
	Imiquimod
	Nitric acid
	Colchicine
	Salicylic acid
	Cidofovir
Intralesional	Interferons
Systemic	Interferon
	Isotretinoin
Miscellaneous	Excision and autogenous vaccination
	Topical BCG

*virus in plume
†anal stricture reported: leave viable skin bridges
#genome is not eradicated
(After: Allen & Siegfrie 1998; Ammori & Ausobsky 2000; Anon 2, 1992; Aynaud et al 1992; Ballaro et al 2001; Bohle et al 2001; Cardamakis et al 1995; Heaton et al 1993; Hengge & Tietze 2000; Lassus et al 1994; Lenk et al 1991; Martinelli et al 2001; Maw 1999; McMillan 1999; Olsen et al 1989; Sand Petersen & Menne 1993; Schurmann et al 2000; Simmons et al 1981; Taylor et al 1994; von Krogh & Ruden 1980; von Krogh & Wikstrom 1991; von Krogh 1978; von Krogh 1991; Wiltz et al 1995).

Regarding anal warts, Strand et al (1999) have observed that morphology and histology (even when koilocytic atypia is considered a diagnostic hallmark, although specific, it is not a very sensitive discriminating feature) cannot distinguish viral from non-viral lesions and point out that sensitive molecular testing is preferable. Colposcopy, cytology and molecular methods can be used (Sonnex et al 1991).

Patients presenting with warts and their sexual partners should be counseled and screened for HPV, other sexually transmitted diseases, including HIV infection and cervical neoplasia (Kinghorn 1978; Campion et al 1985, 1988; Costa et al 1992).

HPV may be very hard to treat. Subclinical infection is very common, difficult to detect and virtually untreatable so there is ambiguity between ambitions for treatment and achievability. Management of the male ... 'should rely on diagnosing and treating relevant lesions causing illness of his own genitals or psychosexual stress to himself or his partner ...' (van Krogh 1992). Reasonable ambitions '... include: (1) induction of wart cure or wart-free periods; (2) alleviation of symptoms such as dyspareunia; (3) therapy no worse than the disease; and (4) minimizing mortality and morbidity from cervical cancer in females ...' (van Krogh 1992) and minimizing

mortality and morbidity from intraepithelial neoplasia and frank cancer in the patient.

Treatments are summarized in the **Tables 9.12–9.13**. Liquid nitrogen cryotherapy and repeated applications of 20% podophyllin and 0.25–0.5% podophyllotoxin (Beutner et al 1989; Syed & Lundin 1993; Kinghorn et al 1993; von Krogh et al 1994; Goh et al 1998) are popular and effective. These complex substances are obtained from the resins of the plants *Podophyllum palatum* or *Podophyllum emodi* grown in North America and the Himalayas, respectively (von Krogh 1978).

Other commonplace approaches include topical 5-fluorouracil (von Krogh 1978; Krebs 1991), simple surgical techniques (Thomson & Grace 1978) and physical destructive modalities (Simmons et al 1981; Taylor et al 1994). Earlier enthusiasm for local or systemic immunostimulation with various interferons (Douglas et al 1986; Eron et al 1986; Kirby et al 1988; Sand Petersen et al 1991; Handley et al 1992; Hopfl et al 1993; Anon 1993) has been replaced by much interest in local immunomodulation, induction of changes in the local cytokine environment, by agents such as imiquimod (Tyring et al 1998; Gollnick et al 2001; Hengge et al 2001). Many modalities have been used in combination.

Table 9.13 Overview of clearance and recurrence rates in the published literature with different treatments for external genital warts

Treatment	Clearance rates (%) End of treatment	≥3 Months	Recurrence rates
Cryotherapy	63–88	63–92	0–39
Electrocautery/electrotherapy	93–94	78–91	24
Interferons			
intralesional	19–62	36–62	0–33
systemic	7–51	18–21	0–23
topical	6–90	33	6
Laser therapy	27–89	39–86	<7–45
Loop electrosurgical excision procedure	≤90	—	—
Podophyllin*	32–79	22–73	11–65
Podophyllotoxin*	42–88	34–77	10–91
Surgical/scissor excision	89–93	36	0–29
Trichloracetic acid	50–81	70	36
5-fluorouracil	10–71	37	10–13

*Studies using more than one treatment strength have been grouped together.
After Beutner in Maw (1999) by kind permission of Dr Karl Beutner, Vallejo, CA, USA.

Some recommend that anal warts might be aggressively treated, for symptomatic relief, by examination of the anal canal under general anesthesia and eradication of lesions by laser, electrocautery and sharp dissection (Morgan et al 1994).

MOLLUSCA

Mollusca are classically small, flesh-colored, monomorphic, dome-shaped papules indented by a central dell or umbilicus (**Fig. 9.52**). Multiple lesions are usually present (**Figs 9.53–9.55**). Giant and polypoidal lesions (**Fig. 9.56**) may occur in HIV (Kumar & Dawn 1995; Bunker 1996). Inflammation and purulence may be due to infection but is a common phenomenon whilst individual lesions spontaneously involute (**Fig. 9.57**).

Mollusca are due to infection with a human DNA pox virus. Sometimes, but not always (even with genital lesions), this may be sexually acquired. Atopic children are particularly prone to generalized cutaneous mollusca, as are the congenitally, iatrogenically and virally immunocompromised. The histology of mollusca shows ballooning of keratinocytes and eosinophilic inclusion bodies.

Mollusca can usually be diagnosed clinically with accuracy. If there is any doubt as sometimes occurs with solitary lesions or in the immunocompromised a biopsy can be taken. Condylomata lata (secondary syphilis) and lichen planus enter the differential diagnosis of mollusca, as does simple HPV infection and Bowenoid papulosis. Patients presenting with mollusca and their sexual partners should be counseled and screened for other

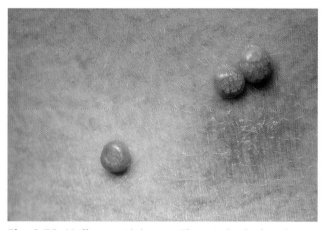

Fig. 9.52 Mollusca. Abdomen. Three individual pocks with central umbilication.

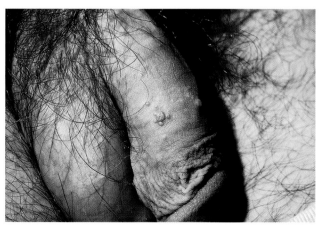

Fig. 9.53 Mollusca. Penis, shaft.

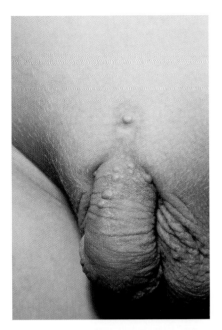

Fig. 9.54 Mollusca. Boy. Penis, shaft. (Reproduced from Bunker CB. Skin conditions on the male genitalia. Medicine 2001; 29:7 by kind permission of the Medicine Publishing Company.)

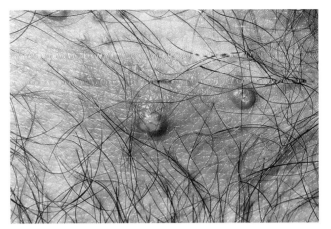

Fig. 9.57 Mollusca. Abdomen. One lesion is involuting with inflammation and purulence.

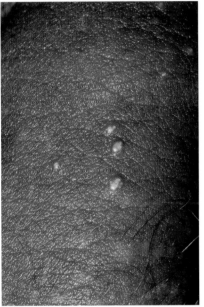

Fig. 9.55 Mollusca. Penis shaft.

sexually transmitted diseases including HIV infection. Solitary lesions have a wider differential diagnosis including many of the other entities discussed in this chapter.

Mollusca respond to cryotherapy, curettage, and cautery or phenolization, but the infection is self-limiting. Severe persistent mollusca, especially in AIDS, have lead to experimentation with numerous topical and systemic modalities (Calista 2000).

DEMODECIDOSIS

The role of the mite *Demodex folliculorum* in human cutaneous diseases such as rosacea is controversial. However, Hwang et al (1998) have described a man with a long-standing pruritic eruption of multiple, mono-morphic, match head-sized, flesh-colored papules on the penis and scrotum (**Fig. 9.58**). Histology demonstrated intrafollicular mites (**Fig. 9.59**) and the patient was cured with topical crotamiton.

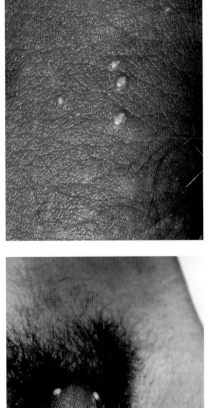

Fig. 9.56 Mollusca/HIV. Penis shaft. (Courtesy of Prof. Bhushan Kumar, Chandigarh, India. Reproduced from Kumar B & Dawn G. Genitourin Med. 1995; 71: 57. With permission from BMJ Publishing Group.)

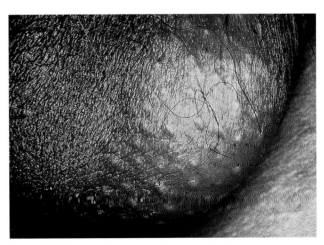

Fig. 9.58 Demodicidosis. Scrotum. Multiple itchy monomorphic white papules. (Courtesy of Dr Sung Ku Ahn, Wonju, South Korea. Reproduced by kind permission of Blackwell Science Ltd from Hwang SM et al. Demodecidosis manifested on the external genitalia. Int J Dermatol. 1998; 37: 634–6.)

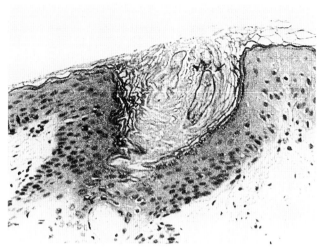

Fig. 9.59 Demodiciosis. Scrotum. Intrafollicular Demodex mites. (Courtesy of Dr Sung Ku Ahn, Wonju, South Korea. Reproduced by kind permission of Blackwell Science Ltd from Hwang SM et al. Demodecidosis manifested on the external genitalia. Int J Dermatol. 1998; 37: 634–6.)

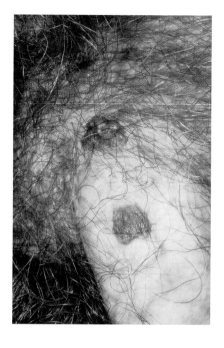

Fig. 9.61 Basal cell papillomas/seborrheic keratoses. Penis shaft, base.

BASAL CELL PAPILLOMA/ SEBORRHEIC KERATOSIS

This most common of all benign skin tumors is not uncommon in and around the anogenital area, including on the penis (**Figs 9.60–9.64**) and in the groins (**Fig. 9.65**). It is rather rare in the perianal area and clinically suggestive lesions at that site (**Fig. 9.66**) should be biopsied to exclude Bowenoid papulosis. Single to multiple, ranging from flesh-colored to black, smooth papule to verrucous plaque, this entity has a wide differential diagnosis and is frequently mistaken for a viral condyloma (Friedman et al 1987).

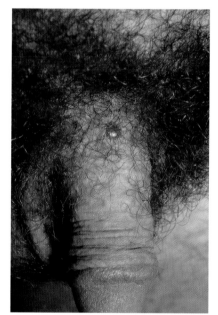

Fig. 9.62 Basal cell papillomas/seborrheic keratoses. Penis shaft, base.

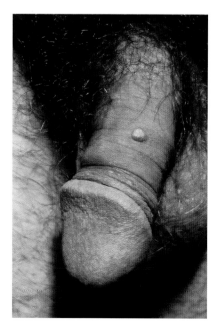

Fig. 9.60 Basal cell papilloma/seborrheic keratosis. Penis shaft.

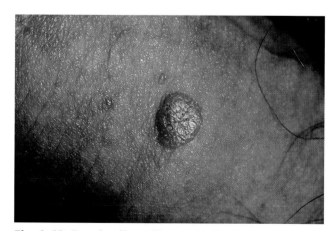

Fig. 9.63 Basal cell papillomas/seborrheic keratoses. Penis shaft.

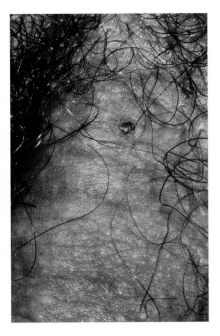

Fig. 9.64 Basal cell papilloma/ seborrheic keratosis. Base dorsal shaft, penis.

VERRUCIFORM XANTHOMA

Verruciform xanthoma is a rare entity that principally involves the mouth. Genitalia are next most frequently affected where it presents as a painless, yellow-brown or red, verrucous, sessile or papillary plaque (**Fig. 9.67**). Less than twenty case reports have appeared (Kraemar et al 1981; Shindo et al 1981; Ronan et al 1984; Balus et al 1991; Lonsdale 1992; Geiss et al 1993; Canillot et al 1994; Cuozzo et al 1995; Mohsin et al 1998). Histologically there is hyperkeratosis, focal parakeratosis, and irregular epidermal acanthosis. Rete ridges are lengthened and extend into the dermis forming areas called dermal papillae and enclosing capillary vessels surrounded by foam cells (**Fig. 9.68**). These stain with CD 68 but not

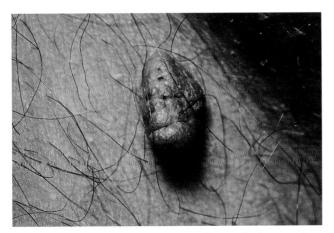

Fig. 9.65 Basal cell papilloma/seborrheic keratosis. Right groin.

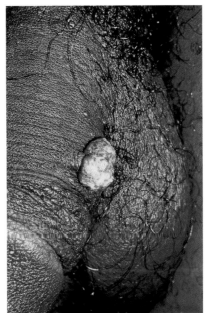

Fig. 9.67 Verruciform xanthoma. Lateral mid-shaft, penis. (Courtesy of Dr Daniel W Cuozzo, Cortland, NJ, USA. Reproduced by kind permission from Cuozzo DW et al. Verruciform xanthoma: a benign penile growth. J Urol. 1995; 153: 1625–7.)

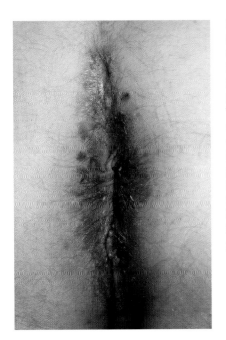

Fig. 9.66 Basal cell papillomas/ seborrheic keratoses. Buttocks and perianal skin. These pigmented warty lesions were suspected to be Bowenoid papulosis in this homosexual man. Repeated histology showed benign basal cell papilloma.

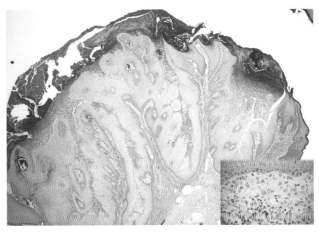

Fig. 9.68 Verruciform xanthoma. Marked hyperkeratosis with irregular and elongated acanthotic epidermis forming a papular lesion. The higher-power view (inset) shows aggregates of pale bland histiocytic cells some of which have prominent single nucleoli filling up the papillary dermis and having a xanthoma cell appearance to them and surrounded by an infiltrate of small numbers of lymphocytes and plasma cells.

193

S100. It is thought that the lesion results from epidermal degeneration and that keratinocyte lipid is taken up by dermal macrophages (Orchard et al 1994) or fibroblasts to form the foam cells. HPV type-6 DNA has been found in one case (Khaskhely et al 2000).

Treatment is by surgical excision.

ACANTHOSIS NIGRICANS

Benign (hereditary, endocrinopathy associated, drug induced (nicotinic acid, fusidic acid, stilboestrol, triazinate, nevoid) and pseudo- (obesity associated) acanthosis nigricans and *malignant* (associated with internal adenocarcinoma) types are recognized. Insulin resistance is a common pathogenic factor. Velvety plaques of confluent, pigmented papillomatous thickened, dry skin are found in the axillae, the anogenitocrural area and around the neck. Almost always the groins are affected (**Figs 9.1, 9.69**).

In pseudo-acanthosis nigricans the obesity is almost always responsible for a compounding intertrigo and associated acrochordons.

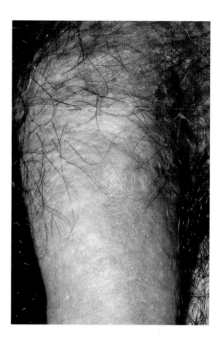

Fig. 9.70 Epidermoid cyst. Penis. Proximal distal shaft.

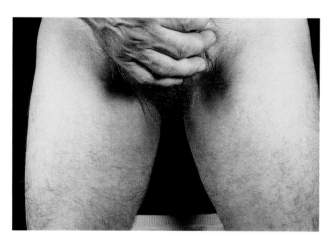

Fig. 9.69 Acanthosis nigricans. Groins. Velvety brown corrugated plaques.

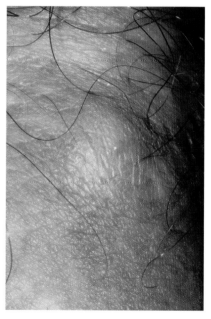

Fig. 9.71 Epidermoid cyst. Penis. Proximal distal shaft. No punctum. Close-up of Fig. 9.70.

EPIDERMOID CYST

This entity is often erroneously termed 'sebaceous cyst'. It is a common flesh-colored lesion that slowly enlarges. The head, neck and back are the most common sites for them to occur but they can be found anywhere (**Figs 9.19, 9.70, 9.71**). Sometimes a central surface punctum can be appreciated – the cysts derive from the hair follicle epithelium. Often they discharge their contents of cheesy-smelling keratin. Occasionally they are traumatized and become infected to form an abscess. Inguinogenital lesions containing mollusca have been described (Park et al 1992).

PILAR CYST

A pilar cyst is similar to an epidermoid cyst but arises from deeper in the hair follicle. Clinically there is no punctum. Epidermoid and pilar cysts are very common at other sites and probably much more common in the anogenital area than the literature attests. Only giant or unusual lesions attract attention (Shah et al 1979).

DERMOID CYST

A dermoid cyst results from epithelial rests along embryological lines of fusion. The head is the most common site (lateral eyebrows, nose and scalp). One case presenting with pain, swelling and suppuration from abscess formation has been reported to have affected the penis (Tomasini et al 1997) but there may be confusion with epidermoid cyst, pilar cyst and pilonidal sinus (see above and page 141).

NEVUS COMEDONICUS

This is a rare, hamartomatous abnormality of the pilosebaceous apparatus characterized by groups of patulous follicles containing dark, horny, comedonal plugs. It is asymptomatic, fixed and unlikely to enlarge. It has even been reported to affect the glans ectopically, which is generally devoid of pilosebaceous structures (Abdel-A'Al & Abdel-Aziz 1975).

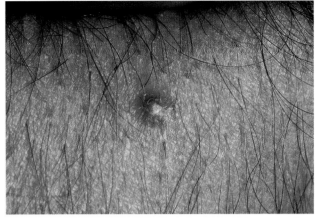

Fig. 9.72 Dermatofibroma/histiocytoma. Arm.

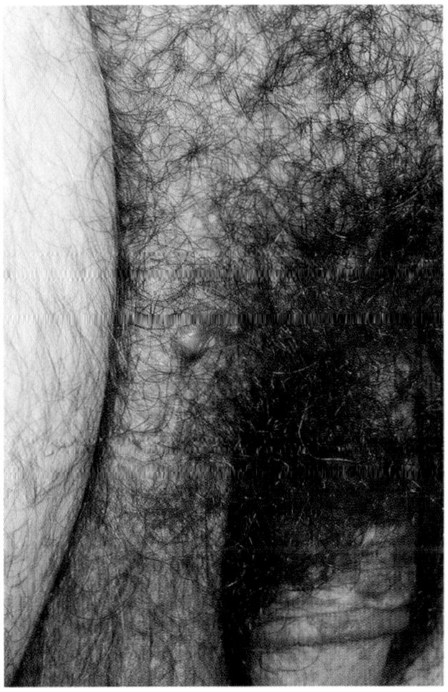

SYRINGOMAS AND BENIGN APPENDAGEAL TUMORS

Appendageal tumors are neoplasms of the appendageal structures (e.g. sweat glands and pilosebaceous apparatus) of skin.

Syringoma is a common benign tumor of eccrine sweat glands usually occurring as multiple symmetrical flesh-colored papules around the eyelids. Rarely there may be a more widespread distribution. Some cases of multiple syringoma focalized at the penis have been described (Lo et al 1990; Casas et al 1995). A man with discrete and grouped, reddish-brown papules of syringoma on the penis has been reported (Zalla & Perry 1971). He was initially misdiagnosed as having lichen planus. Another patient's presentation simulated genital warts (Lipshutz et al 1991).

Apocrine cystadenoma has been described presenting as a slowly growing nodule on the prepuce reaching a maximum size of 3cm. Apocrine fibroadenoma has been proposed as an alternative name (De Dulanto et al 1973). The entity has been described on the scrotum by Flessati et al (1999) who also refer to it as an apocrine hidrocystoma. Sometimes this lesion has been erroneously misdiagnosed for a median raphe cyst (Urahashi et al 2000) or epidermoid cysts (Ahmed & Jones 1969).

A mixed syringocystadenoma papilliferum and papillary eccrine adenoma occurring in a scrotal condyloma has been encountered (Coyne & Fitzgibbon 2000).

DERMATFIBROMA

Dermatofibroma (fibrous histiocytoma) is a very common benign lesion of skin (**Fig. 9.72**) but curiously rather rarely (excluding the upper thigh) found in the anogenital area. Individual lesions are firm dermal nodules (**Figs 9.73–9.77**). Histiocytomas are thought to

Fig. 9.73 Dermatofibroma/histiocytoma. Groin.

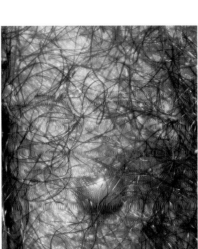

Fig. 9.74 Dermatofibroma/histiocytoma. Groin. Close up of Fig. 9.73.

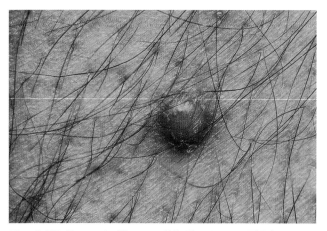

Fig. 9.75 Dermatofibroma/histiocytoma. Thigh.

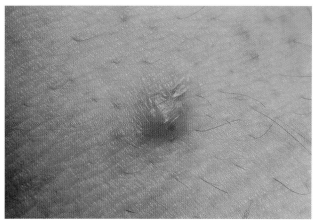

Fig. 9.76 Dermatofibroma/histiocytoma. Thigh.

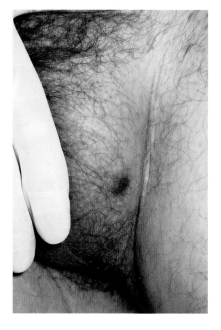

Fig. 9.77 Dermatofibroma/ histiocytoma. Left groin.

represent aberrant healing following an insect bite. One penile case appears in the literature in a 15-year-old boy (Dehner & Smith 1970).

MYXOMA

A patient with long-standing paraparesis who relied on self-catheterization for evacuation of the urinary bladder developed a large, paraurethral, pedunculated nodule (**Fig 9.78**) emerging from the parameatal glans penis. Histologically this was a myxoma. It was excised and has not recurred.

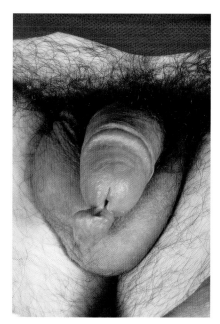

Fig. 9.78 Myxoma. Glans penis. Large pedunculated tumor. Chronically self-catheterizing paraparetic.

GRANULAR CELL TUMOR

This is a benign mesenchymal lesion that can arise at any site, most often the digits, head, oral cavity, neck and chest wall. It can present rarely as a nodule anywhere on or within the penis (Tanaka et al 1991) and may be locally aggressive.

GIANT CELL FIBROBLASTOMA

Giant cell fibroblastoma is a benign, locally recurrent, mesenchymal tumor of young people. Three cases of this neoplasm involving the scrotal wall are recorded where the clinical features were those of a slow-growing nodule in the skin of the scrotal sac (Desanctis et al 1993).

CONNECTIVE TISSUE NEVI

These include a diverse group of hamartomatous lesions that contain abnormal amounts of abnormal collagen, elastin or proteoglycan. A case of elastoma has been described affecting the scrotum (**Fig. 9.79**). The 64-year-old patient presented with slowly enlarging lumps on the scrotal sac described as exophytic grape-like clusters of rubbery papules and nodules (Fork et al 1991).

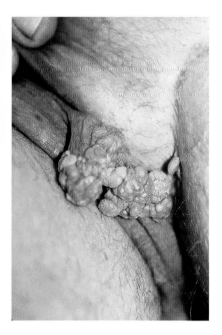

Fig. 9.79 Isolated exophytic elastoma. Scrotum (Courtesy of Dr Richard Wagner Jr, Galveston, Texas, USA. Reproduced from Fork HE et al. A new type of connective tissue nevus: isolated exophytic elastoma. J Cutan Pathol. 1991; 18: 457–63. © 1991 Munksgaard International Publishers Ltd, Copenhagen, Denmark.)

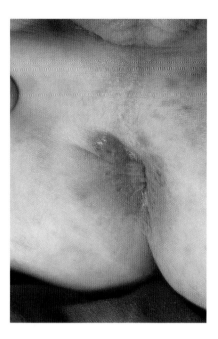

Fig. 9.81 Juvenile xanthogranuloma. Perineum. Infant. No complications.

FIBROUS HAMARTOMA OF INFANCY

This rare benign hamartoma has been reported to have affected the scrotum of a 13-month-old boy (Thami et al 1998)

XANTHOGRANULOMA

Juvenile xanthogranulomas are usually multiple small, orangey-yellowish, flat papules or nodules that are present at birth and then fade in the first year or two of life (Hernandez-Martin et al 1997; Chang 1999). They usually occur on the head and trunk but can involve the genitalia (Nomland 1954). **Figure 9.80** shows a focal penile eruption (Hautmann & Bachor 1993), but I have

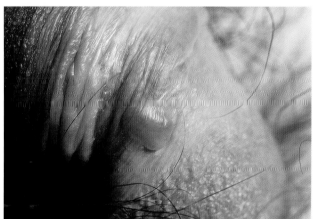

Fig. 9.82 Juvenile xanthogranuloma. Glans penis, right lateral coronal rim. Adult patient.

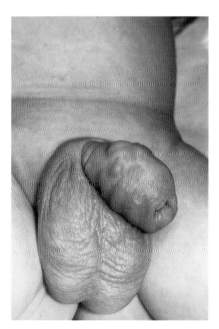

Fig. 9.80 Juvenile xanthogranuloma. Lateral shaft, penis. 2 months old. (Courtesy of Prof Richard Hautmann, Ulm, Germany. Reproduced with permission from Hautmann RE, Bachor R. Juvenile xanthogranuloma of the penis. J Urol. 1993: 150: 456–7.)

seen a solitary perineal papule (**Fig. 9.81**) and Goulding & Traylor (1983) described a scrotal swelling. The histology is of lipid-laden histiocytes and giant cells, negative for CD1 and S100 as found in Langerhans cell histiocytosis. Juvenile xanthogranuloma is not associated with abnormal lipids but there may be a relationship with urticaria pigmentosa, diabetes mellitus, neurofibromatosis, cytomegalovirus infection and leukemia (Cohen & Hood 1989). I have seen a clinically and histologically identical lesion in an adult (**Fig. 9.82**).

LEIOMYOMA

This is another unusual genital tumor presenting as a painless, slow-growing, palpable mass (papule or nodule), and/or difficulty with micturition (Dehner & Smith 1970) if it affects the penis; or swelling of the scrotum – where it arises from the tunica dartos scroti (Siegal & Gaffey 1976; Tomera et al 1981; Newman & Fletcher 1991; Ohtake et al 1997).

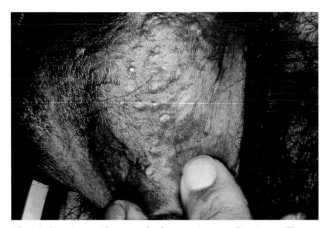

Fig. 9.83 Smooth muscle hamartoma. Scrotum. Firm, flesh-colored papules and nodules. (Courtesy of Guang-Hsiang Hsiao, Taipei, Taiwan. Reproduced with permission from Hsiao GH & Chen JS. Acquired genital smooth-muscle hamartoma. A case report. Am J Dermatopathol. 1995; 17: 67–70.)

GENITAL SMOOTH MUSCLE HAMARTOMA

A case has been described affecting the scrotum (**Fig. 9.83**) where the patient developed several rice grain- to pea-sized, skin-colored, firm papules and nodules over eight years (Hsiao & Chen 1995).

NEUROFIBROMA/ NEURILEMOMA/GRANULAR CELL MYOBLASTOMA

These tumors are rarely encountered on the penis but when they do occur (Dehner & Smith 1970; Maher et al 1988; Chan et al 1990) they present as a non-tender, progressive enlargement of well-circumscribed, doughy

to rubbery, subcutaneous papule or nodule (**Fig. 9.84**) or plexiform mass (Littlejohn et al 2000). Neurofibromas may indicate von Recklinghausen's disease (café au lait spots and Lisch nodules) and in this context are at risk of malignant change. A giant neurilemoma arising from the scrotum has been reported (Fernandez et al 1987).

VARICOSITIES

Varicosities (venous lakes) present as large, blue, distensible folds in the vaginal mucosa and labia. They are not very frequently encountered in men. In the vulva cutaneous venous vessels can become dilated due to the increased venous pressure of pregnancy. Venous varicosities are best left alone if asymptomatic because surgery is complicated by hemorrhage.

HEMORRHOIDS

Hemorrhoids/piles (pila = a ball) refer to dilatations in the venous system of vessels draining the anus or mucosal prolapse or loose tethering of mucosa to the anal wall (Kaufman 1981). Six percent of HIV-positive patients have been found to have piles (Yuhan et al 1998). Symptoms are rectal bleeding, mucous discharge, itch (pruritus ani) and prolapse (**Fig. 9.85**). The complications of piles are thrombosis (**Fig. 9.86**), strangulation, ulceration, fibrosis, infection and abscess, which give rise to pain.

These symptoms should be assessed by a proctologist and by proctoscopy and sigmoidoscopy. Signs depend on the presentation. Perianal skin tags from fibrosed piles are extremely common. The differential diagnosis obviously includes distal bowel cancer, as well as other benign cutaneous lesions such as nevi, Crohn's disease, Kaposi's sarcoma and perianal metastases (Sawh et al 2002). Treatment such as by anal dilatation (Lord 1973; Hancock 1981) is beyond the scope of this book and

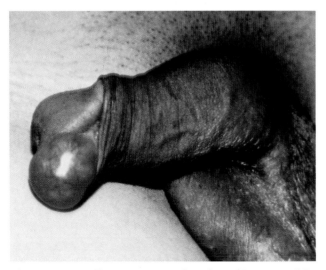

Fig. 9.84 Neurilemoma. Penis frenulum. (Courtesy of Dr Wai Pou Chan, Tainan, Taiwan.)

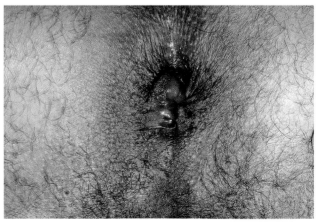

Fig. 9.85 Prolapsing piles. (Courtesy of Prof. Tim Allen-Mersh, London, UK.)

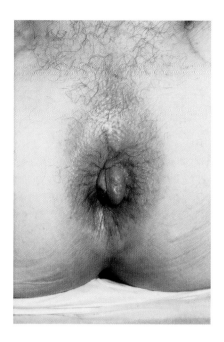

Fig. 9.86 Thrombosed pile. Necrotic portion. (Courtesy of Prof. Tim Allen-Mersh, London, UK.)

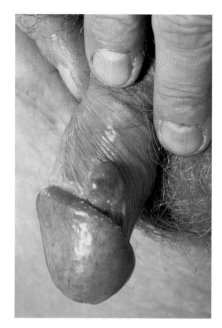

Fig. 9.87 Masson's tumor. Lateral distal shaft, penis. (Courtesy of Mr Alan Paul, Stockport, UK. Reproduced by kind permission of Blackwell Science Ltd from Paul AB et al. Masson's tumour of the penis. Br J Urol. 1994; 74: 261–2.)

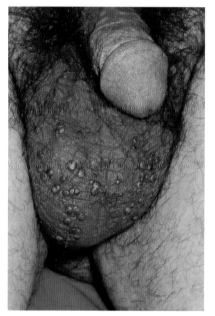

Fig. 9.88 Angiokeratomas. Scrotum.

properly the domain of the colorectal surgeon and gastroenterologist.

HEMANGIOMA

Cherry angiomas are discussed on page 16 and illustrated in Figures 1.56 and 1.57. Acquired capillary and cavernous hemangioma of the penis have been described (Dehner & Smith 1970). Other angiomatous lesions are very much more rare and it is controversial whether they represent a true neoplasm, herniation of the corpus spongiosum or vascularization of a hematoma or thrombus (Senoh et al 1981).

MASSON'S TUMOR

Masson's vegetant, intravascular hemangioendothelioma (Masson 1923) is probably a reactive vascular lesion with characteristic histological appearances of papillary fronds of endothelial cells and organizing thrombus lying in a blood vessel lumen. One case affecting the penis (Fig. 9.87) appears in the literature presenting as a bluish nodule in the coronal sulcus (Paul et al 1994).

ANGIOKERATOMA

Angiokeratomas are commoner in white men and common on the genitalia (where, confusingly, they also have attracted the eponymous epithet of Fordyce, as has ectopic sebaceous glands). They are blue to purple, smooth, 2–5mm papules on the scrotum (**Figs 9.88–9.93**) or penile shaft (**Figs 9.94, 9.95**) or even very

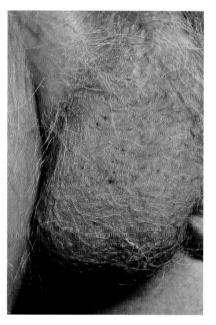

Fig. 9.89 Angiokeratomas. Scrotum.

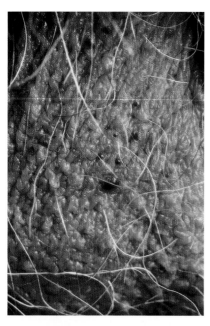

**Fig. 9.90
Angiokeratomas.**
Scrotum. Close-up.
Same case as Fig.
9.89.

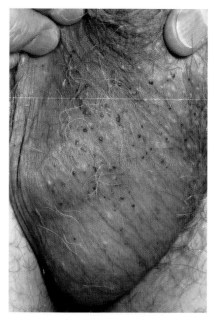

**Fig. 9.93
Angiokeratoma.**
Scrotum.

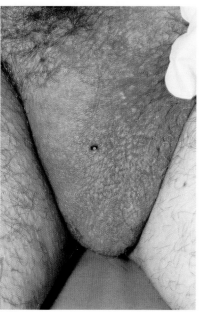

**Fig. 9.91
Angiokeratomas.**
Scrotum.

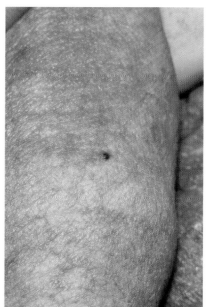

**Fig. 9.94
Angiokeratoma.**
Dorsal shaft,
penis.

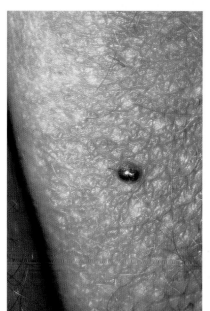

**Fig. 9.92
Angiokeratomas.**
Scrotum. Close-up.
Same case as
Fig. 9.91.

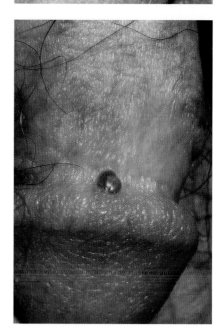

**Fig. 9.95
Angiokeratoma.**
Lateral coronal
sulcus, penis.
Solitary lesion.

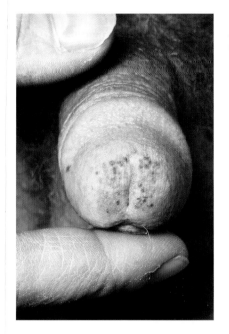

**Fig. 9.96
Angiokeratomas.**
Glans penis.
(Courtesy of
Dr Peter Copeman,
London, UK.)

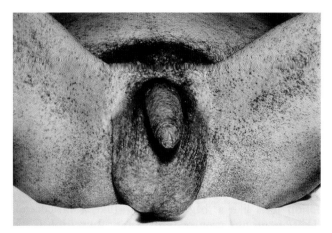

Fig. 9.97 Angiokeratoma corporis diffusum/Anderson-Fabry disease. Anterior pelvic girdle. Numerous pinhead angiokeratomas. (Courtesy of Dr Peter Copeman, London, UK.)

rarely the glans (**Fig. 9.96**, Carrasco et al 2000; Bechara et al 2002) that appear and multiply during life but occasionally present as singletons (Sutton 1911; Imperial & Helwig 1967; Taniguchi et al 1994; Bisceglia et al 1998). Very rarely they are found in the mouth (Karthikeyan et al 2000).

They may bleed following trauma (Hoekx & Wyndaele 1998) and can be mistaken for a nevus or melanoma. Sometimes the suspicion of Kaposi's sarcoma or bacillary angiomatosis is erroneously raised but this is a differential diagnosis that can usually be settled clinically and not require biopsy. However, the histology is characteristic (Gioglio et al 1992). Hyfrecation, electrocautery or laser ablation (Occella et al 1995) can be contemplated but the lesions can recur. Many patients are usually happy to be reassured.

ANGIOKERATOMA CORPORIS DIFFUSUM

This may be a feature of several, very rare congenital diseases affecting lysosomes. The angiokeratomas of Anderson-Fabry disease (α-galactosidase deficiency) are smaller than common angiokeratomas (see page 199), and less hyperkeratotic, and found more extensively around the lower limb girdle and upper thighs (Fig. 9.97), from the navel to the knees.

Apart from the skin signs patients usually present with intermittent, often excruciating pain in the fingers and toes, transient edema; hyperhidrosis and pyrexia are common. Renal damage is detectable early and is often the cause of death. Cerebrovascular and cardiac disturbances also occur and corneal dystrophy is usual. It is sex-linked recessive disorder of sphingolipid metabolism due to galactosidase deficiency. Males are severely affected whilst women may be asymptomatic throughout life (Wallace 1973). Histologically the

angiokeratoma may appear identical to essential angiokeratoma of Fordyce but biorefringent material can be seen in the vessel walls, Sudan black staining demonstrates the glycolipid in the vascular endothelium and electron microscopy shows cytoplasmic inclusion bodies in lysosomes. Birefringent cells are found in urine and blood α-galactosidase levels are reduced (Black 1998).

Other diseases such as fucosidosis may present and progress similarly.

ANGIOKERATOMA CIRCUMSCRIPTUM

Angiokeratoma circumscriptum of Mibelli is a rare, larger (than the angiokeratomas discussed above), local entity (preceded by a chilblain) and has hardly ever been reported to occur in the genital region (Bruce 1960).

GLOMUS TUMOR

This is an uncommon, tender, sometimes painful, vascular tumor. Cases affecting the glans penis have appeared in the literature (Dehner & Smith 1970; Macaluso et al 1985).

PORT WINE STAIN

A capillary nevus, present at birth, is a permanent lesion; flat and non-distensible. If cosmetically necessary then a capillary nevus (port wine stain) can be treated with the tunable dye laser.

HEMANGIOMA OF INFANCY

This may be present at birth but usually appears during the first few weeks and may grow rapidly and ulcerate (Liang & Frieden 2002). It is these features that can

201

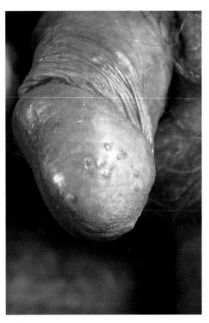

Fig. 9.102 Bowenoid papulosis. Glans penis. Patient with HIV. (Reproduced by kind permission of Blackwell Science Ltd from Bunker CB. Topics in penile dermatology. Clin Exp Dermatol. 2001; 26: 469–79.)

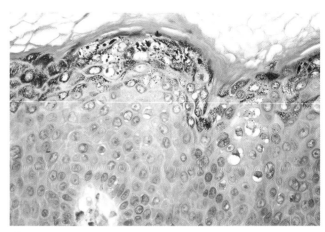

Fig. 9.105 Viral wart. Penis, high-power view. Increased keratohyaline granules; some perinuclear vacuolation; no dysplasia. (Courtesy of Dr Nick Francis, London, UK.)

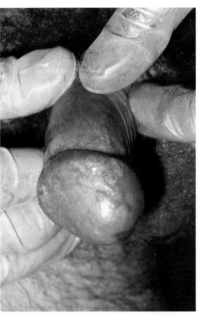

Fig. 9.103 Bowenoid papulosis. Glans penis. Patient with HIV.

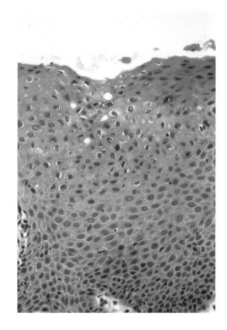

Fig. 9.106 Mild dysplasia. PIN 1/HPV. Penis, high-power view. Viral-type changes in upper epidermis; mild dysplasia in lower half. (Courtesy of Dr Nick Francis, London, UK.)

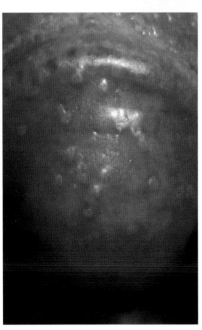

Fig. 9.104 Bowenoid papulosis. Glans penis. Patient with HIV.

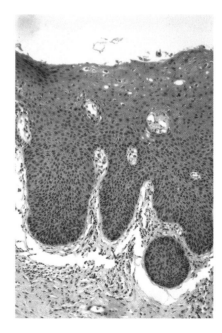

Fig. 9.107 Dysplasia. PIN2/HPV. Penis, medium-power view. Flat lesion; epithelial hyperplasia; superficial viral-type changes; crowding of nuclei; disorganization of maturation of keratinocytes in lower two-thirds of epidermis. (Courtesy of Dr Nick Francis, London, UK.)

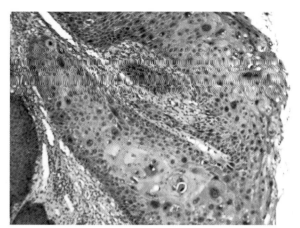

Fig. 9.108 Dysplasia. PIN2/HPV. Penis, high- to medium-power view. Condylomatous lesion with marked viral-type nuclear atypia, dyskeratosis and basal crowding of nuclei. (Courtesy of Dr Nick Francis, London, UK.)

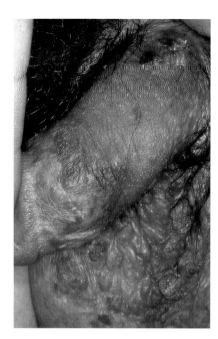

Fig. 9.109 Bowenoid papulosis. Scrotum and penic chaft. Multicentric genital pigmented papules. The patient also had extragenital warts Histology showed Bowenoid papulosis. Treated with surgery and intralesional bleomycin. (Courtesy of Dr Kyoung-C Park, Seoul, Korea.)

Bowenoid papulosis also affects younger, sexually active men. Generally intraepithelial neoplasia can be suspected morphologically (Aynaud et al 1994). If sought, intraepithelial neoplasia can be found in men being screened for HPV infection and has been demonstrated in acetowhite areas of penile skin (Zabbo & Stein 1993).

The condition was first described by Lloyd, who used the term multicentric, pigmented Bowen's disease of the groin (Lloyd 1970). It occurs in young, sexually active patients and in men is most common on the glans over the shaft, prepuce and groins. It can also be seen around the anus. In my practice a significant subgroup of patients has HIV infection. Bowenoid change has been reported in perianal warts associated with ulcerative colitis (Balazs 1991).

Bowenoid papulosis is probably HPV-induced epithelial dysplasia. HPV DNA (principally type 16) is present in most patients with Bowenoid papulosis. HPVs 1, 2, 6, 11, 18, 31, 32 33, 34, 35, 39, 42, 51, 52, 53, 54, 55 and 67, as well as mixed infections, have also been found (Ikenberg et al 1983; Gross et al 1985; Guerin-Reverchon et al 1990; Demeter et al 1993; Cupp et al 1995; Ranki et al 1995; Majewski & Jablonska 1997; Park et al 1998 (**Figs 9.109–9.113**); Salvatore et al 2000; Yoneta et al 2000). HPVs 16, 18 and 33 are considered the most oncogenic.

There may also be associated immunocompromise (Gibbs & Spittle 1995) but I believe a fundamental determinant is a susceptible immunogenotype. Voltz et al (1999) found anogenital warts in 16.5 of all HIV-positive males, nearly half of whom showed histological signs of intraepithelial neoplasia. There is a high prevalence of PIN in male sexual partners of women with cervical intraepithelial neoplasia (Barrasso et al 1987; Kennedy et al 1988) but many patients with PIN have consorts with no evidence of warts or worse.

Mutations of the tumor-suppressor gene *p53* are common in epithelial tumors and may contribute to the development of vulvar cancer. Although aberrant over-

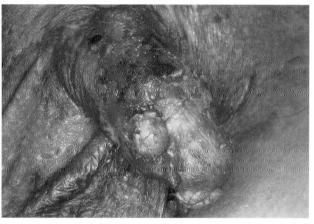

Fig. 9.110 Severe carcinoma in situ. Same patient as Fig. 9.109, six years later. Glans and shaft penis. Multifocal polymorphic change. Multiple biopsies showed Bowen's disease. The darkly pigmented papule at the base of the penis yielded HPV 33. The oozing erythematous plaque mid-shaft yielded HPV 16. (Courtesy of Dr Kyoung-C Park, Seoul, Korea. Reproduced by kind permission of Blackwell Science Ltd from Park KC et al. Heterogenety of human papillomavirus DNA in a patient with Bowenoid papulosis that progressed to a squamous cell carcinoma. Br J Dermatol. 1998; 139: 1087 91.)

expression of *p53* may be found in 40% of lesions of genital warts and Bowenoid papulosis in men (Ranki et al 1995) this does not indicate a *p53* mutation in male genital warts, premalignant lesions or frank squamous carcinoma, suggesting that *p53* mutations are not important at all or at least not in early events in male genital carcinogenesis (Castren et al 1998).

Bowenoid papulosis can be suspected clinically but should be confirmed and graded histologically following a biopsy. Bowenoid papulosis may be mistaken for viral warts, lichen planus, basal cell papilloma, nevi, mollusca and condylomata lata (secondary syphilis). Solitary

205

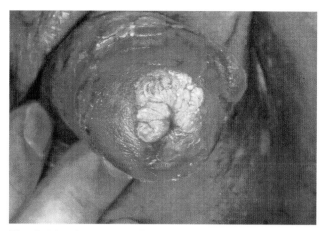

Fig. 9.111 Severe carcinoma in situ. Same case as Figs 9.109, 9.110; same time point as Fig 9.110. Glans penis. Peri meatal verrucous plaque. Biopsy showed Bowen's disease. This lesion yielded HPV 6b. (Courtesy of Dr Kyoung-C Park, Seoul, Korea. Reproduced by kind permission of Blackwell Science Ltd from Park KC et al. Heterogeneity of human papillomavirus DNA in a patient with Bowenoid papulosis that progressed to a squamous cell carcinoma. Br J Dermatol. 1998; 139: 1087–91.)

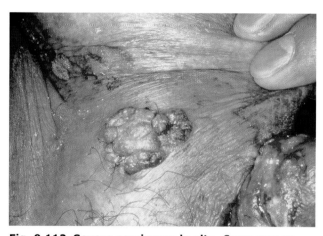

Fig. 9.112 Severe carcinoma in situ. Same case as Figs 9.109, 9.110 and 9.111. Scrotum. Warty nodule. Biopsy showed Bowen's disease. This lesion yielded HPV 18. (Courtesy of Dr Kyoung-C Park, Seoul, Korea. Reproduced by kind permission of Blackwell Science Ltd from Park KC et al. Heterogeneity of human papillomavirus DNA in a patient with Bowenoid papulosis that progressed to a squamous cell carcinoma. Br J Dermatol. 1998; 139: 1087–91.)

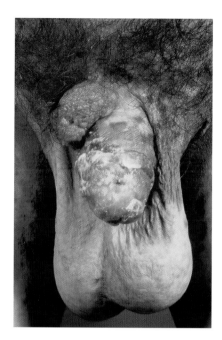

Fig. 9.113 Squamous carcinoma. Same patient as Figs 9.109, 9.112. Four years after Fig. 9.110, having been treated with extensive plastic surgery and grafting. Penis. Large nodule proximal shaft of penis. (Courtesy of Dr Kyoung-C Park, Seoul, Korea. Reproduced by kind permission of Blackwell Science Ltd from Park KC et al. Heterogeneity of human papillomavirus DNA in a patient with Bowenoid papulosis that progressed to a squamous cell carcinoma. Br J Dermatol. 1998; 139: 1087–91.)

The treatment of Bowenoid papulosis may not be straightforward (Gerber 1994). Cryotherapy or curettage and cautery are popular but there may be recurrence. Topical 5-fluorouracil can be useful (Kossow et al 1980). Laser therapy and micrographic surgery are under evaluation. Topical imiquimod is held to be successful (Wigbels et al 2001). Imiquimod and 5-fluorouracil have been used in combination for perianal and anal squamous carcinoma in situ in HIV (Pehoushek & Smith 2001). Topical cidofovir holds promise (Snoeck et al 2001).

The risk of progression to invasive squamous carcinoma is not known but is probably low in the absence of other risk factors especially immunocompromise. However, cases have occurred and **Figs 9.109–9.113** illustrate the fate of one patient (Park et al 1998) over a ten-year period.

ANAL INTRAEPITHELIAL NEOPLASIA

Anal intraepithelial neoplasia is a well-described pathological precursor of invasive squamous cancer of the anus and perianal skin (Zbar et al 2002). It can present relatively asymptomatically as red shiny or scaly

lesions have a wider differential diagnosis including many of the other conditions discussed in this chapter. A biopsy is indicated in most instances. The histology is of squamous carcinoma in situ with full thickness epithelial atypia (see Figs 9.104–9.108 and compare with Figs 6.235–6.237, see pages 115–116).

Patients presenting with Bowenoid papulosis and their sexual partners should be counseled and screened for other sexually transmitted diseases including HIV infection.

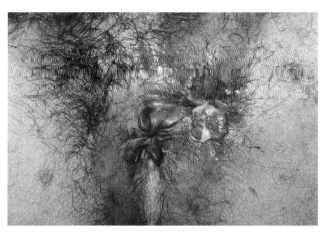

Fig. 9.114 AIN2/HIV. Perianal skin. Erosions and patchy warty change. (Courtesy of Prof Tim Allen-Mersh, London, UK.)

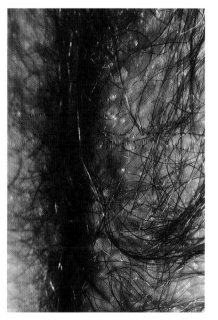

Fig. 9.115 AIN3. Perianal skin. Warty change. Right anal verge. No HPV present. (Courtesy of Prof. Tim Allen-Mersh, London, UK.)

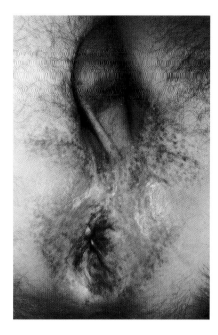

Fig. 9.116 AIN/ radiodermatitis. The AIN has relapsed despite radiotherapy. (Courtesy of Prof. Tim Allen-Mersh, London, UK.)

elicit regression of AIN (Martin & Bower 2001). Expression of Ki-67 may predict which low-grade AIN lesions may recur in patients with AIDS (Calore et al 2001).

KERATOACANTHOMA

Keratoacanthoma is an interesting cutaneous tumor. It is a rapidly growing (2 weeks–2 months) firm, flesh-colored, symmetrical, dome-shaped nodule, centrally umbilicated and plugged with a keratinaceous horn. It remains static for a few weeks and then involutes spontaneously over a similar period to leave a scar. Keratoacanthoma occurs on the sun-exposed skin of elderly people. I have not found an account of a genital presentation but cases have apparently been encountered around the anus. Clinically and histologically it can be difficult if not impossible to differentiate from squamous carcinoma, so complete surgical removal is advised (Küppers et al 2000).

BASAL CELL CARCINOMA

Basal cell carcinoma is a locally invasive hence malignant neoplasm of the pilosebaceous apparatus. Although the most common type of skin cancer it is rare in the anogenital area. only a hundred or so cases have been described (McGregor et al 1982; Gerber 1985; Goldminz et al 1989; Greenbaum et al 1989; Augey et al 1994; Laducsi et al 1998; Gomez et al 1999; Smith & Black 1999; Gibson & Ahmed 2001), because sun exposure is more important as an etiological factor than biological age. However, one case in a black man (Greenbaum et al 1989) and one in a Tunisian (Kort et al 1995) appear in the literature. There has been one

patches (like Bowen's disease of the penis or erythroplasia of Queyrat, see page 110) or as warty lesions like Bowenoid papulosis (**Figs 9.114, 9.115,** see also Fig. 6.234). HPV is strongly implicated in the pathogenesis of AIN and is associated with homosexuality; anal warts and HIV infection are independent risk factors; AIN is common in HIV infection (Palefsky 1991; Carter et al 1995; Zbar et al 2002), although not a prominent feature of other immunosuppressed states in my experience. Routine surveillance of the HIV-positive patient with anal cytology is the ideal (Kotlarewsky et al 2001; Martin & Bower 2001).

Treatment is controversial and problematic with relapse common. Radiotherapy, for example, is frequently complicated by relapse (**Fig 9.116**) The overall risk of progression of AIN associated with anal HPV wart infection to invasive squamous carcinoma is low (Morgan et al 1994) but there is the possibility that immuno-reconstitution with HAART in HIV does not

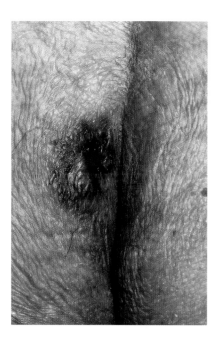

Fig. 9.117 Basal cell carcinoma. Buttocks. Irregular pigmented ulcerating plaque. Malignant melanoma was suspected clinically. Histology confirmed basal cell carcinoma.

case report of the variant fibroepithelioma of Pinkus affecting the base of the penis (Heymann et al 1983).

Prior genital irradiation for cancer or ringworm is a theoretical risk factor that appertains to basal cell carcinoma at other sites. Basal cell carcinoma 'never' metastasizes but this has been very rarely documented, including in the case of multiple erosive scrotal basal cell carcinoma (Staley et al 1983).

Irritation, pain, bleeding, discharge or the discovery of a lump may point to a basal cell carcinoma, which on examination presents as an indolent nodule or ulcer with a pearly edge. Occasionally, pigmented (**Fig. 9.117**) or flat and morpheic morphologies are encountered.

The classical histopathology of basal cell carcinoma consists of foci of basaloid proliferation with peripheral palisading of tumor cells. These foci are separated by clefts of bland stroma (Lucia & Miller 1992).

Basal cell carcinoma can be a straightforward clinical diagnosis elsewhere on the body but less easy in the anogenital area where it may not be suspected because of its rarity.

Surgical excision is the treatment of choice although radiotherapy has been used for the latter (Augey et al 1994). At other sites cryotherapy has its enthusiasts. Moh's micrographic surgery (Brown et al 1988) and intralesional chemosurgery are other options.

SQUAMOUS CELL CARCINOMA

Anogenital squamous carcinoma is sometimes called epidermoid carcinoma. The etiology is not clearly understood but HPV is implicated (McDougall 1994; Kadish 2001). Considerable challenges exist in diagnosis and management.

Carcinoma of the penis accounts for less than 1% of deaths from cancer in the USA. There are approximately 100 deaths per year in the UK and this has been steady over several decades. It is claimed to constitute 10–20% of tumors seen in males in either underdeveloped countries or in areas where early circumcision is not routinely practiced (Muir & Nectoux 1979; Droller 1980; Micali et al 1996; Soria et al 1998).

The earliest stages of penis cancer and precancer form a spectrum of disease (Grossman 1992). Although some penile cancers arise de novo, premalignant states may be misdiagnosed or mismanaged and not followed up, or may be difficult to diagnose, manage and follow up (von Krogh & Horenblas 2000). There are also the issues of multifocality and field change (Cubilla et al 1993) and evolution (the dynamic) to acknowledge.

The precise etiology of the types of penile intraepithelial neoplasia (PIN) (see page 203), verrucous carcinoma (see page 214) and frank invasive squamous cell carcinoma of the penis is unknown, as is their precise relationship to the various types of precursor lesion. However, Cubilla et al (2000) have defined several types of preceeding epithelial abnormality, squamous hyperplasia and SIL: squamous, basaloid or warty, high or low grade).

The presence of a foreskin confers cancer risk. Circumcision appears to protect against penile carcinoma (Wolbarst 1932; Schrek & Lenowitz 1947; Schoen et al 2000) *unless* the circumcision was performed for penile disease (Holly & Palefsky 1993; Maden et al 1993). However, there have been very rare cases in Jews and others circumcised at birth (Melmed & Payne 1967; Boczko & Freed 1979; Rogus 1987).

Carcinoma of the penis is more common in males in either underdeveloped countries or in areas where early circumcision is not routinely practiced (Droller 1980; Schoeneich et al 1999). But the incidence of penis cancer is *low* in Japan and Denmark where circumcision is rare (Williams & Kapila 1993; Frisch et al 1995) so other factors are important in the carcinogenesis

Phimosis and balanitis are known risk factors for penile cancer (Wolbarst 1932; Muir & Nectoux 1979; Reddy et al 1984; Lucia & Miller 1992; Maiche 1992). Poor personal and sexual hygiene (Schrek & Lenowitz 1947) and phimosis may lead to the retention of smegma and balanitis. But the carcinogenicity of human smegma has not been ascertained (Hellberg et al 1987). Also, it has not been widely appreciated that phimosis is a physical sign and not a diagnosis. There may be more in the carcinogenic propensity of phimosis than simply physical retention of smegma.

Lichen sclerosus is a common cause of phimosis in males and lichen sclerosus is a premalignant condition (and predisposes to penile carcinoma (Bart & Kopf 1978; Bingham 1978; Schnitzler et al 1987; Pride et al 1993; Bunker 2001): Powell et al (2001) and Perceau et al (2003) have found that half of patients with penis cancer had a clinical history and/or histological evidence of lichen sclerosus; chronic erosive and hypertrophic lichen planus are premalignant conditions and lichen planus is a cause of phimosis (Worheide et al 1991; Itin et al 1992). An underlying skin disorder was found in 22 out of 23 patients with vulval squamous carcinoma (Derrick et al 2000).

Chronic irritation and inflammation or scarring are all risk factors for squamous carcinoma of the skin generally and the penis is not an exception – penis cancer complicating a burn scar has been reported (Selli et al 1999). Quantifying the malignant potential of the precancerous dermatoses, BDP/EQ/PIN, is not possible but they are acknowledged risks for penile cancer (Blau & Hyman 1955; Graham & Helwig 1973; Gerber 1994).

Smoking is a risk factor independent of phimosis for penile carcinoma (Lucia & Miller 1992) and is also a recognized risk factor for anal cancer (Moore et al 2001) and cervical cancer (Muir & Nectoux 1979). Smoking may cause squamoepithelial cancer not only in parts of the body in contact with smoke but also at distant sites by dissemination of carcinogens in the circulation or in secretions (Winkelstein 1977; Sasson et al 1985). The presence of tobacco-specific nitrosamines in the preputial secretions of rats has been demonstrated (Castonguay et al 1983).

Penile carcinoma is a complication of PUVA photochemotherapy (Perkins et al 1990; Stern et al 1990; Stern et al 2002) and possibly other treatments for psoriasis (de la Brassinne & Richert 1992; Loughlin 1997) and vitiligo (Park et al 2003). The photo dye treatment of genital herpes simplex was curtailed in the 1970s because of the occurrence of Bowen's disease of the penis in young men without other risk factors for erythroplasia (Berger & Papa 1977). However, increased UV exposure of the genitals due to sunlamps and sun beds had not led to an increase in genital skin cancer in the USA by 1986 (Goldoft & Weiss 1992).

Although penis cancer is associated with multiple sexual partners and previous sexually transmitted disease including HIV, the epidemiological features are *not* those characteristic of a sexually transmitted disease (Hellberg et al 1987), unlike carcinoma of the cervix and to a lesser extent anal carcinoma (Bosch et al 1995). In cervical cancer the evidence is that it is a sexually transmitted disease and that HPV is the etiological agent (zur Hausen 1985; Keerti 1997; Walboomers & Meijer 1997). Yet penile cancer puts wives and consorts at risk of cervical cancer (Smith et al 1980); there is a high prevalence of PIN in sexual partners of women with cervical intraepithelial neoplasia (CIN) (Barrasso et al 1987; Kennedy et al 1988) and PIN can be found in men being screened for HPV infection (Zabbo & Stein 1993).

So the role of HPV is still not certain. Many patients with penis cancer have no evidence of viral infection yet giant condylomas should be suspect. Oncogenic HPV particularly types 16 and 18 have been incriminated but also types 6, 31, 33, 35, 45, 52 and 68 (Durst et al 1983; Boshart et al 1984; Villa & Lopes 1986; Löning et al 1988; Strickler et al 1998; Maiche 1992; Cupp et al

1995; Majewski & Jablonska 1997; Griffiths & Mellon 1999; Picconi et al 2000; Bezerra et al 2001; Rubin et al 2001).

The influence of HPV may be variable. In Brazil, Villa & Lopes (1986) found HPV IV in 41% penile squamous carcinomas, and, in Argentina, Picconi et al (2000) found HPV DNA in 71% of 65 penis cancers, 81% of which were 'high risk' HPV with predominance of HPV 18. Gregoire et al (1995) associated HPV with higher-grade, more aggressive, squamous carcinomas of predominantly the glans penis showing basaloid changes.

Specific histological types of penis cancer – warty and basaloid – are consistently associated with HPV whereas only a subset of keratinizing and verrucous penile cancers contains HPV DNA (Rubin et al 2001). The overall low frequency of HPV in penile squamous carcinoma suggests (Gregoire et al 1995; Cubilla et al 2000) that only a small proportion of these cancers can arise from HPV-associated squamous intraepithelial lesions (SILs). Like for vulvar cancer (Leibowitch et al 1990; Jones et al 1997), a bimodal hypothesis of HPV-related and non-HIV-related causation has evolved (Cubilla et al 2000; Horenblas et al 2000; Rubin et al 2001).

Penis cancer has been reported to complicate immunosuppression both congenital and acquired, e.g. iatrogenic, as in renal transplantation (Previte et al 1979) and the treatment of lupus erythematosus (personal experience: see Fig. 9.124), and associated with HIV (Poblet et al 1999).

The historical associations of squamous cancer of the scrotum (Graves & Spencer 1940; Lowe 1983; Gerber 1985; Grossman 1992) afflicting chimney sweeps (exposed to carcinogens in soot (Potts 1779), the carcinogen is 3,4-benzpyrene), mule spinners (exposed to carcinogens in lubricating oils for the spinning jenny that heralded the mechanization of the cloth industry) and other occupations, is well known. Persian nomads developed the disease because they traveled with pots of burning charcoal between their legs. A recent occupational risk in jute oil processing in India has been reported (Murthy 1993). Oil mist exposure in industry is widespread and conjectured to be associated with scrotal cancer and other problems, cutaneous and respiratory (Karube et al 1995).

Other individuals at risk of scrotal squamous carcinoma include those with a history of psoriasis (**Fig. 9.118**) treated with arsenic, coal tar, UVB and PUVA (Ray & Whitmore 1977; McGarry & Robertson 1989; Perkins et al 1990; Stern et al 1990; Gross & Schosser 1991; Loughlin 1997), previous radiotherapy treatment (Ray & Whitmore 1977), scrotal HPV infection, hidradenitis suppurativa and multiple cutaneous keratoses and epitheliomas (Dean 1940; Black & Woods 1982; Andrews et al 1991; Burmer et al 1993). Black men are not exempt although the disease is rare (Lowe 1985).

Anal carcinoma (Vieyra et al 1997) is often associated with a history of anogenital warts. More than 90% of anogenital condylomata contain contain HPV 6 or 11.

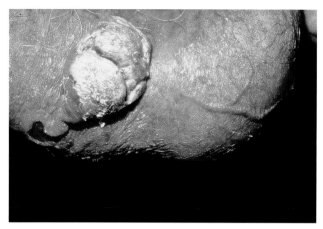

Fig. 9.118 Squamous carcinoma. Scrotum. Long history of psoriasis treated with topical steroids, tar, anthralin and UVB (including a 'home-built' box). (Courtesy of Dr David J Gross, St Augustine, FL, USA. Reproduced by permission from Gross DJ & Schosser RH. Squamous cell carcinoma of the scrotum. Cutis. 1991; 47: 402–4. Copyright 1991 by Quadrant Healthcom Inc.)

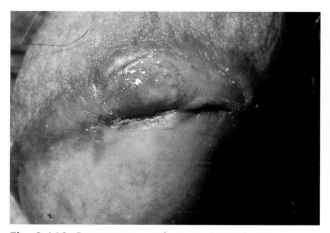

Fig. 9.119 Squamous carcinoma. Coronal sulcus, penis. Nodule and background lichen sclerosus.

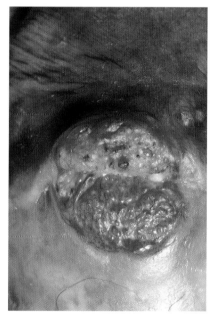

Fig. 9.120 Squamous carcinoma. Coronal sulcus. Ulcer and background lichen sclerosus.

Although these subtypes are not associated with cancer, anogenital HPV infection is a risk factor for anogenital cancer particularly of the anus (and cervix). Yet it is rare for condylomata to contain HPV 16 which has a well-documented association with anal carcinoma. Homosexual men have a higher incidence of both perianal warts and anal carcinoma (both in situ and invasive) and this may be related to receptive anal intercourse, HPV (Gal et al 1987) and other sexually transmitted diseases such as gonorrhea, herpes simplex and *Chlamydia trachomatis* infection.

Warts and these latter listed infections are also risk factors for anal carcinoma in heterosexual men and women, as is cigarette smoking (Daling et al 1987). A role for seminal fluid prostaglandins in homosexual anal cancer has been posited (Kondlapoodi 1982).

Immunosuppression, including by HIV, is a risk factor for AIN and anal cancer (Gibbs & Spittle 1995; Vieyra et al 1997; Aranyi et al 2001). A case of Peutz-Jeghers syndrome associated with anal squamous carcinoma has been reported (Mullhaupt et al 2001).

Itch, irritation, pain, bleeding, discharge, ulceration or the discovery of a lump presage squamous cell carcinoma (**Figs 9.119–9.126**). There is usually a long history of problems with the penis and foreskin amounting to dyspareunia, balanoposthitis or phimosis and dysuria. Irregular nodular and ulcerative morphology is encountered. Background BDP/EQ/BP or lichen sclerosus (or even lichen planus) may be appreciated. Only once has a pigmented squamous carcinoma of the genitalia (scrotum) been reported (Matsumoto et al 1999). Phimosis should be regarded as a sinister situation and impedes complete inspection and palpation of the glans and coronal sulcus. The presence or absence of inguinal lymphadenopathy should be ascertained although in penile cancer only 50% of

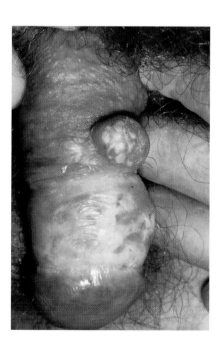

Fig. 9.121 Squamous carcinoma. Distal prepuce. Nodule and background lichen sclerosus.

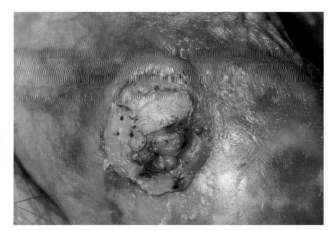

Fig. 9.122 Squamous carcinoma. Coronal rim. Warty nodule with background lichen sclerosus.

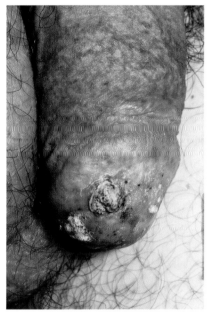

Fig. 9.123 Squamous carcinoma. Glans penis. Unstable glans. Several foci of invasive carcinoma on background field of intraepithelial neoplasia. Note radiodermatitis of penile shaft from prior radiotherapy.

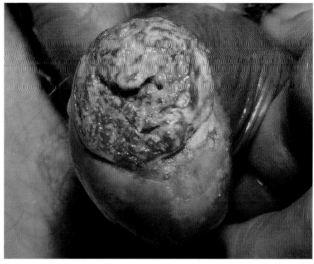

Fig. 9.125 Squamous carcinoma. Glans penis. (Courtesy of Dr Peter Copeman, London, UK).

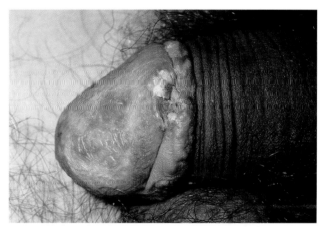

Fig. 9.126 Squamous carcinoma. Coronal rim. (Courtesy of Dr Peter Copeman, London, UK).

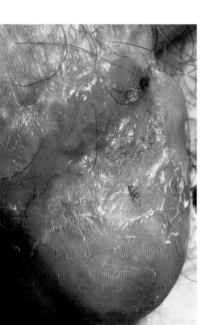

Fig. 9.124 Squamous carcinoma. Lateral glans penis. Nodule in coronal sulcus. Patient with systemic lupus erythematosus and long-standing iatrogenic immunosuppression. Unstable glans with severe intraepithelial neoplasia and previous penile tip carcinoma excised and circumcision performed. Same case as Fig. 6.225.

enlarged glands will be found to contain tumor (Droller 1980). It is important to establish the presence of other disease states, particularly sexually transmitted diseases and immunocompromise (Heyns et al 1997).

Anal carcinoma (Stearns et al 1980; Boman et al 1984; Fenger 1991) often presents with similar symptoms to benign anal lesions such as piles and fissures, i.e. pruritus, discomfort or pain and bleeding.

Squamous carcinoma should be suspected in all nodulo ulcerative anogenital disease especially in the context of lichen sclerosus, lichen planus, hidradenitis suppurativa, intraepithelial neoplasia and immunocompromise. The differential diagnosis includes the manifestations of intraepithelial neoplasia and the differential diagnosis of these: erosive or ulcerative sexually transmitted disease, basal cell carcinoma, Kaposi's sarcoma, pyoderma gangrenosum and artefact.

The differential diagnosis also includes that of ischiorectal or perianal abscess. Genitourinary, urological and/or colorectal assessment should be sought. Procto-

211

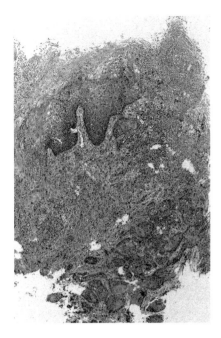

Fig. 9.127 Invasive squamous carcinoma. The surface shows hyperkeratosis and acanthosis. Deep to that there is chronic inflammation and extensive infiltration of the underlying tissue by islands of moderately differentiated squamous carcinoma.

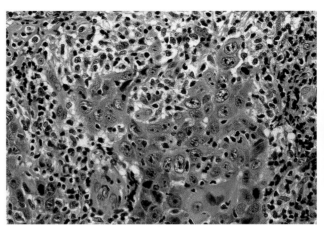

Fig. 9.129 Invasive squamous carcinoma. There is pleomorphism, individual cell apoptotic degeneration and necrosis and some keratinization together with increased numbers of mitotic figures. Same case as Fig. 9.128.

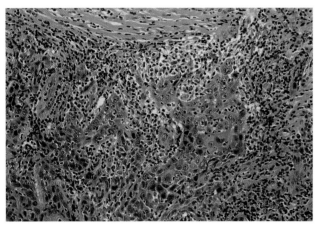

Fig. 9.128 Invasive squamous carcinoma. Invasive, moderately to poorly differentiated squamous carcinoma, showing irregularity of epidermal cell cords with associated chronic inflammation.

scopy and sigmoidoscopy are necessary to exclude anorectal cancer (Drumm et al 1982; Tait & Sykes 1982; Taylor et al 1982). A low threshold for performing a biopsy is essential.

Histologically, in squamous carcinoma, tongues of invasive atypical keratinocytes invade the dermis and contain foci of aberrant and ectopic keratinization called squamous pearls (Lucia & Miller 1992) (Figs 9.127–9.129). Background histological signs of lichen sclerosus are commonly found in vulval carcinoma in women and penis cancer in men (Powell et al 2001).

Verrucous carcinoma is discussed below. Three cases of surface adenosquamous carcinoma of the penis have been encountered by Cubilla et al (1996). Spindle cell carcinoma is a rare variant that has only involved the penis on two or three documented occasions (Patel et al 1982). Telomerase activity is high in penis cancer (Alves et al 2001).

Cubilla et al (1993) studied 66 cases of penis cancer and identified four types: 1) superficial spreading (42%), i.e. a biphasic infiltrative and radially extensive carcinoma in situ contiguously involving several anatomical sites or compartments (glans, coronal sulcus, foreskin even urethra), 2) vertical growth (32%), i.e. unifocal, high grade, deeply invasive, unassociated with carcinoma in situ; 3) verrucous (18%), i.e. low grade, papillary or endophytic (see below); 4) multicentric (8%), i.e. two or more independent primary tumors without contiguous field change. These observations have important applicability in understanding the pathogenesis of the different types and determining management in individual cases.

The treatment of squamous carcinoma is not generally the province of the dermatologist. Generally, it must be treated by adequate surgical excision (including circumcision for disease of the penis). The surgery may need to be radical (Prosvic et al 1997), total or partial (Figs 9.130–9.136), depending on location and extent (Heyns et al 1997; Schoeneich et al 1999). To maximize residual sexual function, conservative plastic techniques are increasingly used (Donnelan & Webb 1998) as are laser treatment (Tietjen & Malek 1998) and Mohs micrographic surgery (Mohs et al 1985; Bernstein et al 1986; Brown et al 1987, 1988) for squamous carcinoma of the penis, but the concepts of field change and infection by HPV and multifocality need to be clearly understood and bargained for.

The management of anal carcinoma requires maximum retention of sphincter function often involving combined radiotherapy and chemotherapy (Chawla & Willett 2001; Esiashvili et al 2002).

Lymphatic or hematogenous dissemination requires individualized multidisciplinary management: management of ilioinguinal lymphadenopathy is controversial (McDougal et al 1986; Heyns et al 1997; Schoeneich et al 1999). Combination chemotherapy has been used for

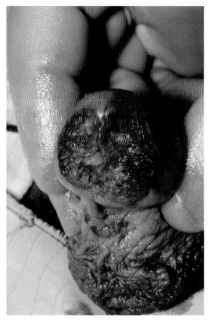

Fig. 9.130 Squamous carcinoma. Glans penis. Prior to partial penile amputation. (Courtesy of Mr Mike Dinneen, London, UK.)

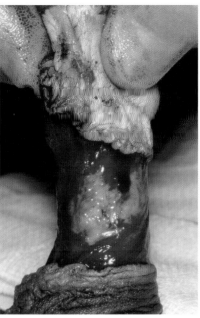

Fig. 9.131 Circumferential incision. (Courtesy of Mr Mike Dinneen, London, UK.)

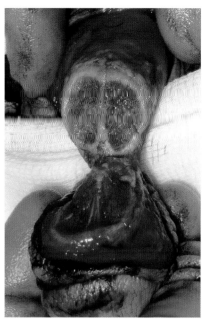

Fig. 9.132 Amputation. (Courtesy of Mr Mike Dinneen, London, UK.)

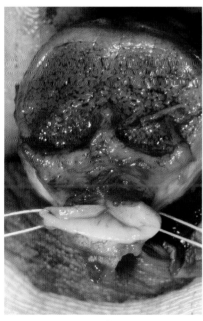

Fig. 9.133 Identification of urethra. (Courtesy of Mr Mike Dinneen, London, UK.)

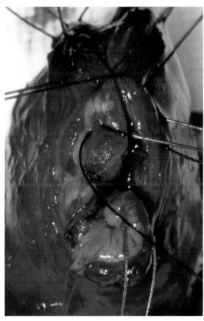

Fig. 9.134 Internal repair. (Courtesy of Mr Mike Dinneen, London, UK.)

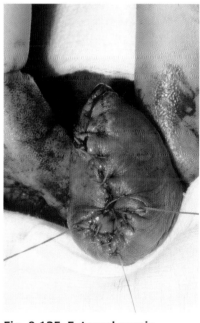

Fig. 9.135 External repair. (Courtesy of Mr Mike Dinneen, London, UK.)

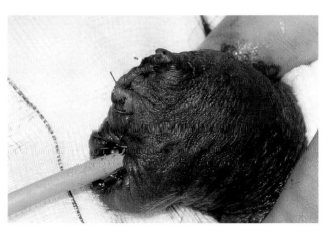

Fig. 9.136 Catheterization. (Courtesy of Mr Mike Dinneen, London, UK.)

palliation and proposed for adjuvant treatment of carcinoma of the penis but remains under evaluation (Dexeus et al 1991; Schoeneich et al 1999; Roth et al 2000).

The prognosis of penis cancer relates to the extent of inguinal lymphadenopathy (Droller 1980; Srinivas et al 1987) and involvement of the corpus (Soria et al 1997). It does not correlate with HPV status (Bezerra et al 2001).

The prognosis for scrotal carcinoma is not good despite apparently adequate primary surgical treatment: the five-year mortality is 50–60% (Lowe 1983; Gerber 1985).

The prognosis for anal carcinoma is variable (Esiashvili et al 2002). Penile cancer puts wives and consorts at risk of cervical cancer (Smith et al 1980). In black men who develop penile cancer there is a substantial risk (18%) of the later development of a second primary malignancy (Hubbell et al 1988).

BUSCHKE-LOWENSTEIN TUMOR/VERRUCOUS CARCINOMA/GIANT CONDYLOMA

Buschke-Lowenstein tumor and verrucous carcinoma can probably be regarded as synonymous; they are rare but probably represent verrucous, low-grade, well-differentiated squamous carcinoma. It is probably more accurate and more clinically useful to consider giant condyloma as a separate HPV-related entity with a better prognosis but controversy exists (Schwartz et al 1991; Niederauer et al 1993; Schwartz 1993; Anadolu 1999; Dogan et al 1998; Codina et al 1999; Cubilla et al 2000).

These are dramatic clinical lesions (**Figs 9.122, 9.137–9.139**, see also Fig 6.233) often polypoid or cauliflower-like. Presentation as a penile cutaneous horn has been described (Yeager et al 1990; Karthikeyan et al 1998). Although locally deeply invasive the tumor is well demarcated from surrounding tissue and probably does not metastasize. Frank squamous carcinoma (Sturm et al 1975; Bertram et al 1995) and foci of invasive squamous carcinoma (Johnson et al 1985) have been reported in some cases of verrucous carcinoma. Women can be affected (Doutre et al 1979).

A specific etiology for verrucous carcinoma of Buschke-Lowenstein has not been irrefutably identified but an apparent origin from genital warts is thought likely. The association of a penile lesion with intraurethral warts in an HIV-positive patient has been reported (Perez et al 1991). HPV types 6 and 11 are most commonly associated (Boshart & zur Hausen 1986; Schwartz et al 1991; Noel et al 1992; Niederauer et al 1993; Grassegger et al 1994; Gonzalez-Lopez et al 1997; Dianzani et al 1998; Yagi et al 1998; Anadolu et al 1999; Haycox et al 1999). A case in a two-month-old

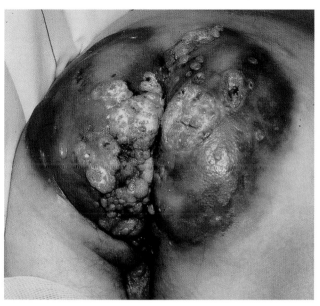

Fig. 9.137 Verrucous carcinoma/Buschke-Loewenstein tumor. Buttocks. Extensive anogenital tumor (with infiltration of pelvic organs). (Courtesy of Dr Alfred Grasseger, Innsbruck, Austria. Reproduced by kind permission of Blackwell Science Ltd from Grassegger A et al. Buschke-Loewenstein tumour infiltrating pelvic organs. Br J Dermatol. 1994; 130: 221 5.)

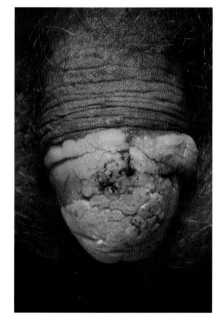

Fig. 9.138 Buschke-Lowenstein tumor/verrucous carcinoma. Circumstantial evidence of prior lichen sclerosus for which the patient had been circumcised several years previously.

Japanese baby boy was HPV 16-associated (Matsumura et al 1992). A patient taking ciclosporin for psoriasis developed a verrucous carcinoma containing HPV 6 and 16 (Piepkorn et al 1993). Multiple HPV types were found in a case obtained from a transplant patient (Soler et al 1992). Tumors containing several HPV types may be mixed verrucous carcinoma containing or adjacent to squamous carcinoma (Noel & de Dobbeleer 1994). Cases emanating from background lichen sclerosus have occurred (Weber et al 1987; Micali et al 2001), yet

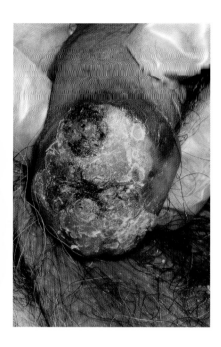

Fig. 9.139
Verrucous
carcinoma.
Glans penis

inanition and death (South et al 1977). Even with treatment recurrence and progressive malignant transformation do occur (Tessler & Applebaum 1982; Croneman et al 1988) so rigorous follow up is advocated.

EXTRA-MUCOSAL ANORECTAL CARCINOMA

Zeinberg & Kays (1957) make the point that there are many cases in the literature of cancers arising from anal glands adjacent to the anorectal wall and not emergent from the mucosa. These frequently present as an inflammatory rather than a malignant condition so are not biopsied (or not biopsied deeply) and the diagnosis is missed or delayed.

Cloacogenic carcinoma constitutes only 2–3% of anorectal cancer but may behave aggressively depending on the histology (Serota et al 1981). They emerge from remnants of the cloacal membrane proximal to the pectinate line where there is an area of mucosa transitional between keratinized and non-keratinized squamous epithelium, penetrated by the anal glands.

Most rectal cancer is adenocarcinoma (derived from columnar epithelium).

MALIGNANT MELANOMA

This is a very rare condition of the penis and there are less than 100 cases in the literature. It is estimated to account for 1–1.5% of all malignancies of the penis (Johnson & Ayala 1973; Stillwell et al 1988) and less than 0.15% of all melanomas (Cascinelli 1969). Sixty to seventy percent of penile lesions occur on the glans.

Melanoma is even rarer on the scrotum with only four cases appearing in the literature (Gerber 1985; Davis et al 1991), whereas vulval melanoma represents 3–7% of melanomas in women and 8–11% of all malignancies, second only to squamous cell carcinoma (Johnson et al 1993). Anorectal melanoma accounts for only 1% of all tumors of this area (Johnson et al 1993); it may occur concomitantly with melanosis of the gastrointestinal tract (Horowitz & Nobrega 1998).

Melanoma presents as a pigmented macule or patch (**Figs 9.140, 9.141**) or as a pigmented or amelanotic papule or nodule 'mole' (possibly developing from a lentiginous area or pre-existing dysplastic nevus) which may ulcerate or bleed (Johnson & Ayala 1973; Bracken & Diokno 1974; Jaeger et al 1982; Jorda et al 1987; Oldbring & Mikulowski 1987; Manivel & Fraley 1988; Stillwell et al 1988; Weiss et al 1992; de Bree et al 1997; Demitsu et al 2000; Honda et al 2001). Estimates for the occurrence of melanoma in pre-existing nevi or developing de novo vary widely. Patients are usually middle-aged or older although it has been reported in a boy (Begun et al 1984). It is exceedingly rare in Asians

lichen sclerosus is not associated with HPV. Chronic hidradenitis suppurativa may rarely be a predisposing factor (Cosman et al 2000).

Suspected verrucous carcinoma demands a deep surgical biopsy. The tumor has a rather different histology from squamous carcinoma, exhibiting deep lobular invaginations of well-defined proliferative epithelium consisting of typical, clear, pale keratinocytes (Lucia & Miller 1992). Frank squamous carcinoma (Sturm et al 1975) and foci of invasive squamous carcinoma (Johnson et al 1985) have been reported in some cases of anogenital verrucous carcinoma. Ultrastructurally verrucous carcinoma is distinct from condyloma acuminatum but similar to squamous cell carcinoma (Hull et al 1981).

It has been argued that clinical, histological and virological differences may distinguish verrucous carcinoma (potential for aggressive lethal behaviour) from Buschke-Lowenstein tumor/giant condyloma (no malignant potential) and that this distinction should direct treatment (Noel et al 1992; Niederauer et al 1993; Gonzalez-Lopez et al 1997; Anadolu et al 1999; Haycox et al 1999).

Surgical excision is the treatment usually recommended, e.g. glansectomy (Hatzichristou et al 2001) or penectomy. Mohs micrographic surgery has been employed successfully (Mohs & Sahl 1979; Brown et al 1987, 1988). Hughes (1979) used cryotherapy in two cases. Laser treatment (Lenk et al 1991), interferon-α (Zachariae et al 1988; Risse et al 1995; Gensau et al 2000, Gomez de la Fuente et al 2000), radiotherapy (Sobrado et al 2000) and bleomycin (Puissant et al 1975) have been used.

The prognosis is poor if untreated because the tumor can continue to grow and invade locally, causing exsanguination from femoral arterial invasion, cachexia,

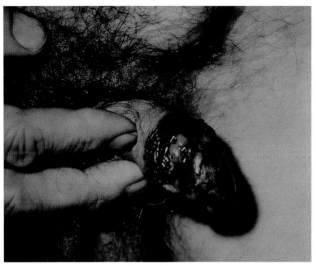

Fig. 9.140 Melanoma. Glans and shaft of penis. This patient had inguinal lymphadenopathy at presentation. (Courtesy of Dr Peter Copeman, London, UK.)

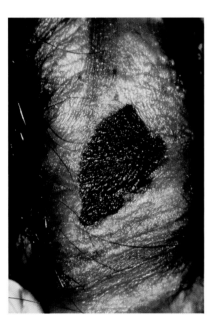

Fig. 9.141 Melanoma in situ. Penis shaft. (Courtesy of Dr Toshio Demitsu, Akita, Japan. Reproduced with permission from Demitsu T et al. Melanoma in situ of the penis. J Am Acad Dermatol. 2002; 42; 386–8.)

and has not been reported in blacks (although melanoma of the urethra has, Sanders et al 1986).

There may be a family history of melanoma and other atypical or 'dysplastic' nevi on examination. The inguinal and other nodes, as well as the abdomen, should be palpated. Forty to fifty percent of patients have lymphatic or other metastatic dissemination at the time of presentation.

Malignant melanoma of any histological subtype may be encountered (Lucia & Miller 1992).

Treatment is by primary excision. Subsequent management depends on the Breslow thickness of the lesion and complete clinical staging. Radical surgery and chemotherapy may be needed but the prognosis is poor for all melanomas that have already metastasized (Johnson & Ayala 1973; Begun et al 1984; Bundrick et al 1991).

MERKEL CELL CARCINOMA

A Merkel cell carcinoma of the scrotum (Best et al 1994) has presented as a rapidly growing tumor. This is a rare but nasty cancer with a high mortality and may be more prevalent in patients on long-term immunosuppressive medication such as azathioprine (Gooptu et al 1997).

MALIGNANT ECCRINE POROMA

Werdin et al (1991) encountered a malignant eccrine poroma at the base of penile shaft. It is a rare malignant appendageal tumor that is treated by wide surgical excision.

MALIGNANT SCHWANNOMA

This is exceedingly rare. Two penile cases have been described in patients with extant or a family history of von Recklinghausen's disease. Clinically they presented as a benign neurogenous tumor (neurofibroma/neurilemoma/granular cell myoblastoma); non-tender, progressive enlargement of well-circumscribed, doughy to rubbery, subcutaneous nodule. Amongst other cases of penile schwannoma that appear in the literature, four were malignant and three of these had von Recklinghausen's disease (Dehner & Smith 1970; Marsidi & Winter 1980). The importance of positive S100 staining in the histological diagnosis has been stressed (Kubota et al 1993).

SARCOMA

Details of only a handful of cases of fibrosarcoma affecting the anogenital area have been published: a well-demarcated, fixed, firm, subcutaneous nodule (Dehner & Smith 1970); a poorly circumscribed, reddish-tan, hemorrhagic pedunculated nodule (Dehner & Smith 1970); and solid, red nodule complicating pre-existing pseudo-epitheliomatous micaceous and keratotic balanitis (Irvine et al 1987); an ill-defined nodule at the base of the penis (Lawrence et al 1983); and another report in the Italian literature (Levi 1930). Dehner & Smith (1970) listed several undifferentiated sarcomas (fascial or embryonal sarcomas, rhabdomyosarcoma, hemangiopericytoma) in their paper; these subcutaneous malignancies of the penis were large, poorly demarcated and fixed to or infiltrating surrounding tissues.

Leiomyosarcoma is a rare tumor that presents painlessly but may differ from the benign and malignant neurogenic tumors in its physical features, usually being poorly circumscribed, firm to stony hard and infiltrative, often with palpable inguinal lymphadenopathy (Dehner & Smith 1970). Well circumscribed preputial cyst-like nodules (Valadez & Waters 1986, Pow-Sang & Orihuela 1994) and a nodule on the penile shaft (Weinberger et al 1982) have been described. Preputial lesions have a lower grade of malignancy and a lesser tendency to metastasize (Pow-Sang & Orihuela 1994).

Malignant fibrous histiocytoma is the most common soft tissue sarcoma in adults (extremities and peritoneum) yet rarely arises in the scrotum. Watanabe et al (1988) describe a case starting as a warty nodule that grew over two years and eventually ulcerated. It was distinctly separate from the testis and spermatic cord; cases have occurred arising from the spermatic cord that have then secondarily invaded the spermatic cord.

Epithelioid sarcoma is a rare mesenchymal neoplasm that is frequently confused with chronic inflammation, necrotizing granuloma and squamous carcinoma. It is an indolent sarcoma that infiltrates insidiously along fasciae or tendons (Iossifides et al 1979). One of Dehner and Smith's (1970) cases meets the criteria for diagnosis of epithelioid sarcoma. A case masquerading as Peyronie's disease has been reported by Moore et al (1975); other cases include one presenting with a nodule at the urethral meatus and pain on urination and erection (Iossifides et al 1979), another with a painful proximal penile mass and dysuria (Pueblitz et al 1986) and one that metastasized to skin (Millan et al 1992).

One case of dermatofibrosarcoma protuberans afflicting the penis exists in the literature and was reported as a mobile non-tender, rubbery, well-circumscribed, subcutaneous mass (Dehner & Smith 1970).

Peritesticular sarcoma presents as a painless, enlarging mass (Berkmen & Celebioglu 1997). A spindle cell sarcoma of the scrotum has been described (Asaadi et al 1980).

Treatment is by circumcision or excision but recurrences occur so Mohs micrographic surgery may become the treatment of choice (Dehner & Smith 1970; Greenwood et al 1972; Blath & Manley 1976; Brown et al 1988). Leiomyosarcoma may affect the scrotum to cause a scrotal tumor and may ulcerate (Johnson 1987; Washecka et al 1989; Echenique et al 1987; Newman & Fletcher 1991).

PRIMARY LYMPHOMA

Although lymphoma of the testis is the most frequent secondary tumor, lymphoma is rare in other parts of the male urogenital tract. Dehner and Smith (1970) included two cases of primary lymphoma in their series of soft tissue tumors of the penis, both presenting as painless subcutaneous nodules without evidence of systemic lymphoma. One case presented with painless priapism and erythematous nodular ulceration of the shaft of the penis (Gonzalez-Campora et al 1981).

Another case presented with progressive swelling of the glans penis (Marks et al 1988) and another with chronic penile ulceration (Gribin et al 1997).

Perineal non-Hodgkin's lymphoma has been reported in HIV-positive AIDS patients (Denis et al 1992; Yuhan et al 1998).

Like at other perineal sites, primary lymphoma of the scrotum is rare. Doll and Diaz-Arias (1994) have described a fungating, nodular tumor of the scrotum in an HIV-negative homosexual that was shown to be an immunoblastic T-cell lymphoma. Despite no evidence of systemic disease and treatment by surgical excision and combination chemotherapy a cutaneous (right hand) relapse occurred, requiring further chemotherapy to achieve remission.

A patient with an atypical presentation of cutaneous T-cell lymphoma has been reported by Hill et al (1995) where for many years there were perianal lesions only.

Treatment is by surgery, radiotherapy and chemotherapy depending on the individual case.

CHRONIC LYMPHOCYTIC LEUKEMIA

There has been a case of this disease presenting with a painless, firm, white mass at the anal orifice associated with weight loss and inguinal lymphadenopathy (Cresson & Siegal 1985).

LANGERHANS CELL HISTIOCYTOSIS

Langerhans cell histiocytosis (LCH, previously histiocytosis X) is a neoplasm of the antigen-presenting cells of the cutaneous immune system (Chu 2001). The Letterer-Siwe variant is characterized by solitary to multiple, pruritic, yellow-reddy brown papules (or nodules), with central foci of ulceration, sometimes in clusters sur-topped by crust or scale, involving the perineum or inguinal regions (but also other skin folds and non-intertriginous sites) in a child (where the differential diagnosis includes juvenile xanthogranuloma) or occasionally an adult (**Figs 9.142–9.144**). Involvement of the penis is very rare. A fleshy papule on the dorsal penis (Meehan & Smoller 1998) and primary penile ulceration (Myers et al 1981) have been reported as presentations. Seseke et al (1999) describe a case (**Fig. 9.145**) and review the literature.

Full assessment should be undertaken to exclude systemic disease manifesting as exophthalmos, lymphadenopathy, hepatosplenomegaly and polyuria. Histology shows infiltrates of histiocytes that stain positive for CD1 and S100. These cells contain Birbeck granules on

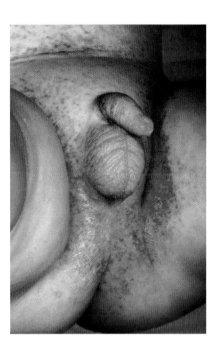

Fig. 9.142 Langerhans cell histiocytosis. Groins. Child.

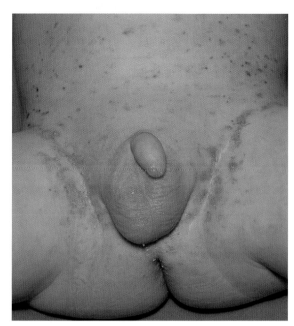

Fig. 9.144 Langerhans cell hsitiocytosis. Genitocrural folds. Intertrigo. (Courtesy of Medical Illustration, UK, Chelsea & Westminster Hospital, London, UK.)

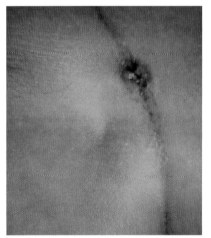

Fig. 9.143 Langerhans cell histiocytosis. Right inguinal fold. 17-month-old boy. Large nodule and some yellow-brown papules. Self-healing. (Courtesy of Dr Ken Hashimoto, Detroit, Michigan, USA. Reproduced with permission from Hashimoto K et al. Immuno-histochemistry and electron microscopy in Langerhans cell histiocytosis confined to the skin. J Am Acad Dermatol. 1991; 25: 1044–56.)

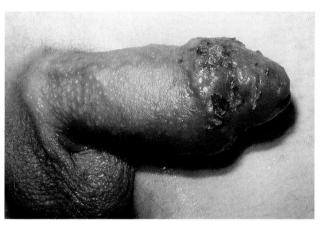

Fig. 9.145 Langerhans cell histiocytosis. Glans and shaft, penis. (Courtesy of Dr Florian Seseke, Gottingen, Germany.)

symmetrically distributed on the trunk and limbs. Confluent plaques can involve the flexures including the groins (**Fig. 9.146**). The mucosae, pharynx, larynx, bronchi and bones can be involved and meningeal disease may cause diabetes insipidus, fits and growth retardation. It is self-limiting but may last for years.

electron microscopy. The disease may be fatal but cases confined to the skin and which remit spontaneously have been described (Hashimoto et al 1991)

XANTHOMA DISSEMINATUM

This is a rare proliferative histiocytic condition of young males complicated by lipid deposition. Classically, erythematous, yellow to brown papules and nodules are

METASTASES

Metastases to the penis are rare but several hundred cases have been reported (Sagar & Retsas 1992). They are usually secondary to cancer of the urogenital tract (e.g. bladder or prostate, Powell et al 1984; Robey & Schellhammer 1984; Ortiz Cabria et al 1999; Miyamato

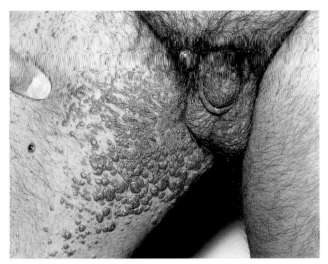

Fig. 9.146 Xanthoma disseminatum. Right groin. Erythematous yellow-brown papules and nodules with confluence in the flexures forming verrucous plaques.

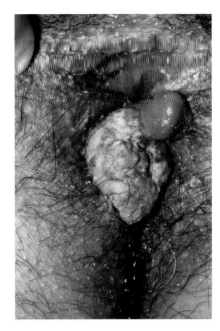

Fig. 9.147 Metastasis. Perineum. Rectal carcinoma. (Courtesy of Prof. Tim Allen-Mersh, London, UK.)

et al 2000) or gastrointestinal system (e.g. rectum), or other common cancers such as of the lung (Ortiz de Saracho et al 1998). They may present with pain, swelling, priapism, urinary symptoms or hematuria. A cutaneous nodule or nodules may be seen or infiltration of the deeper penile structures palpated (Abeshouse & Abeshouse 1961). A very rare cause is secondary melanoma (Sagar & Retsas 1992).

Perineal or perianal metastases from transitional cell carcinoma of the distal urethra (Langlois et al 1992), from rectal carcinoma (Garcia-Armengol et al 1995) and from epidermoid anal canal carcinoma (Nazzari et al 1994) are all recognized (**Fig. 9.147**).

Scrotal metastases are very rare but have been documented to complicate colon and gastric cancer (Boucher & Heymann 2001).

10 Pain and swelling

Presentations of some entities can be painful but generally *pain* is an unusual presentation for a dermatosis. *Swelling* is more common and may be painful or not. A common factor in many but not all causes of swelling may be *edema* or *lymphedema*. Most cutaneous mass lesions (papules and nodules) and the causes of inguinal masses and inguinal lymphadenopathy are not discussed here (see page 173). Orchitis and epididymitis and testicular and epidymal tumors, benign and malignant (e.g. seminoma and teratoma), are beyond the scope of this book.

Anal pain and scrotal pain and swelling are not generally the preserve of the dermatologist but it is useful briefly to consider the differential diagnosis of these symptoms. The causes of anogenital pain and swelling are listed in Tables **10.1–10.5**.

Priapism is discussed on p. 225 (**Table 10.7**).

Table 10.1 Causes of lymphedema

Idiopathic congenital lymphedema (Milroy's disease)

Lipogranuloma and silicone granuloma

Strangulation of the penis

Iatrogenic

Radical abdominopelvic surgery

Radiotherapy

Granulomatous lymphangitis

Post-infectious

Cellulitis and erysipelas

Chancroid

Granuloma inguinale (Donovanosis)

Lymphogranuloma venereum

Tuberculosis

Leprosy

Syphilis

Filariasis/onchocerciasis

Carcinomatosis

Lymphatic involvement

Lymphatic blockage

Lymphoma

IDIOPATHIC CONGENITAL LYMPHEDEMA

Bolt et al (1998) have described three cases of isolated congenital lymphedema of boys. It is extremely rare. Surgical treatment is necessary if persistent.

URETHRAL DIVERTICULUM

Urethral diverticulum is rare in man. It is a pouch opening into the urethra at any point in its course. Diverticula are either congenital or acquired or due to trauma, abscess, schistosomiasis, or calculus. Patients present with a mass or swelling in the penis, scrotum or perineum (Maged 1965). Segmental urethral hypospadias is a rare form of hypospadias where a ventral urethral defect results not in an alternative aperture for urination but in a urethral diverticulum or sac that dilates with urination (Derevyanko & Derevyanko 1998).

ACCESSORY SCROTUM

An accessory scrotum manifesting as a perineal swelling has been reported in association with a Becker's nevus of the buttock (Syzlit et al 1986).

Table 10.2 Causes of penile pain

Common causes	Rare causes
Trauma	Foreign body
Hematoma/fracture	Strangulation of the penis
Priapism	Lipogranuloma and silicone granuloma
Peyronie's disease	Hair strangulation
Sclerosing lymphangitis	Henoch-Schonlein purpura
Cellulitis	Familial Mediterranean fever
Fournier's gangrene	Infected cyst
Herpes simplex	Abscess of corpus cavernosum
Squamous carcinoma	Ecthyma gangrenosum
Fixed drug eruption	Fournier's gangrene
Chronic penile pain syndromes/'penodynia'	Penile necrosis
	Diabetes mellitus (and end-stage renal disease)
	IVC thrombosis (as part of DIC)
	Tuberculosis
	Herpes zoster
	Glomus tumor
	Sarcoma
	Epithelioid hemangioendothelioma
	Penile metastases

Table 10.3 Causes of scrotal pain

Common causes	Rare causes
Trauma	Lipogranuloma and silicone granuloma
Acute scrotum	Scrotal fat necrosis
Cellulitis	Henoch-Schonlein purpura
Herpes simplex	Familial Mediterranean fever
Chronic orchalgia/ scrotodynia syndromes	Polyarteritis nodosa
	Streptococcal dermatitis/perianal cellulitis
	Ecthyma gangrenosum
	Fournier's gangrene
	Tuberculosis
	Herpes zoster
	CMV epidymitis in HIV
	Squamous carcinoma

Table 10.4 Causes of anal and perianal pain

Common causes	Rare causes
Trauma	Hematoma
Rectal prolapse	Foreign body
Piles	Lipogranuloma and silicone granuloma
Proctitis	Streptococcal dermatitis/ perianal cellulitis
Pilonidal sinus	Ecthyma gangrenosum
Cellulitis	Herpes zoster
Perianal abscess	Tuberculosis
Hidradenitis suppurativa	Sarcoma
Herpes simplex	Epithelioid hemangioendothelioma
Squamous carcinoma	Chronic anal pain syndromes
Chronic anal pain syndromes	

RECTAL PROLAPSE

Defects in the pelvic floor or the anal sphincter can cause varying degrees of rectal prolapse (**Fig. 10.1**) and fecal incontinence associated with chronic straining at stool (Farouk & Duthie 1998; Bachoo et al 2000; Karulf et al 2001).

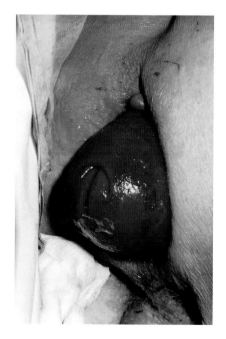

Fig. 10.1 Rectal prolapse.

PENILE HERNIA

Herniation of scrotal contents into the penile shaft can occur, for example after the use of a vacuum erection device (Ganem et al 1998).

Table 10.5 Causes of penoscrotal swelling

Common causes	Rare causes
Paraphimosis	Idiopathic congenital lymphedema
Foreign body	Hemangioma of infancy
Strangulation of the penis	Urethral diverticulum
Iatrogenic	Segmental urethral hypospadias
Continuous ambulatory peritoneal dialysis	Accessory scrotum
Raised right heart filling pressure in ITU	Herniation of scrotal contents into penile shaft
Post-surgical	Foreign body
Post-radiotherapy	Lipogranuloma and silicone granuloma
Varicocele	Aortic aneurysm
Hydrocele	Scrotal fat necrosis
Priapism	Henoch-Schonlein purpura
Peyronie's disease	Familial Mediterranean fever
Epidymitis and orchitis	Acute hemorrhagic edema of childhood
Cellulitis	Anogenital granulomatosis/Granulomatous lymphangitis
Idiopathic penile edema	Sarcoid
Testicular tumors	Infected cyst
	Abscess of corpus cavernosum
	Tuberculosis
	Paracoccidioidomycosis (South American blastomycosis)
	Giant scrotal tumors (e.g. neurilemoma)
	Epithelioid hemangioma
	Kaposi's sarcoma
	Epithelioid hemangioendothelioma
	Lymphoma
	Sarcoma
	Drugs (e.g. angioedema due to lisinopril)

FRACTURE OF THE PENIS/HEMATOMA

There have been a number of reports of this unusual problem, to which the erect penis is prone (Davies & Mitchell 1978; Goh & Trapnell 1980; Uygur et al 1997; Hoekx & Wyndaele 1998; Morris et al 1998; Nouri et al 1998). Pain, swelling and deformity associated with an apposite history (often with the description of a cracking noise) allow the diagnosis. During intercourse the penis may become violently bent or knocked. The tunica albuginea of the corpus cavernosum is split and in 30% a urethral injury occurs. A large hematoma (**Fig. 10.2**) may ensue, as may urinary retention requiring suprapubic catheterization. Otherwise management is conservative with analgesia unless drainage of a hematoma is necessary to prevent gangrene. The prognosis is good for full recovery but Peyronie's disease may be a long-term sequel (Goh & Trapnell 1980).

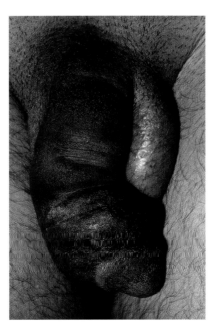

Fig. 10.2 Hematoma. Penis.

STRANGULATION OF THE PENIS

Accidental or intentional strangulation of the penis in boys due to hair is a recognized phenomenon (Alpert et al 1963; Bashir & El-Barbary 1979; Pantuck et al 1997; Silver & Docimo 1997; Pohlman 2000). Presentation is with swelling and edema during the period immediately post-circumcision thus allowing hairs to stick covertly to the wound where they cause a granulomatous reaction similar to pilo-nidal sinus and threaten strangulation (see Fig. 1.67). Complications include urethral fistula, pseudo-ainhum (Novick & Gribetz 1986), gangrene and amputation. Sometimes this presentation is called the tourniquet syndrome.

Other causes of penile strangulation in boys include rubber bands and string or thread used accidentally or to prevent enuresis and incontinence, as an innocent experiment conceived out of ignorance. In adults objects used include rings, nuts, bushes and sprockets, which are placed deliberately on the penis by the patient for masturbation or by his partner to prolong erection (Snoy et al 1984; Bhat et al 1991). Strangulation with swelling and ulceration may occur from the use of external urinary devices employed in the management of urinary incontinence (Fauer & Morrow 1978).

IATROGENIC SWELLINGS AND LYMPHEDEMA

Congenital defects in the inguinal canal and other non-inguinal peritoneal leaks can lead to scrotal, penile (and vulval) swelling as a manifestation of dialysate edema in patients with end-stage renal failure treated by continuous ambulatory peritoneal dialysis (Kopecky et al 1985).

Genital edema is commonplace in intensive care units, due to the practice of maintaining a raised right heart filling pressure (Figs 10.3, 10.4).

Radical surgery to the anogenital area and the draining lymph glands for cancer can cause swelling due to lymphedema, as can radiotherapy. Elephantiasis of the scrotum 30 years after surgery, radiotherapy and chemotherapy for penis cancer has been recorded (Horinaga et al 1998).

Chronic edema resembling keloid on the dorsum of the penis (see Figs 9.21 and 10.5) has been reported to complicate the use of a condom catheter for neurogenic bladder (Bang 1994). The patient also developed a ventral urethral fistula.

Increasingly, patients seek plastic surgery on the penis (Austoni et al 1999) for psychosexual reasons, e.g. dysmorphophobia, but surgery can result in considerable complications. Complications of plastic surgery to the penis, e.g. for penile enlargement, including autologous fat injection are listed in Table 10.6 (Alter 1997).

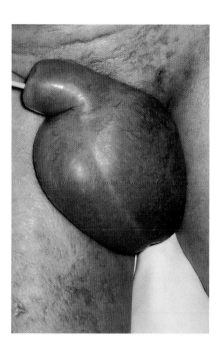

Fig. 10.3 **Penoscrotal edema.** Genitals. ITU patient.

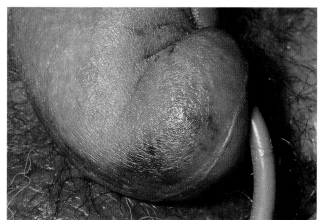

Fig. 10.4 **Preputial penile edema.** ITU patient.

Table 10.6 Complications of plastic surgery to the penis
Hypertrophic scars
Wide scars
Proximal penile hump (thick hair-bearing Y flap)
Low hanging penis
Loss of fat
Nodules
Deformed shaft

ACUTE SCROTUM

Acute scrotum is a clinical syndrome defined as acute painful swelling of the scrotum or its contents, usually in boys, accompanied by local signs and general symptoms (Melekos et al 1988). The important differential diagnosis is torsion of the testis or spermatic cord. Other causes include idiopathic scrotal edema, epididymitis,

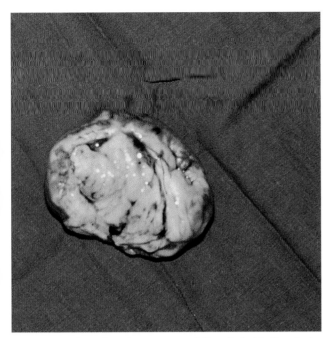

Fig. 10.5 Chronic edema resembling keloid. Surgical specimen. Histology showed focal inflammatory edema, fibrous tissue and vascular proliferation. (Courtesy of Dr Rameshwar Bang, Safat, Kuwait.)

Table 10.7 Causes of priapism

Idiopathic

Os penis

Perineal trauma

Strangulation

Hypertension

Nephrotic syndrome

Sickle cell disease

Coagulopathy

Peyronie's disease

Rheumatoid arthritis

Vasculitis

Tuberculosis

Pelvic tumors

Leukemia

Lymphoma

Penile metastases

Drugs: Papaverine
      Antipsychotics: chlorpromazine, trazodone
      Antihypertensives: hydralazine, guanethidine, prazosin
      Marijuana
      Adrenal corticosteroids
      Warfarin necrosis

(Modified from Levine et al 1991)

orchitis, hernia and hematocele. Thromboangiitis obliterans has been found in two cases (Nesbit & Hodgson 1959).

Acute scrotal swelling may be a physical sign of primary peritonitis in children and infants (Udall et al 1981) or secondary peritonitis due to appendicitis, healed meconium peritonitis in the neonate, hemoperitonitis (ruptured spleen) and pseudo-torsion due to shunts that have migrated into the scrotum from the peritoneum (ventriculoperitoneal shunts inserted for hydrocephalus).

AORTIC ANEURYSM

Inferior venal caval obstruction due to peri-aortic, aneurysmal fibrosis has been reported to cause painless scrotal swelling (Ward et al 1988).

PRIAPISM

Priapism is prolonged painful erection of the penis, unassociated with sexual desire and not relieved by ejaculation. It is not predominantly a dermatological concern but has an important differential diagnosis. The principal causes are listed in Table 10.7. It results in impotence in over 50% of those affected (O'Brien et al 1989) and can lead to gangrenous penile necrosis (Khoriaty & Schick 1980).

Levine et al (1991) distinguish veno-occlusive priapism from arterial priapism. Veno-occlusive priapism results from persistent obstruction to venous outflow from the lacunar spaces. It is a potential vascular emergency because as the corporeal bodies expand to maximal volume and obstructed outflow causes decreased arterial inflow with the potential for ischemia, pain, fibrosis and hence impotence. Arterial priapism is usually secondary to trauma such that a damaged cavernosal artery causes unregulated blood flow to the lacunar spaces; it is thus non-ischemic (Levine et al 1991).

Sickle cell anemia (Tarry et al 1987) is a common cause of veno-occlusive priapism. Leukemia may much more rarely cause priapism, with the mechanism thought to be thrombosis of the venous spaces of the corpus cavernosa due to outflow obstruction from masses of abnormal cells (Pond 1969), as occurs in sickle cell anemia (Tarry et al 1987). Hyperviscosity is another mechanism and in multiple myeloma priapism has been successfully treated with plasmapheresis (Rosenbaum et al 1978). Other hematological causes include lymphoma (Gonzalez-Campora et al 1981) and coagulopathies, e.g. protein C and factor V Leiden mutations and warfarin necrosis (Zimbelman et al 2000). Other drugs incriminated include marijuana, steroids, papaverine (Padma-Nathan et al 1986; Hashmat et al 1991), antipsychotics and antihypertensives. Priapism (see page 225) has been documented as a manifestation of isolated genital vasculitis (Lakanpal et al 1991).

Neurological causes include quadriplegia, spinal canal stenosis (Ramm et al 1987) and cauda equina compression (Ravindran 1979).

Os penis occurs in some mammals (Ruth 1934) but is very rare in man. When found it may be congenital (Champion & Wegrzyn 1964) or acquired (Gerster & Mandlebaum 1913; Vermooten 1933; Bett 1952; Subramanian 1952; Eglitis 1953; Elliott & Fischman 1962). Acquired cases have been attributed to metabolic disease, ageing or trauma.

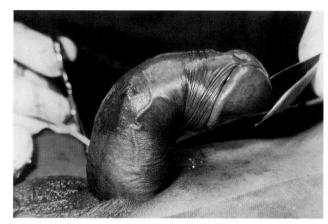

Fig. 10.7 Peyronie's disease. Abdomen, pubis and penis. Perioperative view. (Courtesy of Prof. Bhushan Kumar, Chandigarh, India.)

PEYRONIE'S DISEASE

Peyronie's disease (Billig et al 1975; Bivalacqua et al 2000; Lischer & Nehra 2001; Kadioglu et al 2002) is a localized fibrotic disorder involving tissue immediately adjacent to the erectile tissues. It presents with deformity (**Figs 10.6, 10.7**), pain, and curvature on erection, sensation of a cord within the penis, palpation of a lump or knot, decreased erection distal to the plaque, interference with intercourse and progressive impotence. Middle-aged men and older are affected. It may be subclinical in many men given that 23% of autopsies have shown histological evidence of the condition (Smith 1969). Psychological complications and marital difficulties occur. The penis curves towards the lesion with dorsal curvature being the most common. Plaques range in size and therefore what may be palpated differs. Peyronie (a physician to Louis XIV) described nodules as 'rosary beads'.

Peyronie's disease may be associated with systemic sclerosis (Simeon et al 1994) and these patients may have penile Raynaud's phenomenon (Mooradian et al

1988). It has occurred following the use of a vacuum erection device (Ganem et al 1998) but in most men the cause is unknown. Some evidence has been advanced for an autoimmune pathogenesis (Schiavino et al 1997).

There may be a genetic predisposition: it is associated with HLA B7 and Dupuytren's contracture (Nyberg et al 1982). There is a significant association with risk factors for vascular disease that may also have a bearing on erectile function, such as hypercholesterolemia and diabetes (Kadioglu et al 2002). Associations with beta-blockers, high serotonin levels (as in the carcinoid syndrome) and vitamin E deficiency have been found (Bivalacqua et al 2000; Lischer & Nehra 2001).

The most likely explanation is repeated microvascular trauma with a disproportionate inflammatory response and exaggerated wound healing similar to keloid formation and Dupuytren's contracture (Lischer & Nehra; 2001). Penile blood flow studies show veno-occlusive dysfunction (Bivalacqua et al 2000).

The differential diagnosis is congenital curvature, fibrosis secondary to trauma or urethritis and abscess, syphilitic gumma, lymphogranuloma venereum, and infiltrative tumors, e.g. lipogranuloma. Penile thrombophlebitis – misdiagnosed as Peyronie's disease – as the initial presentation of a paraneoplastic migratory thrombophlebitis due to pancreatic cancer has been reported (Horn et al 1985).

In some men there may be spontaneous regression. Treatment may involve intralesional corticosteroid injection (Desanctis & Furey 1967) including delivery by Dermo-Jet. Surgery is avoided if possible but some specialized techniques are available (Chun et al 2001). Recently good symptomatic relief has been claimed for the technique of iontophoresis of drugs such as dexamethasone, lidocaine and verapamil (Riedl et al 2000). Other treatments that have been used include vitamin E, potassium aminobenzoate, tamoxifen, colchicine and extracorporeal shock-wave lithotripsy (Lischer & Nehra 2001).

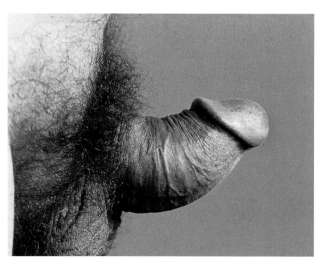

Fig. 10.6 Peyronie's disease. (Courtesy of Dr Nick Soter, New York, NY, USA.)

PROCTITIS

The differential diagnosis of proctitis is not the primary responsibility of the dermatologist or genitourinary physician. Inflammatory bowel disease, cancer, functional disorders, radiotherapy and infections (e.g. herpes simplex, gonorrhea and syphilis) should be considered. Even though the classical chancre of primary syphilis is painless, a proctitis (with pain) can occur (Gluckman et al 1974; Akdamar et al 1977).

ACUTE IDIOPATHIC SCROTAL EDEMA

This usually affects children aged 4–12 years. Allergy, infection (umbilical sepsis), trauma, insect bites, urinary extravasation and Henoch-Schonlein purpura have all been implicated. It is rare in adults but three cases in association with diabetic septic foot have appeared in the literature (Fahal et al 1993).

SCROTAL FAT NECROSIS

This condition is distinct from other causes of the acute scrotum in prepubertal boys. It presents as acute tender, sometimes painful, swelling (classically, but not always, after swimming in cold water). Masses may be palpable in the scrotal wall. The patient is otherwise well, with no fever or leucocytosis. Management is expectant and conservative (Koster & Antoon 1980; Hollander et al 1985).

In adults one case of idiopathic scrotal panniculitis has been reported (Tsurusaki et al 2000) and another associated with pancreatitis (Lin et al 1996).

HENOCH-SCHONLEIN PURPURA/ANAPHYLACTOID PURPURA

This is a systemic neutrophilic leukocytoclastic vasculitis associated with the vascular deposition of IgA. The cause is unknown but some cases in children may be due to a specific viral infection. There may be arthralgia, abdominal pain and renal involvement. In the skin a symmetrical eruption of crops of small, palpable, purpuric lesions is encountered (**Fig. 10.8**). A prodromal, urticarial manifestation is not uncommon.

The genitalia may frequently be affected by the purpura (**Figs 10.9, 10.10**). Renal parenchymal involvement leading to proteinuria and the nephrotic syndrome may not be the limit of the disease in the urogenital system. Ureteritis, renal pelvic hemorrhage and pain and

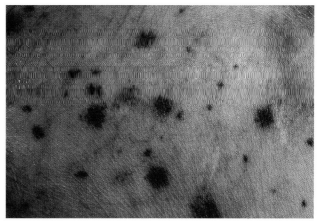

Fig. 10.8 Henoch-Schonlein purpura. Leg. Same case as Fig. 10.6.

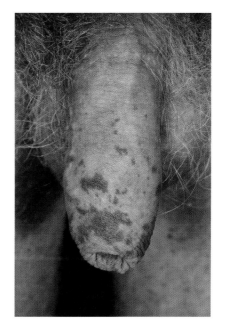

Fig. 10.9 Henoch-Schonlein purpura. Penis shaft.

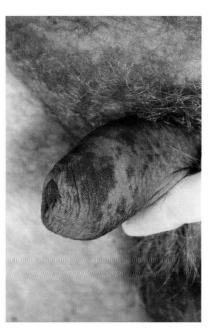

Fig. 10.10 Henoch-Schonlein purpura. Prepuce, penis.

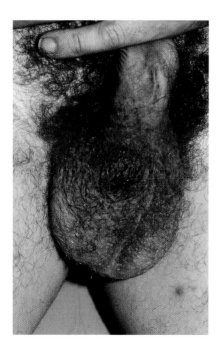

Fig. 10.11 Henoch-Schonlein purpura.
Scrotum. Same case as Fig. 10.8.

swelling of the spermatic cord have been reported. The incidence of scrotal involvement (**Fig. 10.11**) has been quoted as of the order of 2–38%. In some cases the presentation has simulated testicular torsion eliciting unnecessary surgical exploration; ultrasonography can help differentiate (Laor et al 1992). However, testicular torsion can be a serious complication of Henoch-Schonlein purpura (Clark & Kramer 1986).

ACUTE HEMORRHAGIC EDEMA OF CHILDHOOD

This is an unusual variant of leukocytoclastic vasculitis of infants and young children that may present as tenderness, redness and swelling of the penis and scrotum with the development of more widespread hemorrhagic lesions (Dubin et al 1990). Streptococci, staphylococci and adenoviruses have been implicated. The histology shows a leukocytoclastic vasculitis. The differential diagnosis includes acute febrile neutrophilic dermatosis, erythema multiforme, Henoch-Schonlein purpura and child abuse. The prognosis for complete recovery is excellent.

FAMILIAL MEDITERRANEAN FEVER

Acute inflammation of the scrotum in patients with familial Mediterranean fever is not a well-recognized entity (Gedalia et al 1992). It is manifested by unilateral, pain, erythema and swelling, fever, leucocytosis and elevated ESR. It may occur in isolation or alongside

peritonitis. The differential diagnosis includes torsion, orchitis and epidymitis in children.

Other cutaneous presentations of familial Mediterranean fever include erysipelas-like erythema, Henoch-Schonlein purpura (see above) and nodular erythema (Gedalia et al 1992).

POLYARTERITIS NODOSA

Polyarteritis nodosa is a multisystem connective tissue disease. Testicular and epididymal involvement have occurred manifesting as scrotal pain and swelling. In one case these were the sole presenting features: testicular biopsy gave the diagnosis (Dahl et al 1960; Lee et al 1983; Wright & Bicknell 1986). It may be an unrecognized 'cause' of Fournier's gangrene (Downing & Black 1985, see also Fig. 8.61) and it may initiate sclerosing lymphangitis (Coldiron & Jacobson 1988).

GRANULOMATOUS LYMPHANGITIS/ANOGENITAL GRANULOMATOSIS

Granulomas may be found histologically in the investigation and management of penile lymphedema (Mor et al 1997). It can be a rare feature of the Melkersson-Rosenthal syndrome (orofacial granulomatosis). Crohn's disease, sarcoid and Behçet's disease must be excluded (Van de Scheur et al 2003).

STAPHYLOCOCCAL CELLULITIS

Cellulitis may affect the penis and anogenital area as it might any other cutaneous site. An infected piercing site is shown in **Fig. 10.12**. Cellulitis and abscess formation can complicate cysts, sinuses and fistulae (see pages 229–230). It is also unclear what the relationship is between an episode or episodes of acute infection and chronic penile edema (**Fig. 10.13**), which is often complicated by cellulitis (see below). The differential diagnosis is listed in **Table 10.8**.

Anorectal infection in patients with malignant disease is serious and potentially life threatening. Some cases of anorectal cellulitis will respond to antibiotics alone. However, necrotizing fasciitis may occur and external swelling and fluctuance signifying abscess formation may appear late. Deciding when to perform surgery is very difficult. Perianal infiltration, ulceration or abscess occurs in 5% of hematological malignancy and may rarely be the presenting feature (Vanheuverzwyn et al 1980).

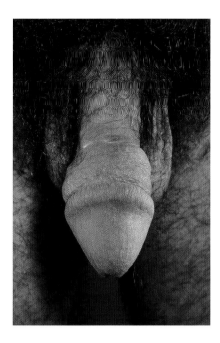

Fig. 10.12 Cellulitis. Glans and distal shaft, penis.

STREPTOCOCCAL DERMATITIS/PERIANAL CELLULITIS

This is a recognized syndrome in children (Brady 1987; Rehder et al 1988; Paradisi et al 1993, 1994a, 1994b; Patrizi et al 1994; Peltola 2000) but probably a similar clinical situation occasionally occurs in adults (Neri et al 1996). A child may present with pruritus, painful defecation, anal soreness and redness (without nappy/diaper rash) and satellite pustulosis of the buttocks. Examination of the anus shows a pronounced, sharply demarcated, boggy erythema (**Figs 10.14, 10.15**) and causes discomfort to the child. Rarely there may be a systemic presentation with fever and rash (Vélez et al 1999). It is much more common in boys in whom, if the penis is involved, there may be dysuria, erythema and swelling of the penis and balanoposthitis. Acute guttate psoriasis has also been observed (Rehder et al 1988; Patrizi et al 1994).

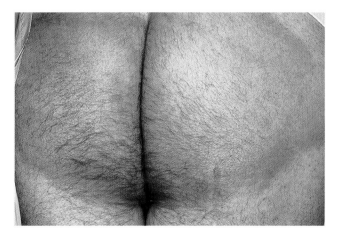

Fig. 10.13 Cellulitis. Buttocks. Acute deterioration with pelvic girdle cellulitis in a patient with idiopathic penile and scrotal edema.

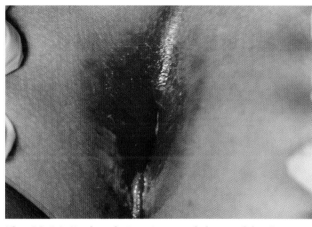

Fig. 10.14 Perianal streptococcal dermatitis. Anus. Child. Associated with guttate psoriasis. (Courtesy of Drs Annalisa Patrizi and Lensko Marzaduri, Bologna, Italy.)

Table 10.8 Differential diagnosis of anogenital cellulitis

Hidradenitis suppurativa

Crohn's disease

Staphylococcal cellulitis

Streptococcal cellulitis

Idiopathic penile edema

Anogenital granulomatosis

Gonococcal cellulitis

Fournier's gangrene and necrotizing fasciitis

Extramammary Paget's disease

Carcinoma erysipeloides (bladder and prostate)

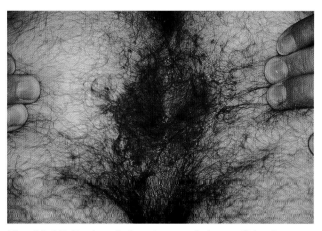

Fig. 10.15 Perianal streptococcal dermatitis. Anus. Adult. Associated with guttate psoriasis. (Courtesy of Drs Annalisa Patrizi and Lensko Marzaduri, Bologna, Italy.)

Group A β-hemolytic streptococci can be isolated and it may be associated with streptococcal infection of the upper respiratory tract in other members of the family. Streptococcal proctocolitis has been reported (Guss et al 1984). *Staphylococcus aureus* has been retrieved from one child who also had satellite pustules on the buttocks (Montemarano & James 1993).

Treatment is generally with systemic penicillin or topical mupiricin or erythromycin if clinically less acute (Amren et al 1966; Hirschfeld 1970; Rehder et al 1988; Paradisi et al 1993, 1994a, 1994b).

Anal disease has been mistaken for sexual abuse and in one case it was fortunate that the penile involvement and isolation of the causative organism led to the correct diagnosis (Duhra & Ilchyshyn 1990).

ABSCESS OF THE CORPUS CAVERNOSUM

This is rare but presents with pain, swelling and dorsal rupture and ulceration (Kaneda et al 1998).

PERIANAL ABSCESS

Perianal/anorectal/ischiorectal abscess presents with painful swelling and purulent discharge. A common complication is fistula in ano. The most common cause of perianal abscess is infection of the anal glands but trauma (e.g. impacted fish bone), diabetes and anal cancer predispose. Twelve percent of HIV-positive patients may develop a perianal abscess (Yuhan et al 1998). Crohn's disease should be considered. Tuberculosis is a rare differential diagnosis and *Enterobius vermicularis* (threadworms) even rarer (Mortensen & Thomson 1984).

CHRONIC IDIOPATHIC PENILE EDEMA

Chronic penile lymphedema (CPL) is a relatively rare condition (Porter et al 2001). It differs from penile venereal edema and acute idiopathic penile edema in several ways; it is persistent, may have no demonstrable infective cause and there is no *documented* effective treatment.

Although it may occur as a consequence of primary hypoplastic lymphatic channels, in my opinion it usually occurs as a result of recurrent unidentified infections and/or another concomitant penile dermatosis and infection thereof, with subsequent damage to the lymphatic vessels. Anogenital granulomatosis should be contemplated as it may be the presenting feature of sarcoid or Crohn's disease (van de Scheur 2003).

CPL is a reactive disfiguring disorder that causes sexual dysfunction and phimosis. It has previously been described as tumorous lymphedema or elephantiasis verrucosa nostra (Luelmo et al 1995). A tentative etiology can usually be identified from the patient's history and examination; for instance, two of my patients had had circumstantial clinical or laboratory evidence of streptococcal infection, whilst two other cases (patients with penile lichen planus and previous treponemal disease) were idiopathic. However, the underlying resultant pathology is presumably the same in all cases, namely 'scarring' of the lymphatics.

No definitive treatment is available although all of our patients have partially responded to long-term antibiotics and/or short courses of prednisolone in the acute phase. This approach stabilizes the process and improves the appearance and function of the penis. Its success rather argues for the importance of infection as a factor in the perpetuation if not initiation of the process. Medical control with antibiotics also allows contemplation of surgical intervention in the form of circumcision. Plastic repair may be necessary after excision of affected tissue (Morey et al 1997; Muehlberger et al 2001).

Only a handful of cases of CPL have been reported before (Thomas et al 1993; Geyer et al 1995) and the etiopathopathogenesis may have been misunderstood. There have been previous reports of penoscrotal edema where the cause has been attributed to continuous ambulatory peritoneal dialysis (Abraham et al 1990), amputation of septic limbs in the context of diabetes (see below: Fahal et al 1993), strangulation, thrombosis, acute necrotizing pancreatitis (Choong et al 1996) and streptococcal infections (Mendelson et al 1997). Penile venereal edema has been associated with gonococcal and herpes infection and scabies infestation, and resolves after treatment of the underlying disease (see above and below, Wright et al 1979). Similarly, childhood penile edema is self-limiting (Brandes et al 1994).

It is probable that cases of CPL are as a result of any of the aforementioned causes or indeed due to temporally unrelated but repetitive venereal disease. Perineal, scrotal, gluteal and penile skin drains to superficial inguinal lymph nodes and deeper structures to the internal iliac nodes. All may be involved in a regional inflammatory process (**Figs 10.13, 10.16–10.24**). Persistent lymphatic insult from whatever cause can lead to this recurrent entity. Hence all cases of penoscrotal edema should be treated aggressively at first presentation.

Not least because the more chronic the genital lymphedema the more difficult it is to treat both medically and surgically (excision and grafting, Malloy et al 1983), the aim of treatment of CPL must be prophylaxis against further infective episodes, aggressive treatment of relapses and in uncircumcised patients, amelioration of signs to enable institution of surgical measures if necessary (for instance, patients with under-

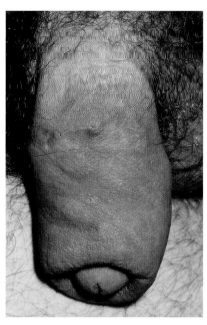

Fig. 10.16 Chronic penile edema. Note chronic penile acne.

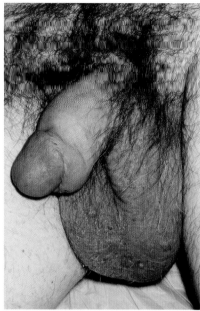

Fig. 10.19 Chronic penile edema.

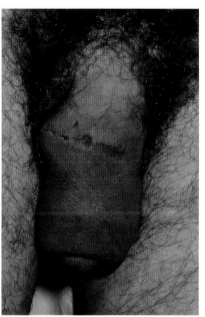

Fig. 10.17 Chronic penile edema. Note chronic penile acne and distal cellulites. Same case as Fig. 10.16.

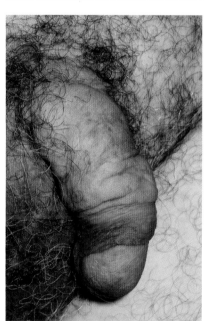

Fig. 10.20 Chronic penile edema.

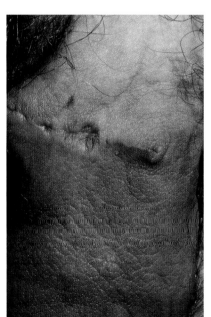

Fig. 10.18 Chronic penile edema. Note chronic penile acne. Enlargement of Fig. 10.17.

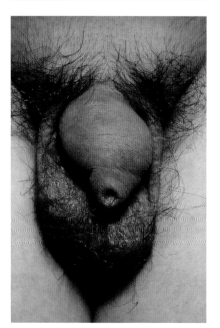

Fig. 10.21 Chronic penile edema. Preputial edema and phimosis.

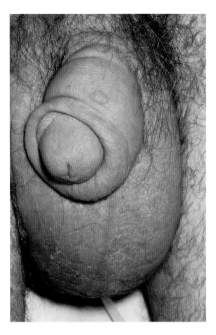

Fig. 10.22 Chronic penoscrotal edema.

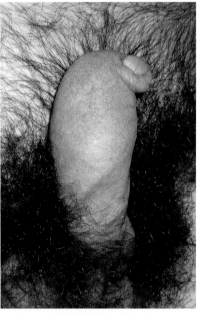

Fig. 10.23 Chronic penile edema. Preputial edema and phimosis.

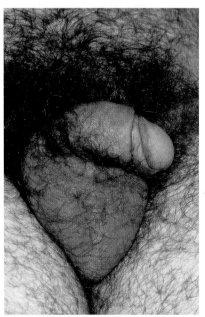

Fig. 10.24 Chronic penile edema. Post protracted medical treatment followed by circumcision. Same case as Fig. 10.23.

lying penile dermatoses who cannot be treated topically due to their CPL). Imaging of lymphatic channels is unlikely to shed further light on the cause of this enigmatic condition though it may be used to differentiate between primary and secondary lymphedema (Samsoen et al 1981).

FILARIAL LYMPHEDEMA

Onchocerciasis can cause a 'hanging groin' and scrotal enlargement (see page 225). Other filarial infections can lead to mild hydrocele or gross elephantiasis. Filariasis can cause secondary lymphangiectasis (**Fig. 10.25**). Excision, grafting and genital reconstruction can be undertaken (Das et al 1983).

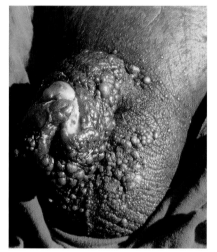

Fig. 10.25 Filariasis. Penis and scrotum. Lymphedema and papules and nodules of lymphangiectasis. (Courtesy of Prof. Bhushan Kumar, Chandigarh, India.)

CARCINOMA ERYSIPELOIDES

This is a term used to describe infiltration of the skin by neoplastic cells such that the clinical appearances of cellulitis or erysipelas are simulated, but if the skin is examined meticulously often small infiltrative papules can be perceived. It is not uncommon in advanced breast cancer but has been observed in the perineum and on the thigh in carcinoma of bladder and prostate (Cohen & Kim 1980; Ng 2000) and also breast cancer (Bunker, personal observation).

EPITHELIOID HEMANGIOENDOTHELIOMA

This very rare tumor can affect the vasculature of the erectile tissue of the penis and can present as a single painful nodule on erection (Dehner & Smith 1970), painful nodules (Quante et al 1998) or asymptomatic swellings (Weiss & Enzinger 1982; Elhosseiny et al

1986). This entity is regarded as a tumor of borderline malignant potential. Treatment is by adequate excision with diligent follow up.

CHRONIC UROGENITAL AND RECTAL PAIN SYNDROMES

These include penile pain 'penodynia', scrotodynia, orchialgia, prostatodynia, coccygodynia, proctalgia fugax, perineal pain, the descending perineum syndrome and vulvodynia (Parks et al 1966; Lark 1982;

Neill & Swash 1982; Luzzi 2002). The neuroanatomy of the pelvis is complicated and the neurophysiological basis of the pathogenesis of these syndromes is poorly understood but their clinical presentations are well recognized. The differential diagnosis is extensively covered in this chapter. Chronic prostatitis may be a cause (Luzzi 2002).

A diagnosis of a chronic pain syndrome carries the possibility of considerable psychological morbidity. The treatment is problematic, at best only empirical: invasive and irreversible procedures should be avoided if at all possible. Multidisciplinary engagement is advocated (Wesselmann et al 1997).

Appendix

Contemporary genital piercings (male)

Place and look of genital piercing	Name	Origin (O), background (B), and myths (M)	Description, peculiarities, and healing time (HT)
*	Ampallang	O: Borneo and supposedly Sulawesi (Celebes) in Indonesia. B: part of ritual initiation. Jewellery was made of bone, ivory, of precious metal. Intended to give sexual pleasure to female sexual partners.	Horizontal pin through the glans (spongeosum). Very bloody and painful. Requires an experienced piercer. If cavernosum is hit by mistake, bleeding can be very hard to stop, loss of erection may follow. HT: 8–10 weeks, sometimes even 6 months. Foreskin has to remain pulled back for adequate circulation of air.
*	Apadravya	O: India. Described in the *Kama Sutra*.	Vertical pin through the glans, mostly between the onset of the frenulum and the top of the glans. Difficult and uncommon piercing that requires an experienced piercer. HT: at least 2 months.
*	Dydoe	O: USA in the 20th century. M: supposed to have originated in the Jewish community. B: intended to sexually stimulate its wearer.	Worn by circumcised men. Through the rim of the glans. Requires a professional piercer. HT: 4–6 weeks.
*	Prince Albert	O: USA in the 20th century. M: supposedly derived from Queen Victoria's husband, who is said to have pierced a ring through his penis tip to attach his penis either to the right or the left of his uniform trousers.	Piercing goes from the opening of the urethra to the frenulum (reverse Prince Albert goes to the top of the glans.) The size of the ring must be chosen correctly – small rings may cleave the glans, large rings may cause pain for the partner. HT: quite fast (aided by sterility of urine).
†	Frenum/ frenulum	O: unpierced penis rings are known from a number of tribal societies (e.g., Tangkhul Nagas in northeast India). Pierced version: Europe and USA in the 20th century. B: used to prevent (frenum) or facilitate erection (frenulum).	Less painful than other penis piercings, easier to execute. A variation of the frenulum is the frenulum ladder – an arrangement of multiple parallel piercings along the bottom of the penis.

Contemporary genital piercings (male) (*Cont'd*)

Place and look of genital piercing	Name	Origin (O), background (B), and myths (M)	Description, peculiarities, and healing time (HT)
*	Guiche (female version fourchette)	O: USA in the 20th century. M: South Pacific Islands (Tahiti). Part of ritual initiation. Adolescent men are cut with a knife and a leather ring is pulled through the opening. Intended to stimulate the perineum.	Piercing canal with a hollow needle through seam between scrotum and anus (raphe). Steel ring, sometimes with additional weights through the opening. HT: at least 6–8 weeks, during which sitting or bicycling may be painful.
†	Hafada	O: USA in the 20th century. M: Arab countries. Part of ritual initiation. Symbolically meant to prevent the testis from re-ascending back into the belly. Sign of wealth and manliness.	Scrotal skin piercing between testis and penis base. Not very painful. Experience needed. Serves rather a decorative than a sexual purpose. Often several rings are worn to which jewellery or weights are attached. HT: short.
†	Pubic	O: Europe in the 20th century. B: serves a decorative rather than a sexual purpose.	To be pierced directly above the penis base, in order to prevent lengthy healing times.
† ‡	Oetang	O: USA in the 20th century. M: it was used as a chastity belt both in Myanmar and in Ancient Rome for slaves and athletes.	Foreskin is pierced on both sides of its edge and is closed with rings. Other foreskin piercing may contain multiple rings. HT: short; more than two piercings should not be done at the same time, since this part may swell considerably.

*Images from Ziegler B, Zoschke B. Body piercing. Rastatt: Pabel Moewig, 1997. Originally in Transfigurations, Quadrillion Publishing Inc.
†Images by Doug Malloy. Courtesy of RE/Search Publications, San Francisco, USA.
‡With permission from Perforations, Brighton, UK (http://www.perforations.com).

Bibliography

A

Abdel–A' Al H, Abdel–Azziz AHM. Nevus comedonicus: report of three cases localized on glans penis. Acta Dermato–Venereologica 1975; 55: 78–80.

Abdul Gaffoor PM. Hypopigmentation of the glans penis. Cutis 1983; 31: 214.

Aberer E, Neumann R, Lubec G. Acrodermatitis chronica atrophicans in association with lichen sclerosus et atrophicans: Tubulo–interstitial nephritis and urinary excretion of spirochete–like organisms. Acta Derm Venereol (Stockh) 1987; 67: 62–91.

Abeshouse BS, Abeshouse GA. Metastatic tumours of the penis: A review of the literature and a report of two cases. J Urol 1961; 86(1): 99–112.

Abraham G, Blake PG, Mathews R et al. Genital swelling as a surgical complication of continuous ambulatory peritoneal dialysis. Surg Gynecol Obstet 1990; 170: 306–308.

Achauer BM, Vander Kam VC. Ulcerated anogenital hemangioma of infancy. Plast Reconstruct Surg 1991; 87(5): 861–868.

Achtstatter T, Moll R, Moore B et al. Cytokeratin polypeptide patterns of different epithelia of the human male urogenital tract: Immunofluorescence and gel electrophoretic studies. J Histochem & Cytochem 1985; 33(5): 415–426.

Acker SM, Sahn EE, Rogers HC et al. Genital cutaneous Crohn disease: two cases with unusual clinical and histopathologic features in young men. Am J Dermatopathol 2000; 22(5): 443–446.

Ackerman AD, Kornberg R. Pearly penile papules. Arch Dermatol 1973; 108: 673–675.

Adams JR Jr, Mata JA, Venable DD et al. Fournier's gangrene in children. Urology 1990; 35: 439–441.

Adeyemi-Doro FAB, Osoba OA, Junaid TA. Perigenital cutaneous schistosomiasis. Br J Venereal Disease 1979; 55: 446–449.

Adjei O, Brenya RC. Secondary bacterial infection in Ghanaian patients with scabies. East Afr Med J 1997; 74(11): 729–731.

Agarwalla A, Agrawal CS, Thakur A et al. Cutaneous horn on condyloma acuminatum. Acta Dermato-Venereologica 2000; 80(2): 159.

Agarwalla B, Mohanty GP, Sahu LK, et al. Tuberculosis of the penis: report of 2 cases. J Urol. 1980; 124(6): 927.

Agostoni C, Migliorini D, Dorigoni N et al. Genital ulcer in an AIDS patient with disseminated leishmaniasis. Eur J Clinical Microbiology & Infectious Diseases 1998; 17(11): 813–814.

Ahmed A, Jones AW. Apocrine cystadenoma. Report of two cases occurring on the prepuce. Br J Dermatol 1969; 81: 899–901.

Akdamar K et al. Syphilitic proctitis. Digest Dis and Sci 1977; 22: 701.

Aki K. Yogurt–induced pruritis ani in a child. Eur J Pediatr 1992; 151(11): 867.

Aki K. Food–induced pruritus ani: A variation of allergic target organ? Eur J Pediatr 1993; 152(8): 701–702.

Akogun OB, Akoh JI, Hellandendu H. Non-ocular clinical onchocerciasis in relation to skin microfilaria in the Taraba River Valley, Nigeria. J Hyg Epidemiol Microbiol & Immunol 1992 36(4): 368–383.

Aksu K, Keser G, Gunaydin G et al. Erectile dysfunction in Behcet's disease without neurological involvement: two case reports. Rheumatol (Oxford) 2000; 39: 1429–1431.

Alberici F, Pagani L, Ratti G et al. Ivermectin alone or in combination with benzyl benzoate in the treatment of human immunodeficiency virus–associated scabies. Br J Dermatol 2000; 142(5): 969–972.

Aldeen T, Lau RK. Genital eczema in an elderly man. Int J STD & AIDS 1999; 10(2): 124–6.

Al–Durazi M, Saleem I, Mohammed AA. Urethral foreign body. Br J Urol 1992; 69(4): 434.

Alessi E, Cusini M. The exanthem of HIV–1 seroconversion syndrome. Int J Dermatol 1995; 34: 238–9.

Alexander RM, Kaminsky DB. Giant condyloma acuminatum (Buschke–Lowenstein tumour) of the anus. Dis Col Rect 1979; 22: 561–565.

Alexander-Williams J. Pruntus ani. Br Med J 1983; 287: 159–160.

Alexander-Williams J, Buchmann P. Perianal Crohn's disease. World J Surg 1980; 4: 203–208.

Aliabadi H, Cass AS, Gleich P et al. Self–inflicted foreign bodies involving the lower urinary tract and male genitals. Urology 1985; 26(1): 12–16.

Alici B, Culha M, Ozkara H et al. Management of buried penis in adults. Urol Int 1998; 61(3): 183–185.

Aljabre SHM, Sheikh YH. Penile involvement in pityriasis versicolor. Tropical and Geographical Medicine 1994; 46(3): 184–187.

Allan A, Ambrose NS, Silverman S et al. Physiological study of pruritus ani. Br J Surg 1987; 74: 576–579.

Allen AL, Siegfried EC. The natural history of condyloma in children. J Am Acad Dermatol 1998; 39(6): 951–955.

Allen-Mersh TG. Pilonidal sinus: finding the right track for treatment. Br J Surg. 1990; 77(2): 123–32.

Allenby CF, Johnstone RS, Chatfield S et al. PERINAL–a new no touch spray to relieve the symptoms of pruritis ani. Int J Colorect Dis 1993; 8(4): 184–187.

Alpert JJ, Filler R, Glaser HH. Strangulation of an appendage by hair wrapping. N Engl J Med 1965; 273(16): 866–867.

Alter GJ. Reconstruction of deformities resulting from penile enlargement surgery. J Urol 1997; 158(6): 2153–2157.

Alter GJ, Ehrlich RM. A new technique for correction of the hidden penis in children and adults. J Urol 1999; 161(2): 455–459.

Bibliography

Altmeyer P, Kastner U, Luther H. Balanitis/ balanoposthitis chronica circumscripta benigna plasmacellularis– entity or fiction? Hautarzt 1998; 49(7): 552–555. German.

Alves G, Fiedler W, Guenther E et al. Determination of telomerase activity in squamous cell carcinoma of the penis. Int J Oncol 2001; 18(1): 67–70.

Amerio PL, Banchieri RF, Provana A et al. Zoon's plasma–cell balanitis. Minerva Urol 1975; 27(5): 232–235. Italian.

Ammini AC, Sabherwal U, Mukhopadhyay C et al. Morphogenesis of the human external male genitalia. Pediatr Surg Int 1997; 12(5–6): 401–406.

Ammori BJ, Ausobsky JR. Electrocoagulation of perianal warts: a word of caution. Digest Surg 2000; 17(3): 296–297.

Amren DP, Anderson AS, Wannamaker LW. Perianal cellulitis associated with Group A Streptococci. Am J Dis Child 1966; 112: 546–552.

Anadolu R, Boyvat A, Calikoglu E et al. Buschke–Loewenstein tumour is not a low-grade carcinoma but a giant verruca. Acta Dermato–Venereologica 1999; 79(3): 253–254.

Anaguchi S, Sinomiya S, Kinebuchi S et al. Solitary reticulohistiocytic granuloma–a report of three cases and a review of the literature. Nippon Hifuka Gakkai Zasshi 1991; 101(7): 735–742.

Andiran F, Tanyel FC, Hicsonmez A. Fraser syndrome associated with anterior urethral atresia. Am J Med Genet 1999; 82(4): 359–361.

Andrews PE, Farrow GM, Oesterling JE. Squamous cell carcinoma of the scrotum: Long–term followup of 14 patients. J Urol 1991; 146(5): 1299–1304.

Anonymous. Drugs that cause sexual dysfunction. Med Lett Drug Therapeut 1980; 22: 108–110.

Anonymous. Recurrent condylomata acuminata treated with recombinant interferon alpha–2a. Acta Dermato–Venereologica (Stockh) 1993a; 73(3): 223–226.

Anonymous. Randomized placebo–controlled double–blind combined therapy with laser surgery and systemic interferon–a2a in the treatment of anogenital condylomata acuminatum. J Infect Dis 1993b; 167(4): 824–829.

Anonymous. Guidance for doctors who are asked to circumcise male children. Gen Med Coun, London. 1997.

Anonymous. Sexually transmitted disease quarterly report: anogenital warts and anogenital herpes simplex virus infection in England and Wales. Communicable Disease Report. CDR Weekly 2000 2000; 10(26): 230–2.

Ansink AC, Krul MRL, de Weger RA et al. Human papillomavirus, lichen sclerosus, and squamous cell carcinoma of the vulva: detection and prognostic significance. Gynecol Oncol 1994; 52: 180–184.

Antman K, Chang Y. Medical Progress: Kaposi's sarcoma. N Engl J Med 2000; 342: 1027–1038.

Arango Toro O, Rosales Bordes A, Vesa Llanes J et al. Plasmocellular balanoposthitis of Zoon. Arch Esp Urol 1990; 43(4): 337–339. Spanish.

Arany I, Evans T, Tyring SK. Tissue specific HPV expression and down–regulation of local immune responses in condylomas from HIV seropositive individuals. Sex Trans Infect 1998; 74(5): 349–353.

Arany I, Muldrow M, Tyring SK. Correlation between mRNA levels of IL–6 and TNF alpha and progression rate in anal squamous epithelial lesions from HIV–positive men. Anticancer Res 2001; 21: 425–8.

Arensmeier M, Theuring U, Franke I et al. Topical therapy of extramammary Paget's disease. Hautarzt 1994; 45(11): 780–782.

Armijo M, Herrera E, De Dulanio F et al. Leiomyosarcome de la verge. Etude ultrastructurale. Annales de Dermatologie et de Venereologie 1978; 105: 267–274.

Armstrong L, Hackett AH. Lipogranuloma of the male genitalia. Austral N Z J Surg 1981; 51(1): 72–73.

Asaadi M, Najmi J, Carter HW et al. Spindle cell carcinoma of the scrotum. Urology 1980; 16(5): 525–526.

Asarch RG, Golitz LE, Sausker WF et al. Median raphe cyst of the penis. Archiv Dermatol 1979; 115: 1084–1086.

Aste N, Pau M, Ferreli C et al. Lichen planus in a child requiring circumcision. Pediatr Dermatol Mar 1997; 14(2): 129–130.

Astori G, Lavergne D, Benton C et al. Human papillomaviruses are commonly founding normal skin of immunocompetent hosts. J Invest Dermatol 1998; 110: 752–755.

Attalla MF. Subcoronal hypospadias with complete prepuce: a distinct entity and new procedure for repair. Br J Plastic Surg 1991; 44: 122–125.

Aubertin E, Roy A, Fenelon J. On a case of thrombosis of the corpus cavernosum in a patient with gout receiving 3 intravenous injections per week of 50mg of heparin. Medecine Bordeaux 1960; 137: 1486–1489.

Audebert C. La gangrene post–operatoire progressive de la peau. Annales de Dermatology et Venereologie 1991; 108: 451–455.

Augey F, Cognat T, Balme B et al. Le carcinome basocellulaire perianal. A propos de 2 observations. Annales de Dermatologie et de Venereologie 1994; 121(6–7): 476–478.

August RJ, Milward TM. Cryosurgery in the treatment of lichen sclerosus et atrophicus of the vulva . Br J Dermatol 1980; 103: 667–670.

Austoni E, Guarneri A, Gatti G. Penile elongation and thickening – a myth? Is there a cosmetic or medical indication? Andrologia 1999; 31(Suppl. 1): 45–51.

Avrach WW, Christensen HE. Metastasizing erythroplasia of Queyrat: report of a case. Acta Dermato–Venereologica 1976; 56: 409–412.

Avram A, Rousselet G, Benazeraf C. Grupper C 'Pityriasis versicolor' de la verge. Bulletin de la Societe Francaise Dermatologie Syphiligraphie 1973; 80: 607–608.

Aynaud O, Casanova JM et al. Interet de la circoncison therapeutique dans la condylomatose diffuse. Annales de Dermatologie et de Venereologie 1992; 119(2): 187–190.

Aynaud O, Ionesco M, Barrasso R. Examen genital masculin: L'utilite de la peniscopie et du test a l'acide acetique pour le despistage des lesions a papillomavirus. Annales D'Urologie 1992; 26(1): 53–57.

Aynaud O, Ionesco M, Barrasso R. Penile intraepithelial neoplasia. Specific clinical features correlate with histologic and virologic findings. Cancer 1994; 74: 1762–1767.

Aynaud O, Casanova JM, Tranbaloc P. CO$_2$ laser for therapeutic circumcision in adults. Eur Urol 1995; 28(1): 74–76.

Aynaud O, Piron D, Casanova JM. Incidence of preputial lichen sclerosus in adults: histologic study of circumcision specimens. J Am Acad Dermatol 1999; 41(6): 923–926.

Aynaud O, Asselain B, Bergeron C et al. Carcinomes intraépithéliaux et carcinomes invasifs de la vulve, du vagin et du pénis en Ile–de–France. Enquête PETRI portant sur 423 cas. Ann Dermatol Venereol 2000; 127: 479–483.

Ayres Jr S, Anderson NP. Persistent nodules in scabies. Archiv Dermatol Syphilol 1932; 25: 485–493.

Azurdia RM, Luzzi GA, Byren I et al. Lichen sclerosus in adult men: a study of HLA associations and susceptibility to autoimmune disease. Br J Dermatol 1999; 140: 79–83.

B

Bachoo P, Brazzelli M, Grant A. Surgery for complete rectal prolapse in adults. Cochrane Database Syst Rev(2):CD. 2000; 001758.

Bailey RC, Muga R, Pouusen R et al. The acceptability of male circumcision to reduce HIV infections in Nyanza Province, Kenya. AIDS Care 2002; 14: 27–40.

Baker H, Ive FA, Lloyd M. Primary irritant dermatitis of the scrotum due to hexachlorophene. Archiv Dermatol 1969; 99: 693–696.

Baker WN, Milton-Thompson GJ. The anal lesion as the sole presenting symptom of intestinal Crohn's disease. Gut. 1971; 12(10): 865.

Balazs M. Bowenoid change in perianal condyloma acuminatum associated with ulcerative colitis. Hepato–Gastroenterology 1991; 38(4): 311–313.

Baldwin HE, Geronemus RG. The treatment of Zoon's balanitis with the carbon dioxide laser. J Dermatol Surg Oncol 1989; 15: 491–494.

Bale TM, Lockhead A, Martin HCO et al. Balanitis xerotica obliterans in children. Pediatr Pathol 1987; 7: 617–617.

Ball LM, Harper JI. Atopic eczema in HIV-seropositive haemophiliacs. Lancet 1987; 2(8559): 627–8

Ballaro A, Webster JJ, Ralph D. Penile resurfacing for extensive genital warts. Int J Impot Res 2001; 13(1): 47–48.

Balus S, Breathnatch AS, O'Grady AJ. Ultrasound observations on 'foam cells' and the source of their lipid in verruciform xanthoma. J Am Acad Dermatol 1991; 24(5 Pt.1): 760–764.

Bang RL. Penile oedema induced by continuous condom catheter use and mimicking keloid scar. Scad J Urol Nephrol 1994; 28: 333–335.

Barbagli G, Lazzeri M, Palminteri E et al. Lichen sclerosis [sic] of male genitalia involving anterior urethra. Lancet 1999; 354(9176): 429.

Bargman H. Pseudoepitheliomatous, keratotic, and micaceous balanitis. Cutis 1985; 35(1): 77–79.

Barnette DJ Jr, Curtin TJ, Yeager JK et al. Asymptomatic penile lesions. Cutis 1993; 51(2): 116–118.

Barnhill RL, Albert LS, Sharma SK et al. Genital lentiginosis: A clinical and histopathologic study. J Am Acad Dermat 1990; 22(3): 453–460.

Barrasso R, De Brux J, Croissant O et al. High prevalence of papillomavirus associated penile intraepithelial neoplasia in partners of women with cervical intraepithelial neoplasia. N Eng J Med 1987; 317: 916–923.

Bart RS, Kopf AW. Tumor conference No. 14: On a dilemma of penile horns: pseudoepitheliomatous, hyperkeratotic and micaceous balanitis. J Dermatol Surg Oncol 1977; 3: 580.

Bart RS, Kopf AW. Tumor conference No 18: Squamous cell carcinoma arising in balanitis xerotica. J Dermatol Surg Oncol 1978; 4: 556–558.

Barth IH, Reshad H, Darley CR et al. A cutaneous complication of Dorbanex therapy. Clin Exp Dermatol 1984; 9: 95–96.

Barton PG, Ford MJ, Beers BB. Penile purpura as a manefestation of lichen sclerosus et atrophicus. Pediatr Dermatol 1993; 10(2): 129–131.

Bashir AY, El–Barbary M. Hair coil strangulation of the penis. J Roy Coll Surg 1979; 25: 47–51.

Baskin LS, Dixon C, Stoller ML et al. Pyoderma gangrenosum presenting as Fournier's gangrene. J Urol 1990; 144(4): 984–986.

Bassi O et al. Primary syphilis of the rectum–endoscopic and clinical features. Report of case. Dis Col Rect 1991; 34: 1024.

Bauer A, Geier J, Elsner P. Allergic contact dermatitis in patients with anogenital complaints. J Reprod Med 2000; 45(8): 649–654.

Baughman RD, Berger P, Pringle WM. Plasma cell cheilitis. Arch Dermatol 1974; 110: 725–726.

Bayne D, Wise GJ. Kaposi sarcoma of the penis and genitalia: A disease of our times. Urology 1988; 31(1): 22–25.

Bechara FG, Huesmann M, Stücker M et al. An exceptional localization of angiokeratoma of Fordyce on the glans penis. Dermatol 2002; 205: 187–188.

Began D, Mirowski G. Perioral and acral lentigines in an African American man. Arch Dermatol 2000; 136(3): 419, 422.

Begun FP, Grossman HB, Dionko AC et al. Malignant melanoma of the penis and male urethra. J Urol 1984; 132: 123–125.

Behçet H. Uber rezidivierende, aphthose, durch ein virus verursachte Geschwure im Mund, am Auge und an denGenitalien. Dermatol Wochenschr 1937; 105: 1152–1157.

Belaich S, Civatte J, Bonvalet D et al. Dermato–fibrosarcome de Darier–Ferrand de la verge. Annales de Dermatologie et de Venereologie 1978; 105: 331–332.

Belisario JC. Topical cytotoxic therapy for cutaneous cancer and precancer. Arch Dermatol 1965; 92: 293.

Beljaards RC, van Dijk E, Hausman R. Is pseudoepitheliomatous, micaceous and keratotic balanitis synonymous with verrucous carcinoma? Br J Dermatol 1987; 117(5): 641–646.

Bendahan J, Paran H, Kolman S et al. The possible role of Chlamydia Trachomatis in perineal suppurative hidradenitis. Eur J Surg 1992; 158: 213–215

Berger TG, Papa CM. Photodye herpes therapy–Cassandra confirmed? J Am Med Ass 1977; 238: 133–134.

Berger TG, Stoner MF, Hobbs ER et al. Cutaneous manifestations of early human immunodeficiency virus exposure. J Am Acad Dermatol 1988; 19: 298–303.

Berger TG, Kaveh S, Becker D et al. Cutaneous manifestations of Pseudomonas infections in AIDS. J Am Acad Dermatol 1995; 32(1 Pt. 1): 279–280.

Berkmen F, Celebioglu AS. Adult genitourinary sarcomas: a report of seventeen cases and review of the literature. J Exp Clin Cancer Res 1997; 16(1): 45–48.

Bernhard JD. Demographic pruritis: Invisible dermographism. J Am Acad Dermatol 1995; 33(2 Pt. 1): 322.

Bernstein G, Forgaard DM, Miller JE. Carcinoma of the glans penis and distal urethra. J Dermatol Surg Oncol 1986; 12: 450.

Bernstein LH, Frank MS, Brant LJ et al. Healing of perineal Crohn's Disease with metronidazole. Gastroenterology 1980; 79(2): 357–365.

Berth–Jones J, Graham–Brown RA, Burns DA. Lichen sclerosus. Arch Dis Child 1989; 64: 1204–1206.

Berth–Jones J, Tan SV, Graham–Brown RAC et al. The successful use of minocycline in pyoderma gangrenosum in a report of seven cases and review of the literature. J Dermatol Treat 1989; 1: 23–25.

Bertram P, Treutnar KH, Rubben A et al. Invasive squamous cell carcinoma in giant anorectal condyloma (Buschke–Lowenstein tumour). Langenbecks Arch Chir 1995; 380: 115–118.

Bessiere L, Allain D, Meleille J. La vaccine ano–genitale. Annales de Dermatologie et de Venereologie (Paris) 1979; 105: 339–341.

Bessman AN, Wagner W. Non–clostridial gas gangrene. Report of 48 cases and a review of the literature. J Am Med Ass 1975; 233: 958–963.

Best TJ, Metcalfe JB, Moore RB et al. Merkel cell carcinoma of the scrotum. Ann Plast Surg 1994; 33(1): 83–85.

Bett WR. The os penis in man and beast. Ann Roy Coll Surg, Engl 1952; 10: 405–409.

Bettloch I, Banuls J, Sevila A et al. Perianal tuberculosis. Int J Dermatol 1994; 33(4): 270–271.

Beutner KR, Conant MA, Friedman–Kien AE et al. Patient applied podofilox for treatment of genital warts. Lancet 1989; i: 831–834.

Bewley AP, Ross JS, Bunker CB et al. Successful treatment of a patient with ocreotide–resistant necrolytic migratory erythema. Br J Dermatol 1996; 134(6): 1101–1104.

Bezerra ALR, Lopes A, Santiago GH et al. Human papillomavirus as a prognostic factor in carcinoma of the penis. Analysis of 82 patients treated with amputation and bilateral lymphadenectomy. Cancer 2001; 91: 2315–2321.

Bhat AL, Kumar A, Mathur SC et al. Penile strangulation. Br J Urol 1991; 68: 618–621.

Bhojwani A, Biyani CS, Nicol A, Powell CS. Bowenoid papulosis of the penis. Br J Urol 1997; 80(3): 508.

Biagi FF, Martuscelli QA. Cutaneous amebiasis in Mexico. Dermato Trop 1963; 2: 129–136.

Bigler LR, Flint ID, Davis LS. Painful ulcers of the scrotum. Archiv Dermatol 1995; 31(5): 609–614.

Billig R, Baker R, Immergut M et al. Peyronie's disease. Urology 1975; 6: 409–418.

Bingham JS. Carcinoma of the penis developing in lichen sclerosus et atrophicus. Br J Vener Dis 1978; 54: 350–351.

Binnick AN, Spencer SK, Dennison WL Jr et al. Glucagonoma syndrome. Report of two cases and literature review. Arch Dermatol 1977; 113(6): 749–754.

Bircher AJ, Hirsbrunner P, Langauer S. Allergic contact dermatitis of the genitals from rubber additives in condoms. Coontact Dermatitis 1993; 28: 125–126.

Birley HDL, Walker MM, Luzzi GA et al. Clinical features and management of recurrent balanitis; association with atopy and genital washing. Genitourinary Med 1993; 69(4): 400–403.

Bisceglia M, Carosi I, Castelvetere M et al. Multiple Fordyce–type angiokeratomas of the scrotum. An iatrogenic case. Pathologica 1998; 90(1): 46–50. Italian.

Biswas M, Godec C, Ireland G et al. Necrotizing infection of the scrotum. Urology 1979; 14(6): 576–580.

Bivalacqua TJ, Purohit SK, Hellstrom WJ. Peyronie's disease: advances in basic science and pathophysiology. Curr Urol Rep 2000; 1: 297–301.

Black MM. In: Textbook of Dermatology RH Champion, JL Burton, DA Burns, SM Breathnach eds Blackwell Science Ltd. Oxford. 1998; 2637–2640.

Black SB, Woods JE. Squamous cell carcinoma complicating hidradenitis suppurativa. J Surg Oncol 1982; 19: 25–26.

Blank AA, Schryder VW. Soft X–ray therapy in Bowen's disease and erythroplasia of Queyrat. Dermatoloxica 1985; 171: 89–94.

Blath RA, Manley CB. Leiomyosarcoma of the prepuce. J Urol. 1976; 115(2): 220–1.

Blau S, Hyman AB. Erythroplasia of Queyrat. Acta Dermato-Venereologica 1955; 35: 341–378.

Blauvelt A, Kerdel FA. Cutaneous cryptococcosis mimicking Kaposi's sarcoma as the initial manifestation of disseminated disease. Int J Dermatol. 1992; 31(4): 279–80.

Boccaletti VP, Ricci R, Sebastio N et al. Penile necrosis. Arch Dermatol 2000; 136(2): 261, 264.

Boczko S, Freed S. Penile carcinoma in circumcised males. NY State J Med 1979; 79: 1903–1904.

Bodey GP et al. Infections caused by Pseudomonas Aeruginosa. Rev Infect Dis 1983; 5: 279.

Boggs Jr HW. Anal lesions of granulomatous (Crohn's) disease of the bowel. South Med J 1970; 63(11): 1265–1267.

Böhle A, Buttner H, Jocham D. Primary treatment of condylomata acuminata with viable bacillus Calmette–Geurin. J Urol 2001; 165(3): 834–836.

Bolt RJ, Peelen W, Nikkels PG et al. Congenital lymphoedema of the genitalia. Eur J Pediatr 1998; 157(11): 943–946.

Boman B, Moertel CG, O'Connell MJ. Carcinoma of the anal canal. Cancer 1984; 54: 114–125.

Boon ME, Schneider A, Hogewoning CJA et al. Penile studies and heterosexual partners. Cancer 1988; 61: 1652–1659.

Borgstrom E. Penile ulcer as complictaion in self-induced papaverine erections. Urology 1988; 32(5): 416–417.

Boshart M, zur Hausen H. Human papillomaviruses in Buschke–Lowenstein tumours: Physical state of the DNA and identification of a tandem duplification in the noncoding region of a human paillomavirus 6 subtype. Virology 1986; 58(3): 963–966.

Boshart M, Gissmann L, Ikenberg H et al. A new type of papillomavirus DNA, its presence in genital cancer biopsies and in cell lines derived from cervical cancer. EMBO J 1984; 3: 1151–1157.

Bottomley WW, Cotterill JA. Acquired zinc deficiency presenting with an acutely tender erythematous scrotum. Br J Dermatol 1993; 129(4): 501–502.

Boucher KW, Heymann WR. Ulcerated papules of the scrotum. Arch Dermatol 2001; 137: 495–500.

Bour J, Steinhardt G. Penile necrosis in diabetes mellitus and end stage renal disease. J Urol 1984; 132: 560–562.

Bouyssou–Gauthier ML, Boulinguez S, Dumas JP et al. Lichen scereux genital masculin: etude de suivi. [Penile lichen sclerosus: follow–up study. Ann Dermatol Venereol 1999; 126: 804–807.

Bowen JT. Precancerous dermatoses: a study of two cases of chronic atypical epithelial proliferation. J Cutan Dis inc Syph 1912; 30: 241–254.

Bowyer A, McColl I. Erythrasma and pruritus ani. Acta Dermato–Venereologie 1971; 51: 444–447.

Boyton KK, Bjorkman DJ. Argon laser therapy for perianal Bowen's Disease: A case report. Lasers Surg Med 1991; 11(4): 385–387.

Bozdag KE, Gül Y, Karaman A. Lipoid proteinosis. Int J Dermatol 2000; 39(3): 203–204.

Bracken RB, Diokno AC. Melanoma of the penis and the urethra: 2 case reports and review of the literature. J Urol 1974; 111: 198–200.

Bradshaw BR, Nuovo GJ, DiCostanzo D et al. Human papillomavirus type 16 in a homosexual man. Archiv Dermatol 1992; 128(7): 949–952.

Brady MT. Cellulitis of the penis and scrotum due to group B streptococcus. J Urol 1987; 137: 736.

Brandes SB, McAninch JW. Surgical methods of restoring the prepuce: a critical review. Br J Urol Int 1999; 83(Suppl. 1): 109–113.

Brandes SB, Chelsky MJ, Hanno PM. Adult acute idiopathic scrotal edema. Urology 1994; 44: 602–605.

Brandt LJ, Bernstein LH, Boley SJ et al. Metronidazole therapy for perianal Crohn's disease. A follow–up study. Gastroenterology 1982; 83: 383–387.

Brassinne de la M, Richert B. Genital squamous-cell carcinoma after PUVA therapy. Dermatology 1992; 185(4): 316–318.

Breathnach SM, Black MM. Atypical tuberculide (acne scrofulosorum) secondary to tuberculous Iymphadenitis. Clin Exp Dermatol 1981; 6: 339–344.

Breen JL, Smith Cl, Gregon CA. Extramammary Paget's disease. Clin Obstet Gynecol 1978; 21: 1107–1115.

Brisson P, Patel H, Chan M et al. Penoplasty for buried penis in children: report of 50 cases. J Pediatr Surg 2001; 36(3): 421–425.

Broaddus SB, Leadbetter GW. Surgical management of persistent, symptomatic nonvenereal sclerosing lymphangitis of the penis. J Urol 1982; 127: 987–988.

Broder SR, Frierson HFJ, Theodorescu D. Unusual case of non-exophytic invasive penile squamous cell cancer arising from a chronic sinus tract. Scand J Urol Nephrol 1999; 33(5): 333–335.

Brodin M. Balanitis circumscripta plasmacellularis J Am Acad Dermatol. 1980; 2(1): 33–35.

Broholm KA. A controllcd trial of a ncw combined preparation for the treatment of constipation in geriatric patients. Gerontology (Basel) 1973; 15: 25–31.

Bronson D, M Barsky R, Barsky S. Acrodermatitis enteropathica. J Am Acad Dermatol 1983; 9: 140–144.

Brown CF, Callup DG, Brown VM. Hidradenitis suppurativa of the anogenital region. Response to isotretinoin. Am J Obstet Gynaecol 1988; 158: 13–15.

Brown MD, Zachary CB, Grekin RC et al. Penile tumours: Their management by Moh's micrographic surgery. J Dermatol Surg Oncol 1987; 13: 1163–1167.

Brown MD, Zachary CB, Grekin RC et al. Genital tumours: Their management by micrographic surgery. J A Dermatol 1988; 18(1): 115–122.

Brown SCW, Kazzasi N, Lord PH. Surgical treatment of penneal hidradenitis suppurativa with special reference to recognition of the perianal form. Br J Surg 1986; 73: 978–980.

Browne SG. Calcinosis circumscripta of the scrotal wall: the etiological role of Onchocerca volvulus. Br J Dermatol 1962; 74: 136–140.

Brownstein MH, Helwig EB. The cutaneous amyloidosis II Systemic Forms. Archiv Dermatol 1970; 102: 20–28.

Bruce DH. Angiokeratoma circumscriptum and angiokeratoma scroti. Archiv Dermatol 1960; 81: 388–393.

Bruynzeel DP. Dermatological causes of pruritis ani. Br Med J 1992; 305: 955.

Bryan JT, Stoler MH, Tyring SK et al. High–grade dysplasia in genital warts from two patients infected with the human immunodeficiency virus. J Med Virol 1998; 54(1): 69–73.

Bryceson ADM, Hay RJ. Cutaneous larva migrans. In: Parasitic worms and protozoa Textbook of Dermatology. Champion RH

Burton JL, Burns DA, Breathnach SM eds. Sixth Edition Blackwell Science Ltd. Oxford 1998; 2: 1392–1393.

Dubrick MP, Hitchcock CR. Necrotizing anorectal and perineal infections Surgery 1979; 86: 655–662.

Buchmann P, Keighley MRB, Allan RN et al. Natural history of perianal Crohn's Disease. Ten year follow-up. A plea for conservatism. Am J Surg 1980; 140: 642–644.

Bundrick WS, Culkin DJ, Mata JH et al. Penile malignant melanoma in association with squamous carcinoma of the penis. 1991; 146(5): 1364–1365.

Bunker CB. Dermatological problems in HIV and AIDS In Miller A, ed. Medical Management of HIV and AIDS London: Springer–Verlag 1996.

Bunker CB. Review of Dermatology Journals. Sex Trans Inf 1999; 75: 281–282.

Bunker CB. Topics in penile dermatology. Clin Exp Dermatol. 2001; 26: 469–79.

Bunker CB, Staughton RCD. Dermatology. Chelsea & Westminster AIDS Care Handbook. Gazzard B, Ed. Mediscript, London; 2002.

Bunker CB et al. Deficiency of calcitonin gene–related peptide in Raynaud's phenomenon. Lancet 1990; 336: 1530–1533.

Bunker CB. Skin conditions of the male genitalia. Medicine. 2001; 29: 9–13.

Bunker CB, Goldsmith PC, Leslie TA et al. Calcitonin gene–related peptide, endothelin–1, the cutaneous microvasculature and Raynaud's phenomenon. Br J Dermatol 1996; 134: 399–406.

Bunney MH, Noble IM. Red skin and Dorbanex. Br Med J 1974; i: 731.

Bureau Y, Barriere H, Evin Y- P. Les erythroplasies benignes a plasmocytes. Annales de Dermatologie et de Syphiligraphie 1962; 89: 271–284.

Burge SM. Hailey-Hailey disease: the clinical features, response to treatment and prognosis.Br J Dermatol. 1992; 126(3): 275–82.

Burmer GC, True LD, Krieger JN. Squamous cell carcinoma of the scrotum associated with human papillomaviruses. J Urol 1993; 149: 374–377.

Burns DA. An outbreak of scabies in a residential home. Br J Dermatol 1987; 117(3): 359–361.

Burns DA, Sarkany I. Tuberculous ulceration of the penis. Proc Roy Soc Med 1976; 69: 883–884.

Burton JL, Burns DA, Breathnach SM. Rook et al. Textbook of dermatology. 6th Edition. Blackwell Science, Oxford. Volume 3, Ch58. 2548–2549.

Buschke A. Ueber die Bedeutung der 'papillen' der corona glandis. Medizinische Klinik 1909; 5: 1621–1623.

Butler JD, Hersham MJ, Wilson CA et al. Perianal Paget's disease. J Roy Sco Med 1997; 90: 688–689.

C

Cabaleiro P, Drut RM, Drut R. Lymphohistiocytic and granulomatous phlebitis in penile lichen sclerosus. Am J Dermatopathol 2000; 22(4): 316–320.

Cabello I, Caraballo A, Millan Y. Leishmaniasis in the genital area. Rev Inst Med Trop Sao Paulo. 2002; 44: 105–107.

Cain C, Seabury-Stone M, Thieburg M et al. Nonhealing genital ulcers. Archiv Dermatol 1994; 130: 1311–1316.

Çalikoglu E. Superficial granulomatous pyoderma of the scrotum: an extremely rare cause of genital ulcer. Acta Dermato–Venereologica 2000; 80(4): 311–312.

Calikoglu E, Soravia-Dunand VA, Perriard J et al. Acute genitocrural intertrigo: a sign of primary human immunodeficiency virus type 1 infection. Dermatology 2001; 203: 171–173.

Calista D. Topical cidofovir for severe cutaneous human papillomavirus and molluscum contagiosum infections in patients with HIV/AIDS. A pilot study. J Eur Acad Dermatol Venereol 2000; 14(6): 484–488.

Calore EE, Nadal SR, Manzione CR et al. Expression of Ki–67 can assist in predicting recurrences of low–grade anal intraepithelial neoplasia in AIDS. Dis Col Rect. 2001; 44(4): 534–537.

Campion MJ, Singer A, Clarkson PK et al. Increased risk of cervical neoplasia in consorts of men with penile condylomata accuminata Lancet 1985; i: 943–946.

Campion MJ, McCance DJ, Mitchell HS et al. Subclinical penile human papilloma virus infection and dysplasia in consorts of women with cervical neoplasia. Genitour Med 1988; 64: 90–99.

Campus GV, Ena P, Scuderi N. Surgical treatment of balanitis xerotica obliterans. Plast Reconst Surg 1984; 73: 652–657.

Campus GV, Alia F, Bosincu L. Squamous cell carcinoma and lichen sclerosus et atrophicus of the prepuce. Plast Reconst Surg 1992; 89(5): 962–964.

Canby JP, Wilde H. Penile venereal edema. N Engl J Med 1973; 289: 108.

Canillot S, Stamm C, Balme B et al. Xanthome verruciforme du gland. Annales de Dermatologie et de Venereologie 1994; 121(5): 404–407.

Cantril ST, Green JP, Schall GL. Primary radiation therapy in the treatment of anal carcinoma. Int J Radiat Oncol Biol Phys 1983; 9: 1271–1278.

Cardamakis E, Kotoulas IG, Relakis K et al. Comparitive study of systemic interferon alfa–2a plus isotretinoin versus isotretinoin in the treatment of recurrent condyloma acuminatum in men. Urology 1995; 45(5): 857–860.

Carli P, Cattaneo A, Pimpinelli N et al. Immunohistochemical evidence of skin immune system involvement in vulvar lichen sclerosus et atrophicus. Dermatologica 1991; 182: 18–22.

Carlson GW, Ferguson CM, Amerson JR. Perianal infections in acute leukaemia. Am Surg 1988; 54: 693–695.

Carlson HE. Sclerosing lipogranuloma of the penis and scrotum. Urology 1968; 100: 656–658.

Carlson JA, Grabowski R, Mu XC et al. Possible mechanisms of hypopigmentation in lichen sclerosus. Am J Dermatopathol 2002; 24(2): 97–107.

Carpenter–Kling JT, Jacyk WK. Anogenital flat papules. Archiv Dermatol 1994; 130: 1311–1316.

Carr ND, Mercey D, Slack WW. Non-condylomatous perianal skin disease in homosexual men. Br J Surg 1989; 76: 1064–1066.

Carrasco L, Izquierdo MJ, Farina MC et al. Strawberry glans penis: a rare manifestation of angiokeratomas involving the glans penis. Br J Dermatol 2000; 142(6): 1256–1257.

Carter PS, DeRuiter A, Whatrup C et al. Human immunodeficiency virus infection and genital warts as risk factors for anal intraepithelial neoplasia in homosexual men. Br J Surg 1995; 82(4): 473–474.

Cartwright LE, Steinman HK. Malignant papillary mesothelioma of the tunica vaginalis testes: Cutaneous metastases showing epidermal invasion. J Am Acad Dermatol 1987; 17(5 Pt.2): 887–890.

Casado M, Jimenez F, Borbujo J et al. Spontaneous healing of Kaposi's angiosarcoma of the penis. J Urol 1988; 139: 1313–1314.

Casale AJ, Beck SD, Cain MP et al. Concealed penis in childhood: a spectrum of etiology and treatment. J Urol 1999; 162(3 Pt 2): 1165–1168.

Cascinelli N. Melanoma maligno del pene. Tumori 1969; 55(5): 313–315.

Castellsague X, Bosch FX, Munoz N et al. The International Agency for Research on Cancer Multicenter Cervical Cancer Study Group. N Engl J Med 2002; 346: 1160–1161.

Castle WN, Wentzell JM, Schwartz BK et al. Chronic balanitis due to pemphigus vegetans. J Urol 1987; 137: 289–291.

Castonguay A, Tjalve H, Hecht SS. Tissue distribution of the tobacco specific carcinogen 4-(methylnitrosamino)-1-(3-pyridyl)– 1 butanone and its metabolites in F344 rats. Cancer Res 1983; 43: 630–638.

Castren K, Vahakangas K, Heikkinen E et al. Absence of p53 mutations in benign and pre-malignant male genital lesions with over-expressed p53 protein. Int J Cancer 1998; 77(5): 674–678.

Bibliography

Catterall RD. In: Symposium on Candida Infections. HL Winner, R Hurley, eds. Edinburgh: Churchill Livingstone. 1966; 113.

Catterall RD. Clinical aspects of Reiter's Disease. Br J Rheumatol 1983; 22(supp 2): 151–155.

Cecchi R, Giomi A. Idiopathic calcinosis cutis of the penis. Dermatology 1999; 198(2): 174–175.

Cerio R, Wilson Jones E. A clinicopathological and immunohistochemical study of angiolymphoid hyperplasia with eosinophili A. Br J Dermatol 1983; 119(Suppl. 33): 36.

Chaikin DC, Volz LR, Broderick G. An unusual presentation of hidradenitis suppurativa: Case report and review of the literature. Urology 1994; 44(4): 606–608.

Chalmers RJ, Burton PA, Bennett R et al. Lichen sclerosus et atrophicus—a distinctive and common cause of phimosis in boys. Br J Dermatol 1982; 22(suppl.): 29–30.

Chalmers RJG, Burton PA, Benett RF et al. Lichen sclerosus et atrophicus: a common and distinctive cause of phimosis in boys. Arch Dermatol 1984; 120: 1025–1027.

Champion R ll, Wegrzyn J. Congenital os penis. J Urol 1964; 91: 663–664.

Chan WP, Chiang SS, Huang AH et al. Penile frenulum neurilemoma: A rare and unusual genitourinary tract tumor. J Urol 1990; 144(1): 136–137.

Chandur-Mnaymneh L, Gonzalez MS. Angiosarcoma of the penis with hepatic angiomas in a patient with low vinyl chloride exposure. Cancer 1981; 47: 1318–1324.

Chang MW. Update on juvenile xanthogranuloma: unusual cutaneous and systemic variants. Semin Cutan Med Surg 1999; 18(3): 195–205.

Chantarasak ND, Basu PK. Fournier's gangrene following vasectomy. Br J Urol 1988; 61(6): 538–539.

Chao SC, Yang MH, Lee JY. Mutation analysis of the ATP2A2 gene in Taiwanese patients with Darier's disease. Br J Dermatol 2002; 146(6): 958–963.

Charthaigh MN, Crowley B, Lynch M et al. Successful treatment of cutaneous cytomegalovirus. Int J STD & AIDS 1993; 4(1): 52–53.

Chawla AK, Willett CG. Squamous cell carcinoma of the anal canal and anal margin. Hematol Oncol Clin North Am 2001; 15(2): 321–344.

Chen YH, Wong TW, Lee JY. Depigmented genital extramammary Paget's disease: a possible histogenetic link to Toker's clear cells and clear cell papulosis. J Cutan Pathol 2001; 28(2): 105–108.

Cherian G. Co-trimoxazole and genital ulceration. Int J Clin Pract 2001; 55(2): 151.

Chernosky ME, Owen DW. Trichorrhexis nodosa: clinical and investigative studies. Arch Dermatol 1966; 94: 577–585.

Chetty R, Bramdev A, Govender D. Cytomegalovirus induced syringosquamous metaplasia. Am J Dermatopathol 1999; 21: 487–900.

Chiewchanvit S, Mahanupab P, Hirunsri P et al. Cutaneous manifestations of disseminated Penicillum marneffei mycosis in five HIV-infected patients. Mycoses 1991; 34: 245–249.

Chiewchanvit S, Thamprasert K, Siriunkgul S. Disseminated cutaneous cytomegalic inclusion disease resembling prurigo nodularis in a HIV-infected patient: a case report and literature review. J Med Assoc Thai 1993; 76(10): 581–584.

Choi GS, Won DH, Lee SJ et al. Divided naevus on the penis. Br J Dermatol 2000; 143(5): 1126–1127.

Choong KK. Acute penoscrotal edema due to acute necrotizing pancreatitis. J Ultrasound Med 1996; 15: 247–248.

Chopra R, Fisher RD, Fencel R. Phimosis and diabetes mellitus. J Urol 1982; 127: 1101–1102.

Chouvet B, Guillet G, Perrot H, et al. [Acquired epidermolysis bullosa with Crohn's disease. Report of two cases and review of literature (author's transl)] Ann Dermatol Venereol. 1982; 109(1): 53–63.

Chu CC, Chen KC, Diau GY. Topical steroid treatment of phimosis in boys. J Urol 1999; 162(3 Pt 1): 861–863.

Chu T. Langerhans cell histiocytosis. Australas J Dermatol 2001; 42(4): 237–242.

Chuang JH, Chen LY, Shieh CS et al. Surgical correction of buried penis: a review of 60 cases. J Pediatr Surg 2001; 36(3): 426–429.

Chun JL, McGregor A, Krishnan R et al. A comparison of dermal and cadaveric pericardial grafts in the modified Horton–Devine procedure for Peyronie's disease. J Urol 2001; 166(1): 185–188.

Chun YS, Chang SN, Park WH. A case of classical Kaposi's sarcoma of the penis showing a good response to high-energy pulsed carbon dioxide laser therapy. J Dermatol 1999; 26(4): 240–243.

CIBA. Foundation Symposium on filariasis. CIBA Found Symp 1987; 127: 1.

Civatte J, Lortat-Jacob E. Balanite pseudo-epitheliomateuse, keratosique et micacee. Bulletin de la Societe Francaise Dermatology et Syphiligraphie 1966; 68: 164–167.

Civatte J, Morel P, Bouhanna P. Canal dysembryoplasique de la verge de revelation tardive. Annales de Dermatologie et de Venereologie 1982; 109: 84–85.

Clark WR, Kramer SA. Henoch-Schonlein purpura and the acute scrotum. J Pediatr Surg 1986; 21: 991–992.

Claudy A, Garcier F, Schmitt D. Sclerosing lipogranuloma of the male genitalia: ultrastructural study. Br J Dermatol 1981; 105: 451–456.

Claudy AL, Dutoit M, Boucheron S. Epidermal and urethroid penile cyst. Acta Dermato-Venereologica 1991; 71(1): 61–62.

Clayden G. Anal appearances and child sex abuse. Lancet 1987; 1(8533): 620–621.

Cleary TL. Overwhelming infection with Group B β–hemolytic streptococcus asssociated with circumcision. Pediatrics 1979; 64(3): 301–303.

Clemmensen OJ, Krogh J, Petri M. The histologic spectrum of prepuces from patients with phimosis. Am J Dermatopathol 1988; 10(2): 104–108.

Cochran RJ, Wilkin JK. An unusual case of calcinosis cutis. J Am Acad Dermatol 1983; 8: 103–106.

Cockburn AG, Krolikowski J, Bariogh K et al. Crohn's disease of penile and scrotal skin. Urology 1980; 15: 596–598.

Cockerell CJ. Human immunodeficiency virus infection and the skin. Arch Intern Med. 1991; 151(7): 1295–303.

Cockerell CJ. Reevaluation of routine histology in the diagnosis of blistering diseases. Semin Dermatol. 1988; 7(3): 171–7.

Coda A, Ferri F. Perianal Verneuil's disease. Minerva Chirurgica 1991; 46(9): 465–467.

Cohen EL, Kim SW. Cutaneous manifestation of carcinoma of urinary bladder: carcinoma erysipelatodes. Urology 1980; 16(4): 410–412.

Cohen EL, Kim SW. Subcutaneous artificial penile nodules. J Urol 1982; 127: 135.

Cohen BA, Hood A. Xanthogranuloma: report on clinical and histologic findings in 64 patients. Pediatr Dermatol. 1989; 6(4): 262–6.

Cohen HA, Ashkenazi A, Nussinovitch M et al. Fixed drug eruption of the scrotum due to methyphenidate. Ann Pharmacother 1992; 26(11): 1378–1379.

Cohen HA, Nussinovitch M, Frydman M. Fixed drug eruption caused by acetaminophen. Ann Pharmacother 1992; 26(12): 1596–1597.

Cohen HA, Barzilai A, Matalon A et al. Fixed drug eruption of the penis due to hydroxyzine hydrochloride. Ann Pharmacother 1997; 31(3): 327–329.

Cohen SM, Schmitt SL, Lucas FV et al. The diagnosis of anal ulcers in AIDS patients. Int J Colorect Dis 1994; 9(4): 169–173.

Cohn M, Loubiere R, Guillaume A et al. Les lesions cutanees de bilharziose: a propos de 14 observations. Annales de Dermatologie et deVenereologie 1980; 107: 759–767.

Cold CJ, Taylor JR. The prepuce. Br J Urol 1999; 83(Suppl 1): 34–44.

Coldiron B, Jacobson C. Common penile lesions. Urol Clin N Am 1988; 15(4): 671–685.

Cole LA, Helwig EB. Mucoid cysts of the penile skin. J Urol 1976; 115: 397–400.

Cole MC, Cohen PR, Satra KH, et al. The concurrent presence of systemic disease pathogens and cutaneous Kaposi's sarcoma in the same lesion: Histoplasma capsulatum and Kaposi's sarcoma coexisting in a single skin lesion in a patient with AIDS. J Am Acad Dermatol. 1992; 26(2 Pt 2): 285–7.

Colebunders R, Blot K, Mertens V, Dockx P. Psoriasis regression in terminal AIDS. Lancet. 1992; 339(8801): 1110.

Coles RB, Wilkinson DS. Necrosis and dequalinium. I Balanitis. Trans St John's Hospital Dermatol Soc 1965; 51: 46–48.

Cook LS, Koutsky LA, Holmes KK. Clinical presentation of genital warts among circumcised and uncircumcised heterosexual men attending an urban STD clinic. Genitour Med 1993; 69(4): 262–264.

Cooke RA, Rodriguez RB. Amoebic balanitis. Med J Austral 1964; 5: 114–117.

Conger K, Sporer A. Kaposi sarcoma limited to the glans penis. Urology 1985; 26(2): 173–175.

Constantain HM, Wyman P. Localized amyloidosis of the urethra: report of a case. J Urol 1980; 124: 728–729.

Cooper C, Pippard EC, Sharp H et al. Is Behçet's disease triggered by childhood infection? Ann Rheum Dis 1989; 16: 12–13.

Cope R, Debou JM. Aids and anorectal pathology. Annales de Chirurgie 1995; 49(4): 310–316.

Coppo P, Salomone R. Pseudoverrucous papules: an aspect of incontinence in children. J Eur Acad Dermatol Venereol. 2002; 16: 409–10.

Corazza M, Ughi G, Spisani L et al. Metastatic ulcerative penile Crohn's disease. J Eur Acad Dermatol Venereol 1999; 13(3): 224–226.

Correia O, Delgado L, Polonia J. Genital fixed drug eruption: cross reactivity between doxycycline and minocycline. Clin Exper Dermatol 1999; 24(2): 137.

Coskunfirat OK, Sayilkan S, Velidedeoglu H. Glans and penile skin amputation as a complication of circumcision. Ann Plast Surg 1999; 43(4): 457.

Cosman BC, O'Grady TC, Pekarske S. Verrucous carcinoma arising in hidradenitis suppurativa. Int J Colorect Dis 2000; 15(5–6): 342–346.

Costa S, Syrjanen S, Vendra C et al. Detection of human papillomavirus infections in the male sexual partners of women attending an STD clinic in Bologna. Int J STD AIDS 1992; 3: 338–346.

Cotterill JA. A dermatological non–disease–a common and potentially fatal disturbance of cutaneous body image. Br J Dermatol 1980; 103(Suppl. 18): 13.

Cotterill JA. A dermatological non–disease–a common and potentially fatal disturbance of cutaneous body image. Br J Dermatol 1981; 104: 611–9.

Cowl CT, Bauer BS. Resection of lymphatic malformation of the scrotum. Plast Reconst Surg 1999; 94(1): 198–201.

Cox NH. Permethrin treatment in scabies infestation: importance of the correct formulation. Br Med J 2000; 320: 37–38.

Coyne JD, Fitzgibbon JF. Mixed syringocystadenoma papilliferum and papillary eccrine adenoma occurring in a scrotal condylom A. J Cutan Pathol 2000; 27(4): 199–201.

Craig MW, Davey WN, Green RA. Conjugal blastomycosis. Am Rev Resp Dis 1970; 102: 86–90.

Crawford SE, Sherman R, Favara B. Pyoderma gangrenosum with response to cyclophosphamide therapy. J Pediatr. 1967; 71(2): 255–8.

Creasman C, Haas PA, Fox TA Jr. et al. Malignant transformation of anorectal giant condyloma acuminatum (Buschke–Loewenstein tumour). Dis Colon Rectum 1989; 32: 481–487.

Cresson DH, Siegal GP. Chronic lymphocytic leukemia presenting as an anal mass. J Clin Gastroenterol. 1985; 7(1): 83–7.

Cribier B, Ndiaye I, Grosshans E. Peno-gingival syndrome. A male equivalent of vulvo–vagino–gingival syndrome. Revue de Stomatologie et de Chirurgie Maxillo–Faciale 1992; 94(3): 148–151.

Cribier B, Lipsker D, Grosshans E et al. Genital ulceration revealing a primary cutaneous anaplastic lymphoma. Genitourin Med 1997; 73(4): 325.

de Crohn Revue generale a propos de deux observations. Annales de Dermatologie et de Venereologie 1982, 109. 53–63.

Crohn NN, Yarnis H. Regional Ileitis 2nd edn. New York: Grune & Stratton; 1958.

Crosby DL, Berger TG, Woosley JT, et al. Dermatophytosis mimicking Kaposi's sarcoma in human immunodeficiency virus disease. Dermatologica. 1991; 182(2): 135–7.

Crow KD. Chloracne and its potential clinical implications. Clin Exper Dermatol 1981; 6: 243–257.

Crudeli F, Cecchi R, Fedi E et al. Zoon's plasma–cell nodular balanitis. G Ital Dermatol Venereol. Nov 1986; 121(6): 431–434.

Csango PA, Skuland J, Nilsen A et al. Papillomavirus among abortion applicants and patients at a sexually transmitted disease clinic. Sex Trans Dis 1992; 19(3): 149–153.

Csonka GW, Murray M. Clinical evaluation of carbenoxolone in balanitis. Br J Venereol 1971; 47: 179–181.

Cubilla AL, Barreto J, Caballero C et al. Pathologic features of epidermoid carcinoma of the penis. A prospective study of 66 cases. Am J Surg Path 1993; 17(8): 753–763.

Cubilla AL, Ayala MT, Barreto JE et al. Surface adenosquamous carcinoma of the penis. A report of three cases. Am J Surg Pathol 1996; 20: 156–160.

Cubilla AL, Meijer CJLM, Young RH. Morphological features of epithelial abnormalities and precancerous lesions of the penis. Scand J Urol Nephrol 2000; 205(Suppl.): 215–219.

Cubilla AL, Velazques EF, Reuter VE et al. Warty (condylomatous) squamous cell carcinoma of the penis: a report of 11 cases and proposed classification of 'verruciform' penile tumors. Am J Surg Pathol 2000; 24(4): 505–512.

Cullen SI Cpt. Incidence of Nevi. Arch Dermatol 1962; 86: 88–91.

Cunningham DL, Persky L. Penile ecthyma gangrenosum. Urology 1989; 34(2): 109–110.

Cuozzo DW, Vachher P, Sau P et al. Verruciform xanthoma: A benign penile growth. J Urol 1995; 153: 1625–1627.

Cupp MR, Malek RS, Goellner JR et al. The detection of human papillomavirus deoxyribonucleic acid in intraepithelial, in situ, verrucous and invasive carcinoma of the penis. J Urol 1995; 154: 1024–1029.

Curtis AC, Cawley EP. Genital histoplasmosis. J Urol 1947; 57: 781–787.

Cusano F, Capozzi M. Photocontact dermatitis from ketoprofen with cross-reactivity to ibuproxam. Cont Dermat 1992; 27(1): 50–59.

Cutler TC. Bowenoid papulosis of the penis. Clin Exper Dermatol 1994; 5: 97–100.

D

Dahl EV, Baggenstoss AH, deWeerd JH. Testicular lesions of periarteritis nodosa, with special reference to diagnosis. Am J Med 1960; 28: 222–228.

Dahlman-Ghozlan K, Hedblad MA, von Krogh G. Penile lichen sclerosus et atrophicus treated with clobetasol dipropionate 0.05% cream: a retrospective clinical and histopathological study. J Am Acad Dermatol 1999; 40(3): 451–457.

Daling JR. History of circumcision, medical conditions, and sexual activity and the risk of penile cancer. J Natl Cacer Inst 1993; 85: 19–24.

Dalton JD. Guidelines on circumcision. Legal position is unclear. Br Med J 1997; 315: 750.

Daneshpouy M, Socie G, Clavel C et al. Human papillomavirus infection and anogenital condyloma in bone marrow transplant recipients. Transplant 2001; 71(1): 167–169.

Daniel GL, Longo WE, Vernava III AM. Pruritis ani. Causes and concerns. Dis Col Rect 1980; 37(7): 670–674.

Bibliography

Daoud MS, Pittelkow MR. Lichen planus. In: Fitzpatrick Dermatology in General Medicine. Greadberg et al eds Vol 1 Sixth edition. McGraw Hill. 2003; 473–474.

Dare AJ, Axelsen RA. Scrotal calcinosis: origin dystrpohic calcification of eccrine duct milia. J Cutan Pathol 1988; 15: 142–149.

Das S, Tunuguntla HSGR. Balanitis xerotica obliterans– a review. World J Urol 2000; 18(6): 382–387.

Das S, Tuerk D, Amar AD et al. Surgery of the male genital lymphedema. J Urol 1983; 129: 1240–1242.

Dasan S, Neill SM, Donaldson DR et al. Treatment of persistent pruritus ani in a combined colorectal and dermatological clinic. Br J Surg 1999; 86(10): 1337–1340.

Datta NS, Kern FB. Silicone granuloma of the penis. J Urol 1973; 109: 840–842.

Datta C, Dutta SK, Chaudhuri A. Histopathological and immunological studies in a cohort of balanitis xerotica obliterans. J Indian Med Assoc 1993; 91(6): 146–148.

Daudén E, Porras JI, Buezo GF et al. Eccrine squamous syringometaplasia and cytomegalovirus. Am J Dermatopathol 2000; 22: 559–561.

Davenport M, Bianchi A, Gough DCS. Idiopathic scrotal haemorrhage in neonates. Br Med J 1989; 298: 1492–1493.

Davenport A, Downey SE, Goel S, Maciver AG. Wegener's granulomatosis involving the urogenital tract. Br J Urol. 1996; 78(3): 354–7.

Davies DM, Mitchell I. Fracture of the penis. Br J Urol 1978; 50: 426.

Davis CM. Granuloma inguinale: a clinical, histological and ultrastructural study. J Am Med Ass 1970; 211: 632–636.

Davis J, Shapiro L, Baral J. Vulvitis circumscripta plasmacellularis. J Am Acad Dermatol 1983; 8: 413–416.

Davis NS, Kim CA, Dever DP. Primary malignant melanoma of the scrotum: case report and literature review. J Urol 1991; 145: 1056–1057.

Davis-Daneshfar A, Trueb RM. Bowen's disease of the glans penis (erythroplasia of Queyrat) in plasma cell balanitis. Cutis 2000; 65(6): 395–8.

Dean AL. Epithelioma of the scrotum. J Urol 1948; 60(3): 508–518.

de Bree E, Sanidas E, Tzardi M et al. Malignant melanoma of the penis. Eur J Surg Oncol 1997; 23(3): 277–279.

de Dulanto F, Armijo-Moreno M, Camacho Martinez F. [Nodular hidradenoma (apocrine cystadenoma) of the penis] Article in French. Ann Dermatol Syphiligr (Paris) 1973; 100: 417–422.

Dehner LP, Smith BH. Soft tissue tumours of the penis. Cancer 1970; 25: 1431–1447.

Dekio S, Jidio J. Tinea of the glans penis. Dermatologica 1989; 178: 112–114.

Dekio S, Qin LM, Jidio J. Tinea of the glans penis: report of a case presenting a crop of papules. J Dermatol 1991; 18: 52–55.

Delacretaz J, Christeler A. Demonstrations. Dermatologica 139. 1969; 313–319.

Delaney TA, Walker NPJ. Penile melanosis successfully treated with the Q-switched ruby laser. Br J Dermatol 1994; 130: 663–664.

Delzotto A, Christol B, Delzotto L et al. Tubercolosi del pene. Urologica 1973; 34: 171–175.

Demeter LM, Stoler MH, Bonnez W et al. Penile intraepithelial neoplasia: clinical presentation and an analysis of the physical state of human Paillomavirus DNA. J Infect Dis 1993; 168: 38–46.

Demir Y, Latifoglu O, Yenidunya S et al. Extensive lymphatic malformation of penis and scrotum. Urology 2001; 58(1): 106.

Demitsu T, Nagato H, Nishimaki K et al. Melanoma in situ of the penis J Am Acad Dermatol. 2000; 42: 386–388.

Denis BJ, May T, Bigard MA et al. Anal and perianal lesions in symptomatic HIV infections. Prospective study of a series of 190 patients. Gastroenterologie Clinique et Biologique 1992; 16(2): 148–154.

Derevianko TI, Derevianko IM. A rare and little known variant of hypospadias. Urol Nefrol (Mosk) (4); 1998: 45–47. Russian.

Derrick EK, Ridley CM, Kobza-Black A, et al. A clinical study of 23 cases of female anogenital carcinoma. Br J Dermatol. 2000; 143(6): 1217–23.

DeSanctis DP, Maglietta R, Miranda R et al. Giant cell fibroblastoma of the scrotum. A case report. Tumori 1993; 79: 367–369.

Desanctis PN, Furey CA Jr. Steroid injection therapy for peyronie's disease: A 10–year summary and review of 38 cases. J Urol 1967; 97: 114–116.

Desruelles F, Lacour JP, Mantoux F et al. Divided nevus of the penis: an unusual location. Arch Dermatol 1998; 134(7): 879–880.

Dexeus FH, Logothetis J, Sella A et al. Combination therapy with methotrexate, bleomycin and cisplatin for advanced squamous cell carcinoma of the male genital tract. J Urol 1991; 146(5): 1284–1287.

Dianzani C, Bucci M, Pierangeli A et al. Association of human papilloma virus type 11 with carcinoma of the penis. Urology 1998; 51: 1046–1048.

Di Silverio A, Serri F. Generalized bullous and haemorrhagic lichen sclerosus et atrophicus. Br J Dermatol 1975; 93: 215–217.

Dixon RS, Mikhail GR. Erythroplasia (Queyrat) of conjunctiva. J Am Acad Dermatol 1981; 4: 160–165.

Dogan G, Oram Y, Hazneci E et al. Three cases of verrucous carcinoma. J Derm 1998; 39(4): 251–254.

Doll DC, Diaz-Arias AA. Peripheral T–cell lymphoma of the scrotum. Acta Haematologica 1994; 91(2): 77–79.

Donnellan SM, Webb DR. Management of invasive penile cancer by synchronous penile lengthening and radical tumour excision to avoid perineal urethrostomy. Aust N Z J Surg 1998; 68(5): 369–370.

Dootson GM, Lott CW, Moisey CU. Fournier's gangrene and diabetes mellitus: survival following surgery. J Roy Soc Med 1982; 75: 916–917.

Dore B, Grange P, Irani J et al. Atrophicus sclerosis lichen and cancer of the glans. J Urol (Paris 1989; 95(7): 415–418. French.

Dore B, Irani J, Aubert J. Carcinoma of the penis in lichen sclerosus atrophicus. A case report. Eur Urol 1990; 18(2): 153–155.

Douglas JM, Rogers M, Judson F. The effect of asymptomatic infection with HTLV 111 on the response of anogenital warts to intralesional treatment with alpha–2 interferon. J Infect Dis 1986; 154: 331–334.

Doutre M-S, Beylot C, Bioulac P et al. Tumeur de Buschke–Lowenstein 2 cas feminins. Annales de Dermatologie et de Venereologie 1979; 106: 1031–1034.

Dowd PM, Champion RH. Cherry angioma. In Disorders of blood vessels Ch. 45. Rook et al. Textbook of dermatology Sixth edition. Blackwell Science, Oxford. Volume 3, Ch. 45. 2092.

Downing R, Black. Polyarteritis nodosa: an unrecognised cause of Fournier's Gangrene. Br J Urol 1985; 57: 355–356.

Downs AM, Harvey I, Kennedy CT. The epidemiology of head lice and scabies in the UK. Epidemiol Infect 1999; 122(3): 471–477.

Droller MJ. Carcinoma of the penis: An overview. Urol Clin N Am 1980; 7(3): 783–784.

Drumm J, Donovan IA, Clain A. Unusual presentation of anorectal carcinoma. Br J Med 1982; 285: 1393.

Drusin LM, Homan WP, Dineen P. The role of surgery in primary syphilis of the anus. Ann Surg. 1976; 184(1): 65–7.

Drut RM, Gomez MA, Drut R et al. Human papillomavirus is present in some cases of childhood penile lichen sclerosus: an in situ hybridization and SP–PCR study. Pediatr Dermatol 1998; 15(2): 85–90.

Dubin BA, Bronson DM, Eng AM. Acute hemorrhagic edema of childhood: An unusual variant of leukocytoclastic vasculitis. Am J Dermatol 1990; 23(2 Pt.2): 347–350.

Duckett JW, Keating MA. Technical challenge of the megameatus intact prepuce hypospadias variant: the pyramid procedure. J Urol 1989; 141: 1407–1409.

Duhra P, Ilchyshyn A. Perianal streptococcal cellulitis with penile involvement. Br J Dermatol 1990; 123(6): 793–796.

Dundar SV, Gençalp U, Simsek S. Familial cases of Behçet's disease. Br J Dermatol 1985; 113: 319–321.

Dundas SAC, Laing RW. Titanium balanitis with phimosis. Dermatologica 1988; 176: 305–307.

Dunlop EMC. Chlamydial genital infection and its complication. Br J Hosp Med 1983; 30: 6–11.

Dunsmuir WD, Gordon EM. The history of circumcision. Br J Urol Int 1999; 83(Suppl. 1): 1–12.

Duperrat B, Carton F-X. Balanite et ulcère de la verge à trichomonas. Bulletin de la Société Française Dermatologie et Syphiligraphie 1969; 76: 345.

Duperrat B, Labouche F. Le granulome venenen (donovanose) en France. Annales de Dermatologie et de Syphiligraphie 1975; 102: 241–250.

Dupre A, Christol B. Dequalinium necrosis penis. Bulletin de la Societe Francaise Dermatologie et de Syphilographie 1975; 80: 194–196.

Dupre A, Schnitzler L. Plasmocytic proliferative lesions of the foreskin. A variety of Zoon's benign circumscribed balanitis. Ann Dermatol Venereol 1977; 104(2): 127–131. French.

Dupre A, Viraben R. Basal lamina with a garland–like pattern in a case of sclero–atrophic lichen. Ultrastructural study. Ann Dermatol Venereol 1988; 115(1): 19–26. French.

Dupre A, Bonafe J–L, Lassere J et al. Lesions bourgeonnant,es pruputiales a plasmocytes: variante anatomo–clinique de la balanoposthite chronique circonscrite benigne de Zoon. Bulletin de la Societe Francaise Dermatologie et Syphiligraphie 1976; 83: 62–63.

Dupre A, Bonafe J–L, Castel M. Etude immuno–pathologique de 4 cas de balano–posthite de Zoon. Annales de Dermatologie et de Venereologie 1981; 108: 691–696.

Dupre A, Lassere J, Christol B et al. Canaux et kystes dysembryo plasiques du raphe genitopenneal. Annales de Dermatologie et de Venereologie 1982; 109: 81–84.

Dupre MMA, Bonafe JL, Lassere J et al. Lesions boureonnantes preputiales a plasmocytes: variante anatomo–clinique de la balano–posthite chronique circonscrite benigne de zoon. Bulletin de la Societe Francaise de Dermatologie et de Syphiligraphie 1976; 83(1): 62–63.

Durst M, Kleinheinz A, Hotz M et al. The physical state of human papillomavirus type 16 DNA in benign and malignant genital tumours. DHJJ Gen Virol 1985; 6: 1515–1522.

Duvic M, Lowe L. Superficial phaeohypomycosis of the scrotum in a patient with the acquired immunodeficiency syndrome. Arch Dermatol 1987; 123: 1597–1599.

Duvic M, Johnson TM, Rapini RP et al. Acquired immunodeficiency syndrome– associated psoriasis and Reiter's syndrome. Arch Dermatol 1987; 123: 1622–1632.

Duvic M, Friedman-Kien AE, Looney DJ, et al. Topical treatment of cutaneous lesions of acquired immunodeficiency syndrome-related Kaposi sarcoma using alitretinoin gel: results of phase 1 and 2 trials. Arch Dermatol. 2000; 136(12): 1461–9.

Duvic M. Papulosquamous disorders associated with human immunodeficiency virus infection. Dermatol Clin. 1991; 9(3): 523–30.

E

Eastridge RR, Carrion HM, Politano VA. Hemangioma of the scrotum perineum and buttocks. Urology 1979; 14(1): 61–63.

Echenique JE, Tully S, Tickman R et al. A 37 pound scrotal leiomyosarcoma: A case report and literature review. J Urol 1987; 138: 1245.

Ecker RI, Schroeter AL. Acrondermatis and acquired zinc deficiency. Arch Dermatol 1978; 114: 937–939.

Edwards S. Balanitis and balanoposthitis: a review. Genitourin Med 1996; 72(3): 155–159.

Egan CA, Rallis TM, Zone TJ. Multiple scrotal lymphangiomas (lymphangiectases) treated by carbon dioxide laser ablation. Br J Dermatol 1998; 139: 534–562.

Eglitis JA. Occurrence of bone tissue in the human penis. J Urol 1953; 70(5): 749–758.

Eickenberg H, Amin M, Lich R. Blastomycosis of the genitourinary tract. J Urol 1975; 113: 650–652.

El–Gadi S. Biopsy before excision. J Eur Acad Dermatol Venereol 1996; 7: 87–90.

El–Hoshy K, Mizuguchi R. Dermatoses of the glans penis: penile venereal edema. J Am Acad Dermatol 1990, 30(1). 615–616.

El–Zawahry M. Schistosomal granuloma of the glans. Br J Dermatol 1965; 77: 344–8.

Elhosseiny AA, Ramaswamy G, Healy RO. Epitheloid hemangioendothelioma of the penis. Urology 1986; 28(3): 243–245.

Elliot JP, Fischman JL. Os Penis. J Urol 1962; 88: 655–656.

Ellis H. A History of Surgery. Greenwich Medical Media Ltd, London; 2000.

Ellis CN, Gilbert M, Cohen KA et al. Increased muscle tone during etretinate therapy. J Am Acad Dermatol 1986; 14(5 Pt.2): 907–909.

Ellsworth P, Cendron M, Ritland D et al. Hypospadias repair in the 1990s. AORN J 1999; 69(1): 148–53, 155–6, 159–161.

Emory RE, Chester CH. Prepuce pollicization: a reminder of an alternate donor. Plast Reconstr Surg 2000; 105(6): 2100–2111.

Eng AM, Morgan NE, Blekys J. Giant condyloma acuminatum. Cutis 1979; 24: 203–206.

Eng A, Armin A, Massa M et al. Peutz-like melanotic macules associated with oesophageal adenocarcinoma. Am J Dermatopathol 1991; 13(2): 152–157.

Engelkens HJ, Judanarso J, van der Sluis JJ et al. Disseminated early yaws: report of a child with a remarkable genital lesion mimicking venereal syphilis. Pediatr Dermatol 1990; 7: 60–62.

English JC III, Laws RA, Keough GC et al. Dermatoses of the glans penis and prepuce. J Am Acad Dermatol 1997; 37(1):1–24: quiz. 25–26.

English JC III, King DH, Foley JP. Penile shaft hypopigmentation: lichen sclerosus occurring after the initiation of alprostadil intracavernous injections for erectile dysfunction. J Am Acad Dermatol 1998; 39(5 Pt 1): 801–803.

Enriquez JM, Moreno S, Devesa M et al. Fournier's syndrome of urogenital and banogenital origin. A retrospective, comparitive study. Dis Col Rect 1987; 36(1): 33–37.

Erlich KS, Jacobson MA, Koehler IE et al. Foscarnet therapy for severe acyclovir resistant herpes simplex virus type–2 infections in patients with acquired immunodeficiency syndrome. Ann Int Med 1989; 110(9): 710–713.

Eron LJ, Judson F, Tucker S. Interferon therapy for condylomata acuminata. N Engl J Med 1986; 315: 1059–1064.

Escala JM, Rickwood AMK. Balanitis. Br J Urol 1989; 63(2): 196–197.

Esdaile B, Davis M, Portsmouth S, et al. The immunological effects of concomitant highly active antiretroviral therapy and liposomal anthracycline treatment of HIV-1-associated Kaposi's sarcoma. AIDS. 2002; 16(17): 2344–7.

Esen AA, Aslan G, Kazimoglu H et al. Concealed penis: rare complication of circumcision. Urol Int 2001; 66(2): 117–118.

Esiashvili N, Landry J, Matthews RH. Carcinoma of the anus: strategies in management. Oncologist 2002; 7(3): 188–199.

Espana A, Sanchez–Yus E, Serna MJ et al. Chronic balanitis with palisading granuloma. An atypical genital localization of necrobiosis lipoidica responsive to pentoxifylline. Dermatology 1994; 188: 222–225.

Esser AC, Nossa R, Shoji T et al. All–trans–retinoic acid–induced scrotal ulcerations in a patient with acute promyelocytic leukaemia. J Am Acad Dermatol 2000; 43: 316–317.

Estéve E, Gironet N, Barthez JP et al. Case for diagnosis. Herpes rugbiorum. Annales de Derm et de Vener 1998; 1125(8): 527–528.

Eusebio EB. New treatment of intractable pruritis ani. Dis Col Rect 1991; 34(3). 289.

Evans AL, Summerly R. Pseudo-chancre redux with negahve serology. A case report. British Journal of Venereal Disease 1964; 40: 222–224.

Evans LM, Grossman ME. Foscarnet-induced penile ulcer. J Am Acad Dermatol 1992; 27(1): 124–126.

Eyers AA, Thompson JPS. Pruritus ani: is anal sphincter dysfunction important in aetiology? Br Med J 1979; i: 1549–1551.

F

Fagan WA, Skinner SM, Ondo A et al. Bacillary angiomatosis of the skin and bone marrow in a patient with HIV infection. J Am Dermatol 1995; 32(3): 510–512.

Fahal AH, Suliman SH, Sharfi AR et al. Acute idiopathic scrotal oedema in association with diabetic septic foot. Diabetes Res Clin Pract 1993; 21(2–3): 197–200.

Fakjian N, Hunter S, Cole GW et al. An argument for circumcision: prevention of balanitis in the adult. Arch Dermatol 1990; 126: 1046–1047.

Farber EM, Nall L. Perianal and intergluteal psoriasis. Cutis 1992; 50(5): 336–338.

Farina LA, Alonso MV, Horjales M et al. Contact-derived allergic balanoposthitis and paraphimosis through topical application of celandine juice. Actas Urologicas Espanolas 1999; 23(6): 554–555.

Farouk R, Duthie GS. Rectal prolapse and rectal invagination. Eur J Surg 1998; 164(5): 323–332.

Farrell AM, Francis N, Bunker CB. Zoon's balanitis: an immuno-histochemical study. Br J Dermatol 1996; 135(suppl 47): 57.

Farell AM, Trendell-Smith NJ, Francis N, et al. Are 'idiopathic' scrotal cysts 'idiopathic'? An immunohistochemical approach.Br J Dermatl. 1996; 135(Suppl 47): 57.

Farrell AM, Black MM, Bracka A et al. Pyoderma gangrenosum of the penis. Br J Dermatol 1998; 138: 337–340.

Farrell AM, Marren P, Dean D et al. Lichen sclerosus: evidence that immunological changes occur at all levels of the skin. Br J Dermatol 1999; 140: 1087–1092.

Farrell AM, Millard PR, Schomberg KH et al. An infective aetiology for lichen sclerosus re–addressed. Clin Exp Dermatol 1999; 24: 479–483.

Farrell AM, Dean D, Charnock FM et al. Do plasminogen activators play a role in lichen sclerosus? Clin Exp Dermatol 2000; 25: 432–435.

Fauer R, Morrow JW. External urinary devices-use and abuse. Urology 1978; 11: 180–182.

Favarger N, Rist M, Krupp S. Cutaneous reconstruction of external genital organs: an older method still in current use. Helvetica Chirurgica Acta 1991; 58(3): 301–303.

Feingold DS. Gangrenous and crepitant cellulitis: J Am Acad Dermatol. 1982; 6: 289–299.

Feldman RT, Maibach HL. Regional variation in percutaneous penetration of 14c cortisol in man. J Invest Dermatol 1967; 48: 181–183.

Feldmann R, Harms M. Lichen sclerosus et atrophicus. Hautarzt 1991; 42(3): 147–153. German.

Fenger C. Anal neoplasia and its precursors: facts and controversies. Sem Diagnost Pathol 1991; 8(3): 190–201.

Ferenczy A, Richart RM, Wright TC. Pearly penile papules: Absence of human papillomavirus DNA by the polymerase chain reaction. Obst Gynecol 1991; 78(1): 118–122.

Fergusson DM, Lawton JM, Shannon FT. Neonatal circumcision and penile problems: An 8 year longitudinal study. Pediatrics 1988;

Fernandez MJ, Martino A, Khan H et al. Giant Neurilemoma: Unusual scrotal mass. Urology 1987; 30(1): 74–76.

Fernandez Vozmediano JM, Romero Cabrera MA, Lasanta Villar J. Zoon's plasmocytary balanitis. Treatment by circumcision and a review of the literature. Med Cutan Ibero Lat Am 1984; 12(4): 331–335. Spanish.

Ferrandiz C, Ribera M. Zoon's balanitis treated by circumcision. J Dermatol Surg Oncol 1984; 10: 622–625.

Fetherston WC, Fredrich EG. The origin and significance of vulvar Paget's disease. Obstet Gynecol 1972; 39: 735–744.

Fetissof F, Lorette G, Dubois P et al. Endocrine cells in the median raphe cysts of the penis. Path Res Pract 1985; 180: 644–646.

Fielding JF. Perianal lesions in Crohn's Disease. J Roy Coll Surg Edinburgh 1972; 17: 32–37.

Fields T, Drylie D, Wilson J. Malignant evolution of penile horn. Urology 1987; 30(1): 65–66.

Findlay GH, Whiting DA. Mondor's phlebitis of the penis. A condition miscalled 'non–venereal sclerosing lymphangitis.' Clin Exper Dermatol 1977; 2: 65–67.

Fine RM. AIDS-related Kaposi's sarcoma. Int J Dermatol. 1992; 31(7): 471.

Firestein GS, Gruber HE, Weisman MH et al. Mouth and Genital and Inflamed Cartilage: MAGIC syndrome. Am J Med 1985; 79: 65–72.

Fisher AA. Unique reactions of scrotal skin to topical agents. Cutis 1989a; 44: 445–447.

Fisher AA. Unusual condom dermatitis. Cutis 1989b; 44: 365.

Fisher AA. Allergic Contact dermatitis to mitomycin-C. Cutis. 1991; 47: 225.

Fisher BK. The red scrotum syndrome. Cutis 1997; 60(3): 139–141.

Fisher BK, Dvoretsky I. Idiopathic calcinosis of the scrotum. Arch Dermatol 1978; 114: 957.

Fisher JR, Conway Ml, Takeshita RT et al. Necrotizing fasciitis: importance of roentgenographic studies for soft tissue gas. J Am Med Ass 1979; 241: 803–806.

Flanigan RC, Kursh FD, McDougal WS et al. Synergistic gangrene of the scrotum and penis secondary to colorectal disease. J Urol 1978; 119: 369–371.

Fleck F, Fleck M. eds: Organische w. Funktionelle Sexualerkrankungen. Berlin: Verlag und Gesundheit. 1974.

Fleisher G, Hodge D, Cromie W. Penile edema in childhood. Ann Emerg Med 1980; 9. 314–315.

Flentje D, Benz G, Daum R. Lichen sclerosus et atrophicus as a cause of acquired phimosis–circumcision as a preventive measure against penis cancer. Z Kinderchir 1987; 42: 308–311.

Flessati P, Camoglio FN, Bianchi S et al. An apocrine hidrocystoma of the scrotum. A case report. Minerva Chirurgica 1999; 54(1–2): 87–89.

Fork HE, Sanchez RL, Wagner Jr RF et al. A new type of connective tissue nevus: isolated expophytic elastoma. J Cutan Pathol 1996; 18: 457–463.

Forstrom L, Winkelmann RK. Factitial panniculitis. Arch Dermatol 1974; 110: 747–750.

Fortier–Beaulieu M, Thomine E, Mitrofanof P et al. Preputial sclero-atrophic lichen in children. Ann Pediatr (Paris 1990; 37(10): 673–676. French.

Foucar E, Downing DT, Gerber WL. Sclerosing lipogranuloma of the male genitalia containing vitamin E. A comparison with classical 'paraffinoma'. J Am Acad Dermatol 1983; 9: 103–110.

Fournier A, Darier J. Epithelioma benin syphiloide de la verge (epitheliome papilllaire). Bull Soc Franc Dermat et Syph 4: 324. 1893;

Fox PA, Barton SE, Francis N et al. Chronic erosive herpes simplex virus infection of the penis, a possible immune reconstitution disease. HIV Med 1999; 1: 10–18.

Franklin EW, Rutledge FD. Epidemiology of epidermoid carcinoma of the vulva. Obstet Gynecol 1972; 39: 165–172.

Franzblau AH. Itchy urethra: a case report. Rocky Mountain Med J 1973; 70: 35.

Friedman SJ, Fox BJ, Albert HL. Seborrhoeic keratoses of the penis. Urology 1987; 29: 204–206.

Frier BM, Howie AD. Scrotal gangrene in asymptomatic myeloma. Br Med J 1972; iv: 26.

Frisch M, Friis S, Kruger Kjaer S et al. 1943–1990 Falling incidence of penis cancer in an uncircumcised population (Denmark) 1995.

Friter BS, Lucky AW. The perineal eruption of Kawasaki syndrome. Arch Dermatol 1988; 124: 1805–1810.

Frydenberg M. Penile gangrene: A separate entity from Fournier's syndrome? Br J Urol 1988; 61(6): 532–533.

Fueston JC, Adams BB, Mutasim DF. Cicatricial pemphigoid-induced phimosis. J Am Acad Dermatol. 2002; 46(5 Suppl): S128–9.

Fulton JE, Carter DM, Hurley HJ. Treatment of Bowen's disease with topical 5–fluorouracil under occlusion. Arch Dermatol 1968; 97; 178–180.

Fung MA, LeBoit PE. Light microscopic criteria for the diagnosis of early vulvar lichen sclerosus: a comparison with lichen planus. Am J Surg Pathol 1998; 22(4). 473–478.

Fungelso PD, Reed WB, Newman SB et al. Herpes zoster of the anogenital area affecting urination and defecation. Br J Dermatol 1973; 89; 285 288.

Fussell EN, Kaack MB, Cherry R et al. Adherence of bacteria to human foreskins. J Urol 1988; 140: 997–1001.

G

Gaines H, von Sydow M, Pehrson PO et al. Clinical picture of primary HIV infection presenting as a glandular–fever–like illness. Br Med J 1988; 297: 1363–1368.

Gaines H, von Sydow M, von Stedingk L et al. Immunological changes in primary HIV–1 infection. AIDS 1990; 4: 995–999.

Gallant JE, Moore RD, Richman DD et al. the Zidovudine Epidemiology Study Group and Incidence and the natural history of cytomegalovirus disease in patients with advanced human immunodeficiency virus disease treated with Zidovudine. Ndo Y, Mikoshiba H, Mochizuku J Infect Dis 1992; 166: 1223–1227.

Gamulka BD. Index of suspicion. Case #1 Diagnosis: Allergic contact dermatitis. Pediatr Rev 2000; 21(12): 421–426.

Ganem JP, Lucey DT, Janosko EO et al. Unusual complications of the vacuum erection device. Urology 1998; 51(4): 627–631.

Ganem JP, Steele BW, Creager AJ et al. Pseudo-epitheliomatous keratotic and micaceous balanitis. J Urol 1999; 161(1): 217–218.

Garcia-Armengol J, Roig JV, Alos R et al. Perianal cuaneous metastasis of rectal adenocarcinoma. Revista Espanola de Enfermedades Digestivas 1995; 87(4): 342–343.

Garcia Panos JM, Buendia Gonzalez E, Jimenez Leiro F et al. Penile cutaneous horn. Report of a case and review of the literature. Arch Esp Urol 1999; 52(2): 173–174. Spanish.

Gass JDM, Glatzer RJ. Acquired pigmentation simulating Peutz–Jeghers syndrome: initial manifestation of diffuse uveal melanocytic proliferation. Br J Opthalmol 1991; 75: 693–695.

Gasser TC, Lehmann K. Male sexual function is more than erection. Lancet 1995; 346: 706.

Gatto–Weis C, Topolsky D, Sloane B et al. Ulcerative balanoposthitis of the foreskin as a manifestation of chronic lymphocytic leukemia: case report and review of the literature. Urology 2000; 56(4): 669.

Gaveau D et al. [Cutaneous manifestations of zinc deficiency in ethylic cirrhosis]. Ann Dermatol Venereol 1987; 114(1): 39–53. French.

Gbery IP, Dheja D, Kacou DE et al. Chronic genital ulcerations and HIV infection: 29 cases. Medecine Tropicale 1999; 59(3): 279–282.

Gedalia A, Adar A, Gorodischer R. Familial Mediterranean fever in children. J Rheumatol 1992; 19(supp. 35): 1–9.

Geiss DF, Del Rosso RQ, Murphy J. Verruciform xanthoma of the glans penis: a benign clinical stimulant of genital malignancy. Cutis 1993; 51(5): 369–372.

Geniaux B, Lazrak B, Moubid MA. Histiocytoses X. Bulletin de la Societe Francaise Dermatologie et Syphiligraphie 1973; 80: 380–382.

George WM. Papular pearly penile pearls. J Am Acad Dermatol 1989; 20(5 Pt.1): 852.

Gerber GS. Carcinoma in situ of the penis. J Urol 1994; 151: 829–833.

Gerber WL. Scrotal malignancies: The University of Iowa experience and a review of the literature. Urology 1985; 26(4): 337–342.

Gerster AG, Mandlebaum FS. On the formation of bone in the human penis. Ann Surg 1913; 896–901.

Geusau A, Heinz–Peer G, Vole-Platzer B et al. Regression of deeply infiltrating giant condyloma (Buschke–Lowenstein tumor) following long–term intralesional interferon alfa therapy. Arch Derm 2000; 136(6): 707–710.

Geyer H, Geyer A, Schubert J. Erysipelas and elephantiasis of the scrotum. Surgical and drug therapy. Urologe–Ausgabe A 1995; 34(1): 59–61.

Gibbs NF. Anogenital papillomavirus infections in children. Curr Opin Pediatr 1998; 10(4): 393–397.

Gibbs SJ, Spittle MF. Seminoma and squamous cell carcinomas in association with lymphopenia. Clin Oncol 1995; 7(1); 46 47.

Gibson GD, Ahmed I. Perianal and genital basal cell carcinoma. A clinicopathologic review of 51 cases. J Am Acad Dermatol 2001; 45(1): 68–71.

Gilbert J, Drehs MD, Weinberg JM. Topical imiquimod for acyclovir–unresponsive herpes simplex virus 2 infection. Arch Dermatol 2001; 137: 1015.

Gil Garcia JF, Lerida Arias MT, del Pozo Hernando LJ et al. Fixed drug eruption due to amoxicillin. Medicina Clinica 1994; 102(11): 438.

Gilmore WA, Weigand DA, Burgdorf WHC. Penile nodules in south–east asian men. Arch Dermatol 1983; 119: 446–447.

Ginkel van CJW, Rundervoort GJ. Increasing incidence of contact allergy to the new preservative 1,2–dibromo–2,4–dicyanobutane (methyldibromoglutaronitrile). Br J Dermatol 1995; 132(6): 918–920.

Gioglio L, Porta C, Moroni M, et al. Scrotal angiokeratoma (Fordyce): histopathological and ultrastructural findings. Histol Histopathol 1992; 7(1): 47–55.

Gissmann L, De Villiers EM, Zur Hansen H. Analysis of human genital warts (condylomata acuminata) and other genital tumors for human papillomavirus type 6 DNA. Int J Cancer. 1982; 29: 13–16.

Givler RL. Necrotizing anorectal lesions associated with Pseudomonas infection in leukemia. Dis Colon Rectum. 1969; 12(6): 438–40.

Glaziou P, Cartel JL, Alzieu P et al. Comparison of ivermectin and benzyl benzoate for treatment of scabies. Trop Med Parasitol 1993; 44(4): 331–332.

Glenister TW. A consideration of the processes involved in the development of the prepuce in man. Br J Urol 1956; 28: 243–249.

Glickman JM, Freeman RG. Pearly penile papules: a statistical study of the incidence. Arch Dermatol 1966; 93: 56–59.

Gluckman JB, Kleinman MS, May AG. Primary syphilis of rectum. NY State J Med 1974; 74: 2210–2211.

Goedert JJ. Prognostic markers for AIDS. Ann Epidemiol. 1990; 1(2): 129–39.

Goette DK Ltc, Carson TE Cpt. Erythroplasia of Queyrat Treatment with topical 5–fluorouracil. Cancer 1976; 38: 1498–1502.

Goette DK, Elgart M, deVillez RL. Erythroplasia of Queyrat. Treatment with topically applied fluorouracil. J Am Med Acad 1975; 232(9): 934–937.

Goh CL, Ang CB, Chan RK et al. Comparing treatment response and complications between podophyllin 0.5%/0.25% in ethanol vs podophyllin 25% in tincture benzoin for penile warts. Singapore Med J 1998; 39(1): 17–19.

Goh M, Tekchandani AH, Wojno KJ et al. Metastatic Crohn's disease involving penile skin. J Urol 1998; 159(2): 506–507.

Goh SH, Trapnell IE. Fracture of the penis. Br J Surg 1980; 67: 680–681.

Goldberg J, Bernstein R. Studies on granuloma inguinale VI. Two cases of perianal granuloma inguinale in male homosexuals. Br J Vener Dis 1964; 40: 137–139.

Goldman R. The psychological impact of circumcision. Br J Urol Int 1999; 83(Suppl. 1): 93–102.

Goldminz D, Scott G, Klaus S. Penile basal cell carcinoma. Report of a case and a review of the literature. J Am Acad Dermatol 1989; 20(6): 1094–1097.

Goldoft MJ, Weiss NS. Incidence of male genital skin tumours: lack of increase in the United States. Cancer Causes & Control 1992; 3(1): 91–93.

Goldstein HH. Cutaneous horns of the penis. J Urol. 1933; 30: 367.

Goldstein N. Psychological implications of tattoos. J Dermatol Surg Oncol 1979; 5: 883.

Bibliography

Goldstein SM. Advances in the treatment of superficial candida infections. Sem Dermatol 1993; 12(4): 315–330.

Gollnick H, Barasso R, Jappe U et al. Safety and efficacy of imiquimod 5% cream in the treatment of penile genital warts in uncircumcised men when applied three times weekly or once per day. Int J STD AIDS 2001; 12(1): 22–28.

Golomb J, Kopolovic J, Siegel Y. Sclerosing lipogranuloma of the external male genitalia. Br J Urol 1992; 70(5): 575.

Gomes CM, Ribeiro–Filho L, Giron AM et al. Genital trauma due to animal bites. J Urol 2001; 165(1): 80–83.

Gomez De La Fuente E, Castano Suarez E, Vanaclocha Sebastian F et al. Verrucous carcinoma of the penis completely cured with shaving and intralesional interferon. Dermatology 2000; 200: 152.

Gomez JIE, Gonzalez–Lopez A, Velasco E et al. Basal cell carcinoma of the scrotum. Australas J Derm 1999; 40(3): 141–143.

Gonzalez–Campora R, Nogales Jr FF, Lerma E et al. Lymphoma of the penis. J Urol 1981; 126: 270–271.

Gonzalez–Lopez A, Esquivias JI, Miranda–Romero A et al. Buschke–Loewenstein Tumor and immunity. Cutis 1997; 59: 119–122.

Goolamali SK, Barnes EN, Irvine WJ et al. Organ–specific antibodies in patients with lichen sclerosus. Br Med J 1974; 4: 78–79.

Gooptu C, Woolllons A, Ross J et al. Merkel cell carcinoma arising after therapeutic immunosuppression. Br J Dermatol 1997; 137: 637–641.

Gordon A, Collin J. Save the normal foreskin. Br Med J 1993; 306: 1–2.

Gordon JA, Schwartz BB. Delayed extrusion of testicular prosthesis. Urology. 1979; 14(1): 59–60.

Gotoh M, Tsai S, Sugiyama T et al. Giant scrotal hemangioma with azoospermia. Urology 1983; 22: 637–639.

Gotz H, Zabel M, Patiri C. [Lichen sclerosus at atrophicus. First observation on a boy's genitalia] Article in German. Hautarzt 1977; 28: 235–238.

Goulding FJ, Traylor RA. Juvenile xanthogranuloma of the scrotum. J Urol. 1983; 129: 841–842.

Graham JA, Hansen KK, Rabinowitz LG et al. Pyoderma gangrenosum in infants and children. Pediatr Dermatol 1994; 11(1): 10–17.

Graham JH, Helwig EB. Precancerous skin lesions and systemic cancer. Tumours of the Skin eds. Chicago: Yearbook Medical Publishers. 1964; 209.

Graham JH, Helwig EB. Bowen's disease and its relationship to systemic cancer. Arch Dermatol 1959; 80: 133–159.

Graham JH, Helwig EB. Erythroplasia of Queyrat. A clinicopathologic and histochemical study. Cancer 1973; 32: 1396–1414.

Graham JH, Mazzanti GR, Helwig E. Chemistry of Bowen's disease: relationship to arsenic. J Invest Dermatol 1961; 37: 317–329.

Grassegger A, Hopfl R, Hussl H et al. Buschke–Loewenstein tumour infiltrating pelvic organs. Br J Dermatol 1994; 130(2): 221–225.

Graves RC, Flo S. Carcinoma of the scrotum. J Urol 1940; 43: 309–332.

Green J, Monteiro E, Bolton VN et al. Detection of human papillomavirus DNA by PCR in semen from patients with and without penile warts. Genitour Med 1991; 67(3): 207–210.

Greene SL, Su WP, Muller SA. Pseudomonas aeruginosa infections of the skin. Am Fam Physician. 1984; 29(1): 193–200.

Greenbaum SS, Krull EA, Simmons Jr. EB. Basal cell carcinoma at the base of the penis in a black patient. J Am Dermatol 1989; 20(2 Pt.2): 317–319.

Greenberg MJ. Gomco circumcision. Am Fam Physician. May 15;59(10):2724, 2729; discussion. 1999; 2730, 2732.

Greenburg RD, Perry TL. Nonvenereal sclerosing lymphangitis of the penis. Arch Dermatol 1972; 105: 728–729.

Greenwood N, Fox H, Edwards EC. Leiomyosarcoma of the penis. Cancer 1972; 29(2): 481–483.

Gregoire L, Cubilla AL, Reuter VE et al. Preferential association of human papillomavirus with high–grade histologic variants of penile–invasive squamous cell carcinoma. J Natl Cancer Inst 1995; 87(22): 1705–1709.

Gregory N, Sanchez M, Buchness MR. The spectrum of syphilis in patients with human immunodeficiency virus infection. J Am Acad Dermatol. 1990; 22(6 Pt 1): 1061–7.

Greilsheimer H, Groves JE. Male genital self–mutilation. Arch Gen Psychiat 1979; 36(4): 441–446.

Grenvalsky HT, Helwig EB. Carcinoma of the anorectal junction. I Histological considerations. Cancer 1956; 19: 480–488.

Gretzula JC, Hevia O, Schachner LS et al. Ruvalcaba–Myhre–Smith syndrome. Pediatr Dermatol 1988; 5(1): 28–32.

Griffiths TRL, Mellon JK. Human papillomavirus and urological tumours: basic science and role in penile cancer. Br J Urol Int 1999; 84: 579–586.

Grigoriu D, Delecretaz J. Actinomyocose peri-anale pruritive. Annales de Dermatologie et de Venereologie 1981; 108: 159–161.

De Groot AC, Van Ulsen J, Weyland JW. Allergisch contacteczeem rond de anus met dyshidrotisch eczeem van de handen door Kathon CG in vochtige toiletdoekjes. Nederlands Tijdschrift voor Geneeskunde 1991; 135(23): 1048–1049.

De Groot AC, Toon J, Baar M et al. Contact allergy to moist toilet paper. Contact Dermatitis 1999; 24: 135–136.

Gross AJ, Heinzer H, Loy V et al. Unusual differential diagnosis of testis tumor: intrascrotal sarcoidosis. J Urol 1992; 147: 1112–1114.

Gross AS, Dretler RH. Foscarnet–induced penile ulcer in an uncircumcised patient with AIDS. Clin Infect Dis 1993; 17(6): 1076–1077.

Gross DJ, Schosser RH. Squamous cell carcinoma of the scrotum. Cutis 1991; 47(6): 402–404.

Gross G, Hagedorn M, Ikenberg H et al. Bowenoid papulosis. Presence of human papillomavirus (HPV) structural antigens and of HPV 16–related DNA sequences. Arch Dermatol 1985; 121: 858–863.

Gross G, Roussaki A, Ikenberg H et al. Genital warts do not respond to systemic recombinant interferon alfa–2a treatment during cannabis consumption. Dermatologica 1991; 183(3): 203–207.

Grosshans E, Jenn P, Baumann R et al. Manifestations anales der maladies du tube digestif. Annales de Dermatologie et de Venereologie 1979; 106: 25–30.

Grosshans E, Grossmann L. Bowenoid papulosis. Arch Dermatol 1985; 121: 858–863.

Grossklaus DJ, Dutta SC, Shappel S et al. Cutaneous mucormycosis presenting as a penile lesion in a patient with acute myeloblastic leukaemia. Jour of Urol 1999; 161(6): 1906–1907.

Grossman A, Kaplan HI, Grossman M et al. Thrombosis of the penis: interesting facet of thrombangiitis obliterans. J Am Med Ass 1965; 192: 329–331.

Grossman HB. Premalignant and early carcinomas of the penis and scrotum. Urol Clin North Am 1992; 19(2): 221–226.

Gruber F, Stasic A, Lenkovic M, Brajac I. Postcoital fixed drug eruption in a man sensitive to trimethoprim–sulphamethoxazole. Clin Exp Dermatol 1997; 22: 144–145.

Grunwald MH, Amichai B, Halevy S. Purplish penile papule as a presenting sign of Kaposi's sarcoma. Br J Urol 1994; 74: 517.

Grunwald MH, Amichai B, Trau H. Cutaneous leishmaniasis on an unusual site– the glans penis. Br J Urol 1998; 82(6): 928.

Gruwez JA, Christiaens MR, Laquet A. La maladie de Crohn de l'anus. Acta Endoscopica 1983; 13: 285–292.

Guerin–Reverchon I, Chardonnet Y, Viac J et al. Human papillomavirus infection and filaggrin expression in paraffin–embedded biopsy specimens of extragenital Bowen's disease and genital bowenoid papulosis. J Cancer Res Clin Oncol 1990; 116: 295–300.

Gungör E, Karakayali G, Alli N et al. Penile pyoderma gangrenosum. J Eur Acad Dermatol Venereol 1999; 12: 59–62.

Gunn RA, Gallagher S. Vulvar Paget's disease: a topographic study. Cancer 1980; 46: 590–594.

Gupta S, Kumar B. Dorsal perforation of prepuce: a common end point of severe ulcerative genital diseases? Sex Trans Infect 2000; 76(3): 210–212.

Gupta S, Kumar B. Dorsal perforation of prepuce due to locally erosive condylomata acuminata. Sex Trans Infect 2001; 77(1): 77–78.

Gupta S, Radotra BD, Javaher M, et al. Lymphangioma circumcision of the penis mimicking venereal lesions. J Eur Acad Dermatol Venereol. 2003; 17: 598–600.

Gurunluoglu R, Bayramicli M, Dogan T et al. Unusual complications of circumcision. Plast Reconstruct Surg 1999; 104: 1938–1939.

Gurunluoglu R, Bayramicli M, Dogan T et al. Keloid after circumcision. Plast Reconst Surg 1999; 103: 1539–1540.

Guss C et al. Group A beta–hemolytic streptococcal proctocolitis. Pediatr Infect Dis 1984; 3: 442.

Guy M, Singer D, Barzilai N et al. Primary classic Kaposi's sarcoma of glans penis– appearance on magnetic resonance imaging. Br J Urol 1994; 74: 521–522.

H

Haddad FS. Penile strangulation by human hair. Report of three cases and review of the literature. Uroloigicas Internationalis 1982; 37: 375.

Hafner J, Keusch G, Wahl C et al. Calciphylaxis: a syndrome of skin necrosis and acral gangrene in chronic renal failure. Vasa 1998; 27(3): 137–143.

Hahn JM, Meisler DM, Lowder CY et al. Cicatrizing conjunctivitis associated with paraneoplastic lichen planus. Am J Ophthalmol 2000; 129(1): 98–99.

Haim S, Merzbach D. Gonococcal penile ulcer. Br J Vener Dis 1970; 46: 336–337.

Haim S, Sobel JD, Friedman-Birnbaum R. Thrombophlebitis. A cardinal symptom of Bechet's syndrome. Acta Dermato–Venereologica 1974; 54: 299–301.

Haimoff H, Dintsman M, Kessler E. Xanthogranuloma of the peri-anal region. A case report. Am J Proctol. 1971; 22: 123–5.

Halperin DT, Bailey RC. Male circumcision and HIV infection: 10 years and counting. Lancet 1999; 354: 1813–1815.

Hamado T. Granuloma intertriginosum infantum. Arch Dermatol 1975; 111: 1072–1073.

Hamuryudan V, Mat C, Saip S et al. Thalidomide in the treatment of the mucocutaneous lesions of the Behcet syndrome. A randomized, double–blind, placebo–controlled trial. An Inter Med 1998; 128(6): 443–450.

Hamm H, Vroom TM, Czametski BM. Extramammary Paget's cells: Further evidence of sweat gland derivation. J Am Acad Dermatol 1986; 15: 1275–1281.

Hanash KA, Furlow WL, Utz DC et al. Carcinoma of the penis. J Urol 1970; 104: 291–297.

Hancock BD. In: The Haemorrhoid Syndrome. Kaufman HD ed. Tunbridge Wells: Abacus. 1981; 93–104.

Handfield-Jones SE, Cronin E. Contact sensitivity to lignocaine. Clin Exper Dermatol 1993; 18(4): 342–343.

Handley JM, Maw RD, Horner T et al. Non-specific immunity in patients with primary anogenital warts treated with interferon alpha plus cryotherapy or cryotherapy alone. Acta Dermato–Venereologica 1992; 72(1): 39–40.

Handley JM, Maw RD, Horner T et al. A placebo controlled observer blind immunocytochemical and histologic study of epithelium adjacent to anogenital warts in patients treated with systemic interferon alpha in combination with cryotherapy or cryotherapy alone. Genitour Med 1992; 68(2): 100–105.

Handley JM, Maw RD, Lawther H et al. Human papillomavirus DNA detection in primary anogenital warts and cervical low grade intraepithelial neoplasias in adults by in situ hybridization. Sex Trans Dis 1992; 19(4): 225–229.

Handley JM, Maw RD, Bingham EA et al. Anogenital warts in children. Clin Exper Dermatol 1993; 18(3): 241–247.

Hanna NF, Clay JC, Harris JRW. Sarcoptes scabiei infestation treated with malathion liquid. Br J Vener Dis 1978; 54: 354.

Handrick M, Kim OM, Contact allergy to lignocaine with cross–reaction to bupivacaine. Contact Dermatitis 1994; 30(4): 245–246.

Harmanyeri Y, Taskapan O, Dogan B et al. A case of coumarin necrosis with penile and pedal involvement. J Eur Acad Dermatol Venereol 1998; 10(3): 248–252.

Harmon CB, Connolly SM, Larson TR. Condom–related allergic contact dermatitis. J Urol 1995; 153(4): 1227–1228.

Harnes JR. The foreskin saga. J Am Med Ass 1971; 217(9): 1241–1242.

Harrington CI. Lichen sclerosus. Arch Dis Child 1990; 65: 335.

Harrington Cl, Dunsmore IR. An investigation into the incidence of autoimmune disorders in patients with lichen sclerosus et atrophicus. Br J Dermatol 1981; 104: 563–566.

Harrington Cl, Gelsthorpe K. The association between lichen sclerosus et atrophicus and HLA–B40. Br J Dermatol 1981; 104: 561–562.

Harrow BR, Sloane IA. Thrombophlebitis of superficial penile and scrotal veins. J Urol 1963; 89: 841–842.

Harth Y, Hirshovitz B. Topical photodynamic therapy in basal and squamous cell carcinoma and penile Bowen's disease with 20% aminolevulinic acid, and exposure to red light and infrared light. Harefuah 1998; 134(8): 602–5, 672, 671. Hebrew.

Harth Y, Hirshowitz B, Kaplan B. Modified topical photodynamic therapy of superficial skin tumors, utilizing aminolevulinic acid, penetration enhancers, red light, and hyperthermia. Dermatol Surg 1998; 24(7): 723–726.

Harto A, Gutiérrez Sanz–Gadea C, Vives R et al. Pioderma gangrenoso en pene. Actas Urol Esp 1985; 9: 263–6.

Hashimoto K, Kagetsu N, Taniguchi Y et al. Immunohistochemistry and electron microscopy in Langerhans cell histiocytosis confined to the skin. J Am Acad Dermatol 1991; 25(6 Pt.1): 1044–1053.

Hashmat AL, Abrahams J, Fani K et al. A lethal complication of papaverine–induced priapism. J Urol 1991; 145(1): 146.

Hatzichristou DG, Apostolidis A, Tzortzis V et al. Glansectomy: an alternative surgical treatment for Buschke–Lowenstein tumors of the penis. Urology 2001; 57(5): 966–9.

Haustein UF, Hlawa B. Treatment of scabies with permethrin versus lindane and benzyl benzoate. Acta Derm Venereol 1989; 69(4): 348–351.

Hautmann RE, Bachor R. Juvenile xanthogranuloma of the penis. J Urol 1993; 150(2 Pt.1): 456–457.

Hawkswell J, Nathan M. Lichen sclerosus and acute urinary obstruction. Genitourin Med 1992; 68(3): 177–178.

Hay RJ. Paracoccidioidomycosis. In; Manson's Tropical Diseases. Cook GC Saunders, ed. 20th edition. London, 1996; 1068.

Haycox CL, Kuypers J, Krieger JN. Role of human papillomavirus typing in diagnosis and clinical decision making for a giant verrucous genital lesion. Urology 1999; 53: 627–630.

Heaton CL, Lichti HF, Weiner M. The revival of nitric acid for the treatment of anogenital warts. Clin Pharmacol Therapeut 1993; 54(1): 107–111.

Heise H, Flegel H, Helmke R. Treatment of lichen sclerosus et atrophicus with testosterone propionate ointment. Dermatol Monatsschr 1984; 170(2): 135–138. German.

Hellberg D, Valentin J, Eklund T et al. Penile cancer: is there an epidemiological role for smoking and sexual behaviour. Br Med J 1987; 295: 1306–1308.

Helm JD, Hodge IG. Thrombophlebitis of a dorsal vein of the penis: report of a case treated by phenylbutazone (Butazolidin). J Urol 1958; 79(2): 306–307.

Helwig EB, Graham I H. Anogenital (extramammary) Paget's disease: a clinico pathological study. Cancer 1963; 16: 387–403.

Hengge UR, Tietze G. Successful treatment of recalcitrant condyloma with topical cidofovir. Sex Trans Infect 2000; 76(2):143.

Hengge UR, Benninghoff B, Ruzicka T et al. Topical immunomodulators – progress towards treating inflammation, infection, and cancer. Lancet Infect Dis 2001; 1(3): 189–198.

Bibliography

Henseler T, Christophers E, Honigsmann H, Wolff K. Skin tumours in the European PUVA Study. Eight year follow–up of 1,643 patients treated with PUVA for psoriasis. J Am Acad Dermatol 1987; 16(1 Pt.1): 108–116.

Henson EB, Bess DT, Abraham L et al. Penile angioedema possibly related to lisinopril. Am J of Health–System Pharmacy 1999; 56(17): 1773–4.

Hernandez–Graulau JM, Fiore A, Cea P et al. Multiple penile horns. Case report and review. J Urol 1988; 139: 1055.

Hernandez–Martin A, Baselga E, Drolet BA et al. Juvenile xanthogranuloma. J Am Acad Dermatol 1997; 36(31): 355–367.

Heymann WR, Soifer I, Burk PG. Penile premalignant fibroepithelioma of Pinkus. Cutis 1983; 31: 519–521.

Heyns CF, van Vollenhoven P, Steenkamp JW et al. Cancer of the penis–a review of 50 patients. S Afr J Surg 1997; 35: 120–124.

Hibbiss JH, Schofield PF. Management of perianal Crohn's disease. J Roy Soc Med 1982; 75: 414–417.

Hicks RA. Empiric therapy of perianal lesions in a sexually abused child: Medical and forensic implications. Pediatr Emerg Care 1993; 9(6): 346–347.

Highet AS, Warren RE, Weekes AJ. Bacteriology and antibiotic treatment of perineal suppurative hidradenitis. Arch Dermatol 1988; 124: 1047–1051.

Hill J, Blyth WA. An alternative theory of herpes–simplex recurrence and a possible role for prostaglandins. Lancet 1976; i: 397–398.

Hill VA, Hall–Smith P, Smith NP. Cutaneous T–cell lymphoma presenting with atypical perianal lesions. Dermatology 1995; 190(4): 313–316.

Hillman RJ, Harris JRW, Walker MM. Value of performing biopsies in genitourinary clinics. Genitour Med 1991; 67(1): 73.

Hillman RJ, Waldron S, Walker MM et al. Granuloma annulare of the penis. Genitour Med 1992; 68(1): 47–49.

Hillman RJ, Walker MM, Harris JRW et al. Penile dermatoses: a clinical and histopathgological study. Genitour Med 1992; 68(3): 166–169.

Hillman RJ, Ryait BK, Botcherby M et al. Human papillomavirus DNA in the urogenital tracts of men with gonorrhoea, penile warts or genital dermatoses. Genitour Med 1993a; 69(3): 187–192.

Hillman RJ, Ryait BK, Botcherby M et al. Changes in HPV infection in patients with anogenital warts and their partners. 1993b; 69(6): 450–456.

Hillman RJ, Botcherby M, Ryait BK et al. Detection of human papillomavirus DNA in the urogenital tracts of men with anogenital warts. Sex Trans Dis 1993c; 20(1): 21–27.

Hills OW, Liebert E, Steinberg DL et al. Cunical aspects of dietary depletion of riboflavin. Archives of Internal Medicine 1951; 87: 682–693.

Hinchliffe SA, Ciftci AO, Rickwood AMK et al. Compostion of the inflammatory infiltrate in pediatric penile lichen sclerosus et atrophicus (balanitis xerotica obliterans). Pediatr Pathol 1994; 14: 223–233.

Hindson TC. Studies in contact dermatitis. Trans St. John's Hospital Dermatol Soc 1966; 52: 1–9.

Hira SK, Wadhawam D, Kamanga J et al. Cutaneous manifestations of human immunodeficiency virus in Lusaka, Zambia. J Am Acad Dermatol 1988; 19: 451–457.

Hirshfeld AJ. Two family outbreaks of cellulitis associated with group A streptococci. Pediatrics 1970; 46: 799–802.

Hobbs CJ, Wynne JM. Physical signs of sexual abuse in children. J R Coll Phys Lond 1997; 31(5): 580–581.

Hobbs CJ, Wynne JM. How to manage warts. Arch Dis Child 1999; 81(5): 460.

Hoekx L, Wyndaele JJ. Fracture of the penis: role of ultrasonography in localizing the cavernosal tear. Acta Urol Belg 1998; 66(1): 23–25.

Hoekx L, Wyndaele JJ. Angiokeratoma: a cause of scrotal bleeding. Acta Urol Belg 1998; 66(1): 27–28.

Höfs W. Special clinical observations of lichen sclerosus et atrophicans. 2(report): Familiar lichen sclerosus et atrophicans in a married couple and their 9–year–old daughter. Dermatol Monatsschr. 1978; Sep;164(9): 633–639. German.

Höfs W, Quednow C. Special clinical observations of lichen sclerosus et atrophicans. 1(report): Lichen sclerosus et atrophicans penis at 8 boys with phimosis. Dermatol Monatsschr. 1978; Sep;164(9): 625–632. German.

Hogan P. Irritant napkin dermatitis. Austral Fam Phys 1999; 28(4): 385–6.

Hollander JB, Begun FP, Lee RD. Scrotal fat necrosis. J Urol 1985; 134: 150–151.

Holly EA, Palefsky JM. Factors related to risk of penile cancer: New evidence from a study in the Pacific northwest. J Nat Cancer Inst 1993; 85(1): 2–3.

Holmes JG, Kipling MD, Waterhouse IAH. Subsequent malignancies in men with scrotal epithelioma. Lancet 1970; i: 214–215.

Honda S, Yamamoto O, Suenaga Y et al. Six cases of metastatic malignant melanoma with apparently occult primary lesions. J Dermatol 2001; 28(5): 265–271.

Hope–Stone H. Carcinoma of the penis. External radiation mould technique. Proc Roy Soc Med 1975; 68: 777–778.

Hopfl RH, Sandbichler M, Zelger BWH, et al. Adjuvant treatment of recalcitrant genitoanal warts with systemic recombinant interferon–alpha–2c. Acta Dermato–Venereologica 1993; 73(3): 223–226.

Hopsu–Havu VK, Sonck CE. Infiltrative, ulcerative and fistular lesions of the penis due to lymphogranuloma venereum. Br J Vener Dis 1973; 49: 193–202.

Horenblas S, von Krogh G, Cubilla AL et al. Squamous cell carcinoma of the penis: premalignant lesions. Scand J Urol Nephrol 2000; 205(Suppl): 187–188.

Horinaga M, Masuda T, Jitsukawa S. A case of scrotal elephantiasis 30 years after treatment of penile carcinoma. Hinyokika Kiyo 1998; 44(11): 839–841. Japanese.

Horn AS, Pecora A, Chiesa JC et al. Penile thrombophlebitis as a presenting manifestation of pancreatic carcinoma. Am J Gastroenterol 1985; 80(6): 463–465.

Horner AA, Dunn K, Stiehm ER. Penile vasculitis with impending necrosis treated with prostaglandin E1 infusion. Am J Dis Child. 1991; 145(6): 604.

Horowitz M, Nobrega MM. Primary anal melanoma associated with melanosis of the upper gastrointestinal tract. Endoscopy 1998; 30(7): 662–625.

Hrbatý J, Molitor M. Traumatic skin loss from the male genitalia. Acta Chir Plast 2001; 43(1): 17–20.

Hrebinko RL. Circumferential laser vaporization for severe meatal stenosis secondary to balanitis xerotica obliterans. J Urol 1996; 156(5): 1735–1736.

Hsiao GH, Chen JS. Acquired genital smooth–muscle harmartoma. A case report. Am J Dermatopathol 1995; 17(1): 67–70.

Hsu C. The development of the prepuce. J Formosan Med. , Assoc 1983; 82: 314–320.

Hubbell CR, Rabin VR, Mora RG. Cancer of the skin in blacks. V A review of 175 black patients with squamous cell carcinoma of the penis. J Am Acad Dermatol 1988; 18(2 Pt.1): 292–298.

Huesner JN, Pugh RP. Erythroplasia of Queyrat treated with topical 5–fluorouracil. J Urol 1969; 102: 595–597.

Hughes PSH. Cryosurgery of verrucous carcinoma of the penis (Buschke–Lowenstein tumor). Cutis 1979; 24: 43–45.

Hughes–Davies LT, Murray P, Spittle M. Fourniers gangrene: A hazard of chemotherapy in AIDS. Clin Oncol 1991; 3: 241–243.

Hull MT, Eble JN, Priest JB et al. Ultrastructure of Buschke–Loewenstein tumor. J Urol 1981; 126: 485–489.

Hulsebosch HJ, Claessen FAP, van Ginkel CJW et al. Human immunodeficiency virus exanthem. J Am Acad Dermatol 1990; 23: 483–486.

Huminer D, Siegman-Igra Y, Morduchowicz G, et al. Ecthyma gangrenosum without bacteremia. Report of six cases and review of the literature. Arch Intern Med. 1987; 147(2): 299–301.

Hutchins P, Dunlop EMC, Rodin P. Benign transient lymphangiectasis (sclerosing lymphangitis) of the penis. Br J Vener Dis 1977; 53: 17.

Hutchinson J. Sebaceous gland tumours in the scrotum. Plate. LXVIII Illustrations of clinical surgery; vol 2 Philadelphia: Blakiston Son & Co. 1888.

Hwang SM, Yoo MS, Ahn SK et al. Demodecidosis manifested on the external genitalia. Int J Derm 1998, 37(8): 614–616.

I

Ikenberg H, Gissmann L, Gross Grussendorf–Cohen E I zur Hausen H. Human papillomavirus type 16 DNA in genital Bowen's disease and in Bowenoid papulosis. Int J Cancer 1983; 32: 563–565.

Imakado S, Abe M, Okuno T et al. Two cases of genital Paget's disease with bilateral axillary involvement: Mutability of axillary lesions. Arch Dermatol 1991; 127: 1243.

Imperial R, Helwig EB. Angiokeratoma. A clinicopathological study. Arch Dermatol 1967; 95: 166–175.

Inagaaki H, Nonaka M, Eimoto T. Bowenoid papulosis showing polyclonal nature. Diagn Mol Pathol 1998; 70: 122–126.

International Study Group for Behçet's disease. Criteria for diagnosis of Behçet's disease. Lancet 1990; 335: 1078–1080.

Invernizzi R, Ubiali P, Barcella A et al. Kaposi's sarcoma–classic form. A rare familial case. Minerva Chirurgica 1993; 48(5): 237–241.

Iossifides I, Ayala AG, Johnson DE. Epithelioid sarcoma of the penis. Urology 1979; 14(2): 190–191.

Ippen H. Toxizitat und stoffwechsel des cignolins (Wz). Derrmatologica 1959; 119: 211–220.

Irvine C, Anderson JR, Pye RJ. Micaceous and keratotic pseudoepitheliomatous balanitis and rapidly fatal fibrosarcoma of the penis occuring in the same patient. Br J Urol 1987; 116(5): 719–725.

Isa SS, Almaraz R, McGreen J. Leiomyosarcoma of penis. Case report and review of literature. Cancer 1984; 54: 939–942.

Ishida–Yamamoto A, Sato K, Wada T et al. Fibroepithelioma–like changes occurring in perianal Paget's disease with rectal mucinous carcinoma: case report and review of 49 cases of extramammary Paget's disease. J Cutan Pathol 2002; 29: 185–189.

Ishizawa T, Koseki S, Mitsuhashi Y et al. Squamous cell carcinoma arising in chronic perianal pyoderma: a case report and review of Japanese literature. J Dermatol 2000; 27(11): 734–739.

Itin PH, Hirsbrunner P, Buchner S. Lichen planus: an unusual cause of phimosis. Acta Dermato–Venereologica 1992; 72(1): 41–42.

Ito A, Sakamoto F, Ito M. Dystrophic scrotal calcinosis originating from benign eccrine epithelial cysts. Br J Derm 2001; 144(1): 146–150.

Ive FA. The umbilical, perianal and genital regions, Textbook of Dermatology. Rook/Wilkinson/Ebling. Champion RH, Burton JL, Burns DA, Breathnach SM eds. 6th edition. Blackwell Science, Oxford. Volume 4, Ch 72, p. 3191.

Ive FA, Marks R. Tinea incognito. Br Med J 1968; i: 149–152.

Ivker RA, Woosley J, Briggaman R. Calciphylaxis in three patients with end–stage renal disease. Arch Dermatol 1995; 131(1): 63–68.

Iwakawa A, Hammo K. Intrascrotal sclerosing lipogranuloma: A case report. Acta Urologica Japonica 1989; 35: 357.

Iwamura H, Horri Y, Tokuchi H et al. A case of genital Paget's disease with severe dermal invasion and early dissemination. Acta Urologica Japonica 1999; 45(4): 281–284.

Izquierdo MJ, Pastor MA, Carrasco L et al. Epithelioid blue naevus of the genital mucosa: report of four cases. Br J Dermatol 2001; 145: 496–501.

J

Jacobs EC. Oculo–oro–genital syndrome: a deficiency disease. Ann Intern Med 1951; 35: 1049–1054.

Jaeger N, Wirler H, Tschubel K. Acral lentiginous melanoma of the penis. Eur J Urol 1982; 8(3): 182–184.

Jaisanker TJ, Garg BR, Reddy BS et al. Penile lupus vulgaris. Int J Dermatol 1994; 33(4): 272–274.

Jakhmola RSi, Subhash SM, Sabharia Z et al. Idiopathic vulvar calcinosis: The counterpart of idiopathic scrotal calcinosis. Cutis 1988; 41: 273–275.

James O, Mayes RW, Stevenson CJ. Occupational vitiligo induced by p–tert–butylphenol, a systemic disease? Lancet 1977; ii: 1217–1219.

Jansen GT, Dillaha CJ, Honeycutt WM. Bowenoid conditions of the skin: treatment with topical 5–Fluorouracil. S Med J 1967; 60: 185–188.

Jayalakshmi P, Goh KL. Disseminated histoplasmosis presenting as penile ulcer. Aust NZ J Med 1990; 20: 175–176.

Jemec GBE, Baadsgaard O. Effect of cyclosporin on genital psoriasis and lichen planus. J Am Acad Dermatol. 1993; 29: 1048–9.

Jensen SL. A randomised trial of simple excision of non–specific hypertrophied anal papillae versus expectant management in patients with chronic pruritus ani. Ann Roy Coll Surg (England) 1988; 70: 348–349.

Jenkins IL. Extra–mammary Paget's disease of the penis. Br J Urol 1989; 63(1): 103–104.

Jenny C, Kirby P, Fuquay D. Genital lichen sclerosus mistaken for child sexual abuse. Pediatrics 1989; 83: 597–599.

Jensen SL, Sjolin KE, Shokouh–Amiri MH. Paget's disease of the anal margin. Br J Surg 1988; 75: 1089–1092.

Jeyakumar W, Ganesh R, Mohanram F et al. Papulonecrotic tuberculids of the glans penis: case report. Genitourin Med 1988; 64: 130–132.

Jimenez I, Anton E, Picans I et al. Fixed drug eruption from amoxycillin. Allergol Immunopathol (Madr 1997; 25: 247–248.

Johnson A, Mathai G, Robinson WA. Malignant melanoma of the perineum. J Surg Oncol 1993; 54(3): 185–189.

Johnson BL, Baxter DL. Pearly penile papules. Arch Dermatol 1964; 90: 166–167.

Johnson DE, Ayala AG. Primary melanoma of the penis. Urology 1973; 2: 174–177.

Johnson DE, Lo RK, Srigley J et al. Vererucous carcinoma of the penis. J Urol 1985; 133: 216–218.

Johnson H. Jr. Leiomyosarcoma of scrotum. Urology 1987; 29(4): 436–438.

Johnson HD, Thin RNT. Disease of the median raphe of the penis. Report of two cases. Br J Vener Dis 1972; 49: 467–468.

Johnson WT. Cutaneous chylous reflux, 'The weeping scrotum'. Arch Dermatol 1979; 115: 464–466.

Journal of the American Journal of Dermatology 29(6. 1993;

Jolly BB, Krishnamurty S, Vaidyanathan S. Zoon's balanitis. Urol Int 1993; 50(3): 182–184.

Jones DH, Cunliffe W, King K. Hidradenitis suppurativa—lack of success with cis–retinoic acid. Br J Dermatol 1982; 107: 252.

Jones DJ. Pruritis ani. Br Med J 1992; 305: 575–577.

Jones RB, Hirschmann JV, Brown GS et al. Fournier's syndrome: necrotizing subcutaneous infection of the male genitalia. J Urol 1979; 122: 279–282.

Jones RW, Baranyai J, Stables S. Trends in squamous cell carcinoma of the vulva: the influence of vulvar intraepithelial neoplasia. Obstet Gynecol 1997; 90: 448–452.

Jonquieres EDL. Balanitis pseudoeritroplasicas. Archivos Argentinos de Dermatologica 1971; 21: 85–95.

Jonquieres EDL, de Lutzky FK. Balanites et vulvites pseudo–erythroplasiques chroniques. Aspects histopathologiques. Annales de Dermatology et de Venereology 1980; 107(3): 173–180.

van Joost TH, Faber WR, Manuel HR. Drug–induced anogenital cicatricial pemphigoid. Br J Dermatol 1980; 715: 718.

Jorda E, Verdeguer JM, Moragon M et al. Desmoplastic melanoma of the penis. J Am Acad Dermatol 1987; 16: 619–620.

Jørgensen ET, Svensson A. The treatment of phimosis with a potent topical steroid (clobetasol propionate 0.05%) cream. Acta Derm Venereol 1993; 73: 55–56.

Jørgensen ET, Svensson A. Problems with the penis and prepuce in children. Lichen sclerosus should be treated with corticosteroids to reduce need for surgery. Br Med J 1996; 313(7058): 692.

Joshi UY. Carcinoma of the penis preceded by Zoon's balanitis. Int J STD AIDS 1999; 10(12): 823–825.

K

Kadish AS. Biology of anogenital neoplasia. Cancer Treat Res 2001; 104: 267–286.

Kadioglu A, Tefekli A, Erol B et al. A retrospective review of 307 men with Peyronie's disease. J Urol 2002; 168: 1075–1079.

Kadunce DP, Piepkorn MW, Zone JJ. Persistant melanocytic lesions associated with cosmetic tanning bed use: "Sunbed lentigines". J Am Acad Dermatol 1990; 23(5 Pt. 2): 1029–1031.

Kalis BJ. Case presentations. In: 16th International Congress on Dermatology. Tokyo: Univ of Tokyo Press. 1982; 841.

Kalsi JS, Arya M, Peters J et al. Grease–gun injury to the penis. J R Soc Med 2002; 95: 254.

Kamalam A, Senthamilselvi G, Ajithadas K et al. Cutaneous trichosporosis. Mycopathologia 1988; 101(3): 167–175.

Kameda K, Hayashi N, Arima K et al. Abscess of corpus cavernosum: a case report. Hinyokika Kiyo 1998; 44(12): 893–895. Japanese.

Kandil E, Al–Kashlan IM. Non–venereal sclerosing lymphangitis of the penis. Acta Dermato–Venereologica 1970; 50: 309–312.

Kanerva L, Kousa M, Niemi KM et al. Ultrahistology of balanitis circinata. Br J Vener Dis 1982; 58: 188–195.

Kanwar AJ, Bharija SC, Singh M et al. Ninety–eight fixed drug eruptions with provocation tests. Dermatologica 1988; 177: 274–279.

Kanzler MH, Rasmussen JE. Isotretinoin therapy for recurrent herpes simplex lesions. Arch Dermatol 1988; 124: 232–235.

Kapdagli H, Gunduz K, Ozturk G et al. Pseudo–Kaposi's sarcoma (Mali type). Int J Dermatol 1998; 37: 223–225.

Kaplan C, Katoh A. Erythroplasia of Queyrat (Bowen's disease of the penis). J Surg Oncol 1973; 5: 281–290.

Kaplan GW. Complications of circumcision. Urol Clin N Am 1983; 10(3): 543–549.

Kaporis A, Lynfield Y. Penile lentiginosis. J Am Acad Dermatol 1998; 38(5 Pt 1): 781.

Kappel TJ, Abenoza P. Mucinous syringometaplasia. Am J Dermatopathol 1993; 15(6): 562–567.

Kartamaa M, Reitamo S. Treatment of lichen sclerosus with carbon dioxide laser vaporization. Br J Dermatol 1997; 136(3): 356–359.

Karthikeyan, Thappa DM, Jaisankar TJ et al. Cutaneous horn of glans penis. Sex Transm Infect 1998; 74: 456–457.

Karthikeyan K, Sethuraman G, Thappa DM. Angiokeratoma of the oral cavity and scrotum. J of Derm 2000; 27(2): 131–132.

Karube H, Aizawa Y, Nakamura K et al. Oil mist exposure in industrial health– a review. Sangyo Eiseigaku Zasshi 1995; 37(2): 113–122.

Karulf RE, Madoff RD, Goldberg SM. Rectal prolapse. Curr Probl Surg 2001; 38(10): 771–832.

Kashima M, Mori K, Kadono T et al. Tuberculide of the penis without ulceration. Br J Derm 1999; 140(4): 757–759.

Katsas AG. Diabetic scrotal gangrene. J Roy Soc Med 1982; 75: 988.

Kaufman HD. In: The Haemorrhoid Syndrome. Kaufman HD, ed, Tunbridge Wells: Abacus. 1981; 61.

Kaufman RH, Adam E, Mirkovic RR et al. Treatment of genital herpes simplex virus infection with photodynamic inactivation. Am J Obst Gynecol 1978; 132: 861–869.

Kavak A, Akman RY, Alper M et al. Penile Kaposi's sarcoma in a human immunodeficiency virus–seronegative patient. Br J Dermatol 2001; 144: 207–208.

Kawada A. Morbus Kimura Darstellung der Erkrankung und ihre Differentialdiagnose. Der Hautarzt 1976; 27: 309–317.

Kawatsu T, Miki Y. Triple extramammary Paget's disease. Arch Derm 1971; 104: 316–319.

Kearney GP, Carling PC. Fournier's gangrene: and approach to its management. J Urol 1983; 130: 695–698.

Keat A. Reiter's syndrome and reactive arthritis in perspective. N Engl J Med 1983; 309(26): 1606–1615.

Keerti VS. Human papillomaviruses and anogenital cancers. N Engl J Med 1997; 337: 1386–1387.

Kennedy CTC. Pressure ulcer. In: Rook/Wilkinson/Ebling: Textbook of Dermatology, Champion RH, Burton JL, Burnns DA, Breathnach SM eds. Blackwell Science Ltd. Oxford 1998; 1: 897–901.

Kennedy CTC, Lyell A. Perianal orf. J Am Acad Dermatol 1984; 11: 72–74.

Kennedy L, Buntine DW, O'Connor D et al. Human papillomavirus– a study of male sexual partners. Med J Aust 1988; 149: 309–311.

Kern AB, Kaufman JJ, Combes FC. Granular cell myoblastoma: report of a case simulating granuloma inguinale. Arch Dermatol Syphilol 1950; 62: 109–116.

Kessler R. Complications of inflatable penile prostheses. Urology 1981; 18(5): 470–472.

Khaskhely NM, Uezato H, Kamiyama T et al. Association of human papillomavirus type 6 with a verruciform xanthoma. Am J of Dermatopathol 2000; 22(5): 447–452.

Khoriaty N, Schick E. Penile gangrene: An unusual complication of priapism. How to avoid it? Urology 1980; 16: 280.

Khoubehi B, Schofield A, Leslie M et al. Metastatic in situ perianal Paget's disease. J Roy Soc Med 2001; 94(3): 137–138.

Kiene P, Folster–Holst R. No evidence of human papillomavirus infection in balanitis circumscripta plasmacellularis Zoon. Acta Derm Venereol 1995; 75(6): 496–497.

Kim SW, Choi SW, Cho BK et al. Tuberculosis cutis orificialis: An association with Evan's syndrome. Acta Dermato–Venereologie 1995; 75(1): 84–85.

Kimura S. Verruciform xanthoma of scrotum. Arch Dermatol 1984; 120: 1378–1379.

Kimura S, Hirai A, Harada R et al. So–called multicentric pigmented Bowen's disease. Dermatologica 1978; 157: 229–237.

King DT, Brosman S, Hirose FM et al. Idiopathic calcinosis of scrotum. Urology 1979; 14(1): 92–94.

Kinghorn GR. Genital warts: incidence of associated genital infections. Br J Dermatol 1978; 99: 405–409.

Kinghorn GR, Abeywickrame I, Jeavons M et al. Efficacy of combined treatment with oral and topical acyclovir in first episode genital herpes. Genitourin Med 1986; 62: 186–188.

Kinghorn GR, McMillan A, Mulcahy F et al. An open, comparitive, study of the efficacy of 0.5% podophyllotoxin lotion and 25% podophyllotoxin solution in the treatment of condylomata acuminata in males and females. Int J STD AIDS 1993; 4: 194–199.

Kinloch de Loës S, de Saussure P, Saurat J et al. Symptomatic primary infection due to Human Immunodeficiency Virus Type 1: Review of 31 cases. Clin Infect Dis 1993; 17: 59–65.

Kirby B, Whitehurst C, Moore JV et al. Treatment of lichen planus of the penis with photodynamic therapy. Br J Derm 1999; 141(4): 765–766.

Kirby KA, Cohen R, Upson CV. Fixed drug eruption to papaverine. Urology 1994; 43(6): 886–887.

Kirby PK, Kiviat N, Beckman A et al. Tolerance and efficacy of recombinant human interferon gamma in the treatment of refractory genital warts. Am J Med 1988; 85: 183–188.

Kirkali Z, Yigitbasi O, Sasmaz R. Urological aspects of Bechet's disease. Br J Urol 1991; 67(6): 638–639.

Kirtschig G, Gieler U, Happle R. Treatment of Hailey–Hailey disease by dermabrasion. J Am Acad Dermatol 1993; 28(5 Pt.1): 784–786.

Kirtschig G, Mengel R, Mittag H et al. Desquamative gingivitis and balanitis–linear IgA disease or cicatricial pemphigoid? Clin & Exp Derm 1998; 23(4): 173–177.

Kirtschig G, Murrell D, Wojnarowska F, et al. Interventions for mucous membrane pemphigoid and epidermolysis bullosa acquisita. Cochrane Database Syst Rev. 2003; (1). CD004056.

Kim M, Han S, Sung J et al. Papillomavirus DNA hybridisation in condyloma acuminatum patients and their consorts. Acta Dermato–Venereologie 1993; 73(5): 352–355.

Klein E, Milgrum H, Helm F et al. Effects of local use of cytotoxic agents. 1962, Skin 1 : 81 [OR on back page range]

Knight EL, Post GJ, Morabito RA et al. Leukemic infiltration of penis. Urology 1979; 14(1): 83–84.

Kocsard E. Pruritus ani. A symptom of fecal contamination. Cutis 1981; 27: 518.

Koga F, Gotoh S, Suzuki S, et al. Congestion of the corpus spongiosum and necrosis of the glans penis in systemic vasculitis. Br J Urol. 1996; 78(5): 796–7.

Koh FBH, Nazarina AR. Paget's disease of the scrotum: report of a case with underlying carcinoma of the prostate. Br J Dermatol 1995; 133: 306–307.

Kohler S, Rouse RV, Smoller BR. The differential diagnosis of Pagetoid cells in the epidermis. Mod Pathol 1998; 11(1): 79–92.

Kokx NP, Comstock J, Facklam RR. Streptococcal perianal disease in children. Pediatrics 1987; 80: 659–663.

Kolligian ME, Franco I, Reda EF. Correction of penoscrotal transposition: a novel approach. J Urol. Sep;164(3 Pt 2):994–996; discussion. 2000; 997.

Konstantinov D, Stanoeva L, Yawalkar SJ. Crotamiton cream and lotion in the treatment of infants and young children with scabies. J Int Med Res 1979; 7(5): 443–448.

Kopecky RT, Funk MM, Kreitzer PR. Localized genital edema in patients undergoing continous ambulatory peritoneal dialysis. J Urol 1985; 134: 880–884.

Kopf AW, Bart RS. Tumor conference No 11: Multiple bowenoid papules of the penis: a new entity? J Dermatol Surg Oncol 1977; 3: 265–269.

Kopf AW, Bart RS. Tumor conference 43: Penile lentigo. J Dermatol Surg Oncol 1982; 8: 637–639.

Kormoczy I. Enormous keloid (?) on a penis. Br J Plas Surg 1978; 31: 268–269.

Kort R, Fazaa B, Bouden S et al. Perianal basal cell carcinoma. Int J Dermatol 1995; 34(6): 427–428.

Kossard S et al. Necrobiotic granulomas localised to the penis: a possible variant of subcutaneous granuloma annulare. J Cutan Pathol 1990; 17: 101–104.

Kossard S, Shumack S. Lichen aureus of the glans penis as an expression of Zoon's balanitis. J Am Acad Dermatol 1989; 21(4 Pt.1): 804–806.

Kossow AS, Cotelingham JD, Macfarland F. Bowenoid papulosis of the penis. J Urol 1980; 125: 124–126.

Koster LH, Antoon SJ. Fat necrosis in the scrotum. J Urol 1980; 123: 599–600.

Kotlarewsky M, Freeman JB, Cameron W et al. Anal intraepithelial dysplasia and squamous carcinoma in immunosuppressed patients. Can J Surg 2001; 44: 450–454.

Koyuncuoglu M, Yalçin N, Özkan S et al. Primary Kaposi's sarcoma of the glans penis. Br J Urol 1996; 77: 614–615.

Kraemer BB, Schmidtb WA, Foucar E et al. Verruciform xanthoma of the penis. Arch Dermatol 1981; 177: 516–518.

Kraus FT, Perez-Mesa C. Verrucous carcinoma: clinical and pathological study of 105 cases involving oral cavity, larynx and genitalia. Cancer 1966; 19: 26–38.

Kraus S, Ludecke G, Weidner W. Mondor's disease of the penis. Urol Int 2000; 64(2): 99–100.

Krebs HB. Treatment of genital condylomata with topical 5–fluorouracil. Dermatol Clin 1991; 9(2): 333–341.

Kristensen JK, Scheibel J. Sclerosing lymphangitis of the penis: a possible Chlamydia aetiology. Acta Dermato–Venereologie 1981; 61: 455–456.

von Krogh G. Topical treatment of penile condylomata acuminata with podophyllin, podophyllotoxin and colchicine: a comparative study. Acta Dermato–Venereologie 1978; 58: 163–168.

von Krogh G. The beneficial effect of 1% 5–fluorouracil in 70% ethanol on therapeutically refractory condylomas in the preputial cavity. Sex Trans Dis 1978; 5(4): 137–140.

von Krogh G. Genitoanal papillomavirus infection: diagnostic and therapeutic objectives in the light of current epidemiological observations. Int J STD AIDS 1991; 2(6): 391–404.

von Krogh G. Clinical relevance of evaluation of genitoanal papilloma virus infection in the male. Sem Dermatol 1992; 11(3): 229–240.

von Krogh G, Horenblas S. Diagnosis and clinical presentation of premalignant lesions of the penis. Scand J Urol Nephrol Suppl.(205). 2000; 201–214.

von Krogh G, Ruden A–K. Topical treatment of penile condylomata acuminata with colchicine at 48–72 hour intervals . Acta Dermato–Venereologica 1980; 60: 87–89.

von Krogh G, Szpak E, Andersson M et al. Self–treatment using 0.25%–0.50% podophyllotoxin–ethanol solutions against penile condylomata acuminata: a placebo–controlled comparative study. Genitourin Med 1994; 70(2): 105–109.

von Krogh G, Wilkstrom A. Efficacy of chemical and/or surgical therapy against condylomata acuminata: A retrospective evaluation. Int J STD AIDS 1991; 2(5): 333–338.

Kubota Y, Nakada T, Yaguchi H et al. Schwannoma of the penis. Urologia Internationalis 1993; 51: 111–113.

Kumar A, Kossard S. Band–like sebaceous hyperplasia over the penis. Australas J Dermatol 1999; 40(1): 47–48.

Kumar B, Dawn G. Polypoidal and giant molluscum contagiosum in an AIDS patient. Genitourin Med 1995; 71(1): 57.

Kumar B, Talwar P, Kaur S. Penile tinea. Mycopathologia 1981; 75: 169–172.

Kumar B, Sharma V, Bakaya V et al. Isolation of anaerobes from bulbo associated with chancroid. Genitourinary Medicine 1991; 67(1): 47–48.

Kumar B, Sharma R, Rajagopalan M et al. Plasma cells balanitis: clinical and histopathological features–response to circumcision. Genitourin Med 1995; 71: 32–34.

Kumar B, Kaur I, Rai R et al. Involvement of male genitalia in leprosy. Lepr Rev 2001; 72: 70–77.

Kuniyuki S, Asada T, Yasumoto R. A case of vulvitis circumscripta plasmacellularis positive for herpes simplex type II antigen. Clin Exp Dermatol 1998; 23: 230–231.

Kuppers F, Jongen J, Bock JU et al. Keratoacanthoma in the differential diagnosis of anal carcinoma: difficult diagnosis, easy therapy. Report of three cases. Dis Col Rect 2000; 43(3): 427–429.

Kurokawa I, Nishijima S, Suzuki K, et al. Cytokeratin expression in pilonidal sinus. Br J Dermatol. 2002; 146(3): 409–13.

Kurwa AR, Vickers HR. Benign familial chronic pemphigus. Br J Dermatol 1985; 113(supp. 29): 64.

Kyriazi NC, Costenbader CL. Group A β–hemolytic streptococcal balanitis: it may be more common than you think. Pediatrics 1991; 88(1): 154–156.

L

Lambropoulou V, Balamotis A, Tosca A et al. Typing of human papillomavirus in condylomata acuminata from Greece. J of Med Virol 1994; 43(3): 259–263.

Labrune P, Assathiany R, Penso D et al. Progressive vitiligo, mental retardation, facial dysmorphism, and urethral duplication without chromosomal breakage or immunodeficiency. J Med Genet 1992; 29(8): 592–594.

Ladocsi LT, Siebert CF Jr, Rickert RR et al. Basal cell carcinoma of the penis. Cutis 1998; 61(1): 25–27.

Laird SM. Granuloma annulare of the penis. Genitourin Med 1992; 68(4): 277.

Lakhanpal S, Lie JT, Karper RE, et al. Priapism as a manifestation of isolated genital vasculitis. J Rheumatol. 1991; 18(6): 902–3.

Lal S, Nicholas C. Epidemiological and clinical features in 165 cases of granuloma inguinale. Br J Vener Dis 1970; 46: 461.

Bibliography

Lambert D, Laurent R, Bouilly D et al. Oedeme aigu hemorragique du nourrisson. Donnees immunologiques et ultra structurales. Annales de Dermatologie et de Syphiligraphie 1979; 106: 975–987.

Landergren G. Gonorrheal ulcer of the penis: report of a case. Acta Dermato–Venereologica 1961; 41: 320–323.

Lands RH, Ange D, Hartman DL. Radiation therapy for classic Kaposi's sarcoma presenting only on the glans penis. J Urol 1992; 147: 468–470.

Langenburg J. Am Acad Dermatol 1992; 26: 951–955.

Langlois NEI, McClinton S, Miller ID. An unusual presentation of transitional cell carcinoma of the distal urethra. Histopathol 1992; 21(5): 482–484.

Langtry JA, Ostlere LS, Hawkins DA, et al. The difficulty in diagnosis of cutaneous herpes simplex virus infection in patients with AIDS. Clin Exp Dermatol. 1994; 19(3): 224–6.

Laor T, Atala A, Teele RL. Scrotal ultrasonography in Henoch–Schonlein purpura. Pediatr Radiol 1992; 22(7): 505–506.

Lapins J, Lindback S, Lidbrink P et al. Mucocutaneous manifestations in 22 consecutive cases of primary HIV–1 infection. Br J Dermatol 1996; 134: 257–261.

Lapins NA, Willoughby C, Helwig EB. Lichen nitidus. A study of 43 cases. Cutis 1978; 21: 634–637.

Lark B. Chronic perianal pain. J Roy Soc Med 1982; 75: 370.

Lassus A, Niemi KM, Valle S–L et al. Sclerosing lymphangitis of the penis. Br J Vener Dis 1972; 38: 545–548.

Lassus A, Karvonen J, Iuvakoski T. Dextran polymer particles (Debrisani) in the treatment of penile ulcers. Acta Dermato–Venereologica 1977; 57: 361–363.

Lassus J, Niemi KM, Syrjanen S, et al. A comparison of histopathologic diagnosis and the demonstration of human papillomavirus–specific DNA proteins in penile warts. Sex Trans Dis 1992; 19(3): 127–132.

Lassus J, Happonen HP, Niemi KM et al. Carbon dioxide (CO$_2$)–laser therapy cures macroscopic lesions, but viral genome is not eradicated in men with therapy resistant HPV infection. Sex Trans Dis 1994; 21(6): 297–302.

Latifoglu O, Yavuzer R, Demir Y et al. Surgical management of penoscrotal lymphangioma circumscriptum. Plast Reconstr Surg 1999; 103(1): 175–178.

La Touche CJ. Scrotal dermatophytosis. An insufficiently documented aspect of tinea. Br J Dermatol 1967; 79: 339–344.

Laumann A. Appropriate controls are essential in assessing the relationship between circumcision and penile dermatoses. Arch Dermatol 2001; 137(4): 503.

Laumann EO, Masi CM, Zuckerman EW. Circumcision in the United States. Prevalence, prophylactic effects, and sexual practice. JAMA 1997; 277: 1052–1057.

Lautenschlager S, Eichmann AR. Chancoid. In: Fitzpatrick: Dermatology in General Medicine Sixth edition. Vol 2 Freedberg et al eds. McGraw Hill. 2003; 2193–97.

Law C, Merianos A, Thompson C et al. Manifestations of anogenital HPV infection in the male partners of women with anogenital warts and/or abnormal cervical smears. Int J STD AIDS 1991; 2(3): 188–194.

Lawrence D, Howard ER, Harris RF. A case of congenital urethral duplication cyst and its embryological significance. Br J Surg. 1983; 70(9): 565–6.

Leal SM, Novsam N, Kacks SI. Case report: amyloidosis presenting as a penile mass. J Urol. 1988; 140(4): 830–831.

Leal–Khouri S, Hruza GJ. Squamous cell carcinoma developing within lichen planus of the penis. Treatment with Mohs micrographic surgery. J Dermatol Surg Oncol 1994; 20(4): 272–276.

Le Bourgeois PC, Poynard T, Modai l et al. Ulceration perianale. Ne pas oublier la tuberculose. La Presse Medicale 1984; 13: 2507–2509.

Lecroq C, Thomine E, Bouillie MC et al. Necrobiose lipoidique atypique genitale. Ann Dermatol Venereol 1984; 111: 717–718.

Ledwig PA, Weigand DA. Late circumcision and lichen sclerosus et atrophicus of the penis. J Am Acad Dermatol 1989; 20(21): 211–214.

Lee JY. Cytomegalovirus infection involving the skin in immunocompromised hosts. A clinicopathologic study. Am J Clin Pathol 1989; 92: 96–100.

Lee LM, Moloney PJ, Wong HCG et al. Testicular pain: an unusual presentation of polyarteritis nodosa. 1983; 129: 1243–1244.

Lee SJ, Phillips SMA. Recurrent lichen sclerosus et atrophicus in urethroplasties from multiple skin grafts. Br J Urol 1994; 74(6): 802–803.

Lee WR, Alderson MR, Downes JE. Scrotal cancer in the North–West of England. Br J Industr Med 1972; 29: 188–195.

Leeuwen van TM. Vereenigingsverslagen. 1938; 82(3): 4758–4759.

Lehn H, Ernest T–M, Sauer G. Transcription of episomal papillomavirus DNA in human condylomata acuminata and Buschke–Lowenstein tumours. J Gener Virol 1984; 65: 2003–2010.

Lehrman SN, Douglas JM, Corey L et al. Recurrent genital herpes and suppressive oral acyclovir therapy. Ann Intern Med 1986; 104: 786–790.

Lehrnbecher T, Kontny HU, Jeschke R. Metastatic Crohn's disease in a 9–year–old boy. J Pediatr Gastroenterol Nutr 1999; 28(3): 321–323.

Leiberman DA. Common anorectal disorders. Ann Intern Med 1984; 101: 837–846.

Leibowitch M, Neill S, Pelisse M et al. The epithelial changes associated with squamous cell carcinoma of the vulva: a review of the clinical, histological and viral findings in 78 women. Br J Obstet Gynaecol 1990; 97: 1135–1139.

Leicht S, Youngberg G, Diaz–Miranda C. Atypical pigmented penile macules. Arch Dermatol 1988; 124: 1267–1270.

Leighton JA, Valdovinos MA, Pemberton JH et al. Anorectal dysfunction and rectal prolapse in progressive systemic sclerosis. Dis Col Rect 1993; 36(2): 182–185.

Lejman K, Starzycki Z. Syphilitic balanitis of Follmann developing after the appearance of the primary chancre. A case report. Br J Vener Dis. 1975; 51(2): 138–40.

Lenane P, Keane CO, Connell BO et al. Genital melanotic macules: clinical, histologic, immunohistochemical, and ultrastructural features. J Am Acad Derm 2000; 42(4): 640–644.

Lenk S, Oesterwitz H, Audring H. Laser surgery in superficial penile tumours. Int Urol Nephrol 1991; 23: 357–363.

Lestringant GG, Khalil I, Fletcher S. Is the incidence of trichomycosis of genital hair underestimated? J Am Acad Dermatol 1991; 24: 297–298.

Levell NJ, Bewley AP, Levene GM. Porokeratosis of Mibelli on the penis, scrotum and natal cleft. Clin Exper Dermatol 1994; 19: 77–78.

Lever WF, ed. Pemphigus and Pemphigoid. Springfield: Thomas; 1965.

Levine FJ, de Tejada IS, Payton TR et al. Recurrent prolonged erections and priapism as a sequela of priapism: pathophysiology and management. J Urol 1991; 145: 764–767.

Lewis RJ, Bendl BJ. Erythroplasia of Queyrat–Report of a patient successfully treated with topical 5–fluorouracil. Can Med Assoc J 1971; 104: 148–149.

Lejman K, Starzycki Z. Syphilitic balanitis of Follmann developing after the appearance of the primary chancre. A case report. Br J Vener Dis 1975; 51: 138–140.

Liatsikos EN, Perimenis P, Dandinis K et al. Lichen sclerosus et atrophicus. Findings after complete circumcision. Scand J Urol Nephrol 1997; 31: 453–456.

Liang MG, Frieden IJ. Perineal ulcerations as the presenting manifestations of hemangioma. Arch Dermatol. 2002; 138: 126–7.

Lim KB, Tulip T, Daniel M et al. Artificial penile nodules: case reports. Genitourin Med 1986; 62: 123–125.

Lin RY, Smith JK Jr. Hyper-IgE and human immunodeficiency virus infection. Ann Allergy. 1988 Oct;61(4):269–72.

Lin Y, Lin M, Huang C et al. Acute epididymitis masquerading as testicular torsion. Am J Emerg Med 1996; 14: 654–655.

Lindhagen T. Topical clobetasol propionate compared with placebo in the treatment of unretractable foreskin. Eur J Surg 1996; 162: 969–972.

Lipscombe TK, Wayte J, Wojnarowska F et al. A study of clinical and aetiological factors and possible associations of lichen sclerosus in males. Australas J Dermatol 1997; 38(3): 132–136.

Lipshultz RL, Kantor GR, Vonderheid EC. Multiple penile syringomas mimicking verrucae. Int J Dermatol 1991; 30: 69.

Lischer GH, Nehra A. New advances in Peyronie's disease. Curr Opin Urol 2001; 11: 631–636.

Litt JL. Drug eruption reference manual DERM. Parthenon, New York; 2001.

Littlejohn JO, Belman AB, Selby D. Plexiform neurofibroma of the penis in a child. Urology 2000; 56(4): 669.

Litwin MA, Williams CM. Cutaneous Pneumocystis carinii infection mimicking Kaposi sarcoma. Ann Intern Med. 1992; 117(1): 48–9.

Livden JK, Thunold S, Schsonsby. Epidermolysis bullosa acquisita and Crohn's disease. Acta Dermato–Venereologica 1978; 58: 241–244.

Lloyd KM. Multicentric pigmented Bowen's disease of the groin. Arch Dermatol 1970; 101: 48–51.

Lo JS, Dijkstra JW, Bergfeld WF. Syringomas on the penis. Int J Dermatol 1990; 29: 309–310.

Lockhard–Mummery HE. Non–venereal lesions of the anal region. Br J Vener Dis 1963; 39: 15–17.

Lockhart–Mummery HE. Anal lesions of Crohn's disease. Clin Gastroenterol 1972; 1(2): 377–382.

Loening–Baucke V. Lichen sclerosus et atrophicus in children. Am J Dis Child 1991; 145: 1058–1061.

Löning T, Riviere A, Henke RP et al. Penile/anal condylomas and squamous cell cancer. A HPV DNA hybridization study. Virchows Arch A Pathol Anat Histopathol 1988; 413: 491–498.

Lonsdale RN. Verruciform xanthoma of the penis. British J Urol 1992; 70(5): 574–575.

Lord PH. Diverse methods of managing haemorrhoids: dilatation. Dis Col Rect 1973; 16: 180–192.

Lord PH. Anorectal problems: Etiology of pilonidal sinus. Dis Col Rect 1975; 18: 661–664.

Lord PH, Millar DM. Pilonidal sinus: a simple treatment. Br J Surg 1965; 52: 298–300.

Lord PH, Sakellariades P. Perianal skin gangrene due to amoebic infection in a diabetic. Proc Roy Soc Med 1973; 66: 677–678.

Lortat–Jacob, Civatte J. Balanite pseudo–epithiliomateuse, keratosique et micacee. Bulletin de la Societe Francaise de Dematologie et de syphilographie 1961; 68: 164–167.

Lortat–Jacob, Civatte J. Balanite pseudo–epithiliomateuse, keratosique et micacee. Bulletin de la Societe Francaise de Dematologie et de syphilographie 1966; 73: 931.

Loughlin KR. Psoriasis: association with 2 rare cutaneous urological malignancies. J Urol 1997; 157(2): 622–623.

Lowe FC. Squamous cell carcinoma of the scrotum. J Urol 1983; 130: 423–427.

Lowe FC. Squamous cell carcinoma of scrotum. Urology 1985; 25(1): 63–65.

Lowe FC, Brendler CB. Penile gangrene: a complication of secondary hyperparathyroidism from chronic renal failure. J Urol 1984; 132: 1189–1191.

Lowe FC, McCullough AR. Cutaneous horns of the penis: An approach to management. J Am Acad Dermatol 1985; 13(2 Pt.2): 369–373.

Lowe FC, Lattimer DG, Metroka CE. Kaposi's sarcoma of the penis in patients with acquired immunodeficiency syndrome. J Urol 1989; 142: 1475–1477.

Lowhagen GB, Bolmstedt A, Ryd W et al. The prevalence of the "high risk" HPV types in penile condylomata–like lesions: correlation between HPV type and morphology. Genitourin Med 1993; 69(2): 87–90.

Lu S, Bodemer W, Ostwald C et al. Anal verrucous carcinoma and penile condylomata acuminata. Dermatology 2000; 200(1) 320–323.

Lucia MS, Miller GJ. Histopathology of malignant lesions of the penis. Urol Clin North Am 1992; 19: 227–246.

Lucke T, Fallowfield M, McHenry P. Idiopathic calcinosis cutis of the penis. Br J Dermatol 1997; 137(6): 1025–1026.

Lucke TW, Fleming CJ, McHenry P. Clothing dye dermatitis of the scrotum. Contact Dermatitis 1998; 38(4): 224.

Lucker GPH, Hulsmans R–FHJ, van der Kley AMJ et al. Evaluation of the frequency of contact allergic reactions to kathon CG in the Maastricht area–1987–1990 Dermatology. 1992; 184(2): 90–93.

Luelmo J, Tolosa C, Prats J et al. Tumorous lymphoedema of the penis. Report of verrucous elephantiasis A brief case. Preliminary note. Actas Urol Esp 1995; 19: 585–587.

Luger A, Gschnait F. Condylomata acuminata. Weiner Klinische Wochenschrift 1981; 93: 746–750.

Luzzi GA. Chronic prostatitis and chronic pelvic pain in men: aetiology, diagnosis and management. J Eur Acad Dermatol Venereol. 2002; 16(3): 253–6.

Lynch JL. Erythroplasia of Queyrat. Arch Dermatol 100: 782. 1969;

Lyon CC, Kulkarni J, Zimerson E et al. Skin disorders in amputees. J Am Acad Derm 2000; 42(3): 501–507.

M

Mabogunje O. Kaposi sarcoma of glans penis. Urology 1981; 27(5): 476–478.

Macaluso JN, Sullivan JW, Tomberlin S. Glomus tumor of the glans penis. Urology 1985; 25(4): 409–410.

MacKie RM. Tumours of the skin. In: Textbook of Dermatology Rook A J Wilkinson D S Ebling F J et al eds, 4th edn., Vol 3 Oxford: Blackwell Scientific Publications. 1986; 2428–2430.

MacMillan RW, MacDonald BR, Alpern HD. Scrotal lymphangioma. Urology 1984; 23(1): 79–86.

Madden JF. The Balanitides. J Am Med Ass 1935; 195: 420–427.

Maden C, Sherman KJ, Beckmann AM et al. History of circumcision, medical conditions, and sexual activity and the risk of penile cancer. J Nat Cancer Inst 1993; 85(1): 19–24.

Maden C, Sherman KJ, Beckmann AM et al. Lichen sclerosus et atrophicus. Findings after complete circumcision. Scand J Urol Nephrol 1997; 31: 453–456.

Madison JF, Haserick JR. Topically applied mechlorethamine on twelve dermatoses. Arch Dermatol 1962; 86: 663–667.

Maekawa Y, Sakazaki Y, Hayashibara T. Diaper area granuloma of the aged. Arch Dermatol 1978; 114: 382–383.

Maged A. Urethral diverticula in males (with a report of eight cases). Br J Urol 1969; 37: 560–568.

Maher JD, Thompson GM, Loening S et al. Penile plexiform neurofibroma: Case report and review of the literature. J Urol 1988; 139: 1310.

Mahmood N, Afzal N, Joyce A. Sarcoidosis of the penis. Br J Urol 1997; 80: 155.

Maiche AG. Epidemiological aspects of cancer of the penis in Finland. Eur J Cancer Prevent 1992; 1(2): 153–158.

Maiche AG, Holsti P, Gröhn P et al. Kaposi's sarcoma of penis. Br J Urol 1986; 58: 557.

Majewski S, Jablonska S. Human papillomavirus–associated tumors of the skin and mucosa. J Am Acad Dermatol 1997; 36: 659–685.

Makino T, Nakamura S, Nakayama H et al. Genital Paget's disease with clear cells in the epidermis of the axilla. J Cut Path 1998; 25(10): 560–571.

Mallon E, Ross JS, Hawkins DA et al. Biopsy of male genital dermatosis. Genitourin Med 1997; 73(5): 421.

Mallon E, Young D, Bunce M et al. HLA–Cw*0602 and HIV associated psoriasis. Br J Dermatol 1998; 139:527–533.

Bibliography

Mallon E, Bunce M, Savoie H et al. HLA–C and guttate psoriasis. Br J Dermatol 2000; 143: 1177–1182.

Mallon E, Hawkins D, Dinneen M et al. Circumcision and genital dermatoses. Arch Dermatol 2000; 136: 350–354.

Mallon E, Bunker C. Management of penile erosions and ulcers. Postgraduate Doctor Middle East. 1998; 21: 163–8.

Malloy TR, Wein AJ, Gross P. Scrotal and penile lymphedema: surgical considerations and management. J Urol 1983; 130: 263–265.

Manivel JC, Fraley EE. Malignant melanoma of the penis and male urethra: 4 case reports and literature review. J Urol 1988; 139: 813.

Mankodi RC, Kanvinde MS, Mohapatra LN. Penile histoplasmosis. A case report. Indian J Med Sci 1970; 24: 354–356.

Mansfield P. The Arabs, 3rd edn. Penguin, London 1992.

Manzano de Arostegui JA, Borbujo Martinez J, Juez Juez AA et al. Bowenoid papulosis. Review of 4 cases in a health center. Atencion Primaria 1994; 13(7): 367–371.

Markos AR. The male genital skin burning syndrome (dysaesthetic peno/scroto–dynia). Int J STD AIDS 2002; 13: 271–272.

Markowitz J, Daum F, Aiges H et al. Perianal disease in children and adolescents with Crohn's disease. Gastroenterol 1984; 86(5 Pt.1 of 2): 829–833.

Marks CG, Ritchie JK, Lockhard–Mummery HE. Anal fistulas in Crohn's disease. B J Surg 1981; 68: 525–527.

Marks D et al. Therapy of primary diffuse large cell lymphoma of the penis with preservation of function. J Urol 1988; 139: 1057.

Markus HS, Bunker CB, Kouris K et al. rCBF abnormalities detected and sequentially followed by SPECT in neuro–Behçet's syndrome with normal CT and MRI imaging. J Neurol 1992; 239: 363–366.

Marquart KH, Oehlschlaegel G, Engst R. Disseminated Kaposi's sarcoma that is not associated with acquired immunodeficiency syndrome in a bisexual man. Arch Pathol Lab Med 1986; 110: 346–347.

Marquart KH, Engst R, Oehlschlaegel G. An 8–year history of Kaposi's sarcoma in an HIV–negative bisexual man. AIDS 1991; 5(3): 346–348.

Marshescu S, Braun–Falco O, Konz B. Communications sur les dermatoses precancereuses. Bulletin de la Societe Francaise Dermatologie et Syphiligraphie 1975; 83: 293–294.

Marsidi PJ, Winter CC. Schwannoma of penis. Urology 1980; 16: 303.

Martenstein H. Induratio penis plastica und dupuytrensche contractur. Medizinische Klinik 1920; 8: 1–4.

Martin F, Bower M. Anal intraepithelial neoplasia in HIV positive people. Sex Transm Infect 2001; 77(5): 327–331.

Martinelli C, Farese A, Del Mistro A et al. Resolution of recurrent perianal condylomata acuminata by topical cidofovir in patients with HIV infection. JEADV 2001; 15: 568–569.

Martinez F, Gil–Albarellos R, Cabezudo JI et al. Primary tuberculosis of the penis. Actas Urolog Espan 1994; 18(3): 245–248.

Martinez L. Relationship of squamous cell carcinoma of the cervix uteri to squamous cell carcinoma of the penis among Puerto Rican women married to men with penile carcinoma. Cancer 1969; 24: 777–780.

Mascaro JM, Torras H, Bou D. Papulosis bowenoide de los genitales. Comentario sobre su significado. Actas Dermo–Sifilographicas 1980; 71: 119–128.

Masih AS, Stoler MH, Farrow GM et al. Human papillomavirus in penile squamous cell lesion. Arch Pathol Lab Med 1993; 117(3): 302–307.

Massa MC, Jason SM, Gradini R et al. Lichenoid drug eruption secondary to propanolol. Cutis 1991; 48(1): 41–43.

Massmanian A, Valis GS, Sempere FJV. Fordyce spots on the glans penis. Br J Dermatol 1995; 133: 498–499.

Masson P. Bulletin de la Societe Anatomie de Paris. 1923; 93: 517, 523.

Matis WL, Triana A, Shapiro R et al. Dermatologic findings associated with the human immunodeficiency virus. J Am Acad Dermatol 1987; 17: 746–751.

Matsuda O, Mitsukawa S, Ishii N et al. A case of Wegener' granulomatosis with necrosis of the penis. Tohuku J Exper Med 1976; 118: 145–151.

Matsuda T, Shichiri Y, Hida S et al. Eosinophilic sclerosing lipogranuloma of the male genitalia not caused by exogenous lipids. J Urol 1988; 140: 1021.

Matsumoto M, Sonobe H, Takeuchi T et al. Pigmented squamous cell carcinoma of the scrotum associated with a lentigo. Br J Dermatol 1999; 141: 132–136.

Matsumura N, Kumasaka, Maki H et al. Giant condyloma acuminatum in a baby boy. J Dermatol 1992; 19(7): 432–435.

Matsushima M, Takanami M, Tajima M et al. Primary lipogranuloma of male genitalia. Urology 1988; 31(1): 75–77.

Maw R. National guideline for the management of anogenital warts. Clinical Effectiveness Group (Association of Genitourinary Medicine and the Medical Society for the Study of Venereal Diseases) Sexually Transmitted Infections should be added to the Fp & LP 1999. 1999; 75(Suppl 1): 71–75.

Mazuecos J, Rodriguez–Pichardo A, Camacho F. Pubic trichotillomania in an adult man. Br J Dermatol. 2001; 145(6): 1034–5.

Mazzatenta C, Andreassi L, Biagioli M et al. Detection and typing of genital papillomaviruses in men with a single polymerase chain reaction and type specific DNA probes. J Am Acad Dermatol 1993; 28(5 Pt. 1): 704–710.

McAninch JW. Management of genital skin loss. Urol Clin N Am 1989; 16(2): 387–390.

McAninch JW, Moore CA. Precancerous penile lesions in young men. J Urol 1970; 104: 287–290.

McCallum DI, Kinmont PDC. Dermatological manifestations of Crohn's disease. Br J Dermatol 1968; 80: 1–8.

McCann J, Voris J. Perianal injuries resulting from sexual abuse: A longitudinal study. Pediatrics 1993; 91(2): 390–393.

McCarley ME, Cruz PD, Sontheimer RD. Chancroid: Clinical variants and other findings from an epidemic in Dallas County 1986–87. J Am Acad Dermatol. 1988; 19: 330–344.

McConnell EM. Squamous carcinoma of the anus–a review of 96 cases. Br J Surg 1970; 57: 89–92.

McDonald MW. Carcinoma of scrotum. Urology 1982; 19(3): 269–274.

McDougal WS, Kirchner FR, Edwards RH et al. Treatment of carcinoma of the penis: case for primary lymphadenectomy. 1986; 136: 38–41.

McDougall JK. Immortalization and transformation of human cells by human papillomavirus. Curr Topics Microbiol Immunol 1994; 186: 101–119.

McElroy JA, Mehregan DA, Roenigk RK. Carbon dioxide laser vaporization of recalcitrant symptomatic plaques of Hailey–Hailey disease and Darier's disease. J Am Acad Dermatol 1990; 23(5 Pt.1): 893–897.

McGarry GW, Robertson JR. Scrotal carcinoma following prolonged use of crude coal tar ointment. Br J Urol 1989; 63: 211–219.

McGregor D. Distribution of pubic hair in sample of fit men. Br J Dermatol 1961; 73: 61–64.

McGregor DH, Tanimura A, Weigel JW. Basal cell carcinoma of the penis. Urology 1982; 20(3): 320–323.

McKinlay JR, Graham BS, Ross EV. The clinical superiority of continuous exposure versus short–pulsed carbon dioxide laser exposures for the treatment of pearly penile papules. Dermatol Surg 1999; 25(2): 124–126.

McLeod R, Davis NC, Herron JJ et al. A retrospective survey of 498 patients with malignant melanoma. Surg Gynecol Obstet 1968; 126: 99–108.

McMahon JE, Simonsen PE. Filiariases. Onchocerciasis. In: Manson's Tropical Diseases, 20th edn. Cook GC, Saunders eds. London. 1996; 1338–1351.

McMillan A. Lymphocoele and localized lymphoedema of the penis. Br J Vener Dis 1976; 52: 409–411.

McMillan A. The management of difficult anogenital warts. Gen Trans Infect 1999; 75(3): 192–194.

McMillan A, Smith IW. Painful anal ulceration in homosexual men. Br J Surg 1984; 71: 215–216.

Mc Partland N, Grove JS, Chomet B. Actinomycosis of penis. J Urol 1961, 86(1). 95–97.

Meehan SA, Smoller BR. Cutaneous Langerhans cell histiocytosis of the genitalia in the elderly: a report of three cases. J Cut Path 1998; 25(7): 370–374.

Meffert JJ, Davis BM, Grimwood RE. Lichen sclerosus. J Am Acad Dermatol 1995; 32: 393–416.

Melekos MD, Asbach HW, Markou SA. Etiology of acute scrotum in 100 boys with regard to age distribution. J Urol 1988; 139: 1023.

Meleney FL. Hemolytic streptococcus gangrene. Arch Surg 1924; 9: 317–364.

Melmed EP, Payne JR. Carcinoma of the penis in a Jew circumcised in infancy. Br J Surg 1967; 54: 729–731.

Mendelson J, Miller M. Streptococcal venereal edema of the penis. Clin Infect Dis 1997; 24: 516–517.

Mendelson J, Clecner BYA, Eiley S. Effect of recombinant interferon alpha 2 on clinical course of first episode genital herpes infection and subsequent recurrences. Genitourin Med 1986; 62: 97–101.

Menzel E. Diagnostische gesichtspunkte bei der penistuberkulose. Journal of Urology and Nephrology 1966; 59: 287–291.

Merot Y, Harms M. Circumscribed urethritis plasmacellularis (Zoon) of the navicular fossa. Hautarzt 1983; 34(1): 18–19. German.

Metcalf JS, Lee RE, Maize JC. Epidermotropic urothelial carcinoma involving the glans penis. Arch Dermatol 1985; 121: 532–534.

Meuli M, Brinker J, Hanimann B et al. Lichen sclerosus et atrophicus causing phimosis in boys: a prospective study with 5–year followup after complete circumcision. J Urol 1994; 152(3): 987–989.

Meyer T, Arndt R, Christophers E et al. Association of rare human papillomavirus types with genital premalignant and malignant lesions. J Infect Dis 1998; 178: 252–255.

Meyrick-Thomas RH, Ridley CM, Black MM. The association of lichen sclerosus et atrophicus and autoimmune–related disease in males. Br J Dermatol 1983; 109: 661–664.

Meyrick-Thomas RH, Ridley CM, Black MM. Clinical features and therapy of lichen sclerosus et atrophicus affecting males. Clin Exper Dermatol 1987; 12: 126–128.

Meyrick-Thomas RH, Ridley CM, Sherwood F et al. The lack of association of lichen sclerosus with HLA–A & B tissue antigens. Clin Exper Dermatol 1984; 9: 290–292.

Micali G, Innocenzi D, Nasca MR et al. Squamous cell carcinoma of the penis. J Am Acad Dermatol 1996; 35: 432–451.

Micali G, Nasca MR, Innocenzi D. Lichen sclerosus of the glans is significantly associated with penile carcinoma. Sex Trans Infect 2001; 77(3): 226.

Michalowski R. Balano–posthites a tnchomonas: a propos de 16 observations. Annales de Dermatologie et de Venereologie 1981; 108: 731–738.

Millan JA, Santiago Gonzalez de Garibay AM, Idigora Planas X et al. Cutaneous metastases of epitheliod sarcoma of the penis: report of a case. Actas Urol Espan 1992; 16(3): 254–256.

Millar DM. Aetiology of post anal pilonidal disease. Proc Roy Soc Med 1970; 63: 1263–1264.

Millet P, Sonneck J–M, Lanternier G et al. Actinomyocose perineo fessiere et deficit en G6 PD. Annales de Dermatologie et de Venereologie. 1982; 109: 789–790.

Milstein HG. Erythroplasia of Quevrat in a partially circumcised man. J Am Acad Dermatol 1982; 10(6): 398

Mindel A, Faherty A, Hindley D et al. Prophylactic oral acyclovir in recurrent genital herpes. Lancet 1984; i: 57–59.

Minkin W, Frank SB, Cohen HJ. Penile granuloma. Arch Dermatol 1972; 106: 756.

Miranda–Romero A, Sanchez–Sambucety P, Bajo C et al. Genital oedema from contact allergy to prednicarbate. Contact Dermatitis 1999, 30(1): 228–229.

Mirande LM, Valera JA, Perroni CA et al. Variable pseudoerythroplasic telangiectasis balanitis. Med Cutan Ibero Lat Am 1975; 3(4): 293–296. Spanish.

Mitchell NJ, Gamble DR. Clothing design for operating room personnel. Lancet 1974, 1. 1133–1136.

Miyamoto T, Ikehara A, Araki M et al. Cutaneous metastatic carcinoma of the penis: suspected metastasis implantation from a bladder tumor. J Urol 2000; 163(5): 1519.

Mohs FE, Blanchard I. Microscopically controlled surgery for extra–mammary Paget's disease. Arch Dermatol 1979; 115: 706–708.

Mohs FE, Sahl WJ. Chemosurgery for verrucous carcinoma. J Dermatol Surg Oncol 1979; 5: 302.

Mohs FE, Snow SN, Messing EM et al. Microscopically controlled surgery in the treatment of carcinoma of the penis. J Urol 1985; 133: 961–966.

Mohsin SK, Lee MW, Amin MB et al. Cutaneous verruciform xanthoma: a report of five cases investigating the etiology and nature of xanthomatous cells. Am J Surg Pathol 1998; 22(4): 479–487.

Mollard P, Basset T, Mure PY. Male epispadias: experience with 45 cases. J Urol 1998; 160(1): 55–59.

Monro PAG, ed. Sympathectomy. Oxford: Clarendon Press. 1959; 146.

Montemarano AD, James WD. Staphylococcus aureus as a cause of perianal dermatitis. Pediatr Dermatol. 1993; 10(3): 259–262.

Mooradian AD, Viosca SP, Kaiser FE et al. Penile Raynaud's phenomenon: a possible cause of erectile failure. Am J Med 1988; 85: 748–750.

Moore SW, Wheeler JE, Hefter LG. Epitheloid sarcoma masquerading as Peyronie's disease. Cancer. 1975; 35(6): 1706–10.

Moore TO, Moore AY, Carrasco D et al. Human papillomavirus, smoking and cancer. J Cutan Med Surg 2001; 5(4): 323–328.

Mor Y, Zaidi SZ, Rose DS et al. Granulomatous lymphangitis of the penile skin as a cause of penile swelling in children. J Urol 1997; 158(2): 591–592.

Morelli AE, Ronchetti RD, Secchi AD et al. Assessment by planimetry of Langerhans' cell density in penile epithelium with human papillomavirus infection: changes observed after topical treatment. J Urol 1992; 147(5): 1268–1273.

Morestin H. Deux cas de cancer du penis. Bul Soc Anat Paris 1903; 5: 387.

Morey AF, Meng MV, McAninch JW. Skin graft reconstruction of chronic genital lymphedema. Urology 1997; 50(3): 423–6.

Morgan AR, Miles AJ, Wastell C. Anal warts and squamous–in–situ of the anal canal. J Roy Soc Med 1994; 87(1): 15.

Morgan MB, Viloria J, Morgan JD et al. Human immunodeficiency virus infection and hypereosinophilic syndrome. J Florida Med Ass 1994; 81(6): 401–402.

Morgan WP, Harding KG, Richardson G et al. The use of Silastic foam dressing in the treatment of advanced hidradenitis suppurativa. Br J Surg 1980; 67: 277–280.

Moritz DL, Lynch WS. Extensive Bowen's disease of the penis shaft treated with fresh tissue Mohs micrographic surgery in two separate operations. J Dermatol Surg Oncol 1991; 17(4): 374–378.

Morris SB, Miller MAW, Anson K. Management of penile fracture. J Roy Soc Med 1998; 91: 427–428.

Morris–Jones R, Fearfield L, Nelson M et al. Acute stridor and phimosis secondary to Kaposi's sarcoma. Retinoids 2000, 16: 41–42.

Morrissette DL, Goldstein MK, Raskin DB et al. Finger and penile tactile sensitivity in sexually functional and dysfunctional diabetic men. Diabetologia 1999; 42(3): 336–342.

Morson BC. Histopathology of Crohn's disease. Proc Roy Soc Med 1968; 61: 79–81.

Mortensen NJ, Thomson JP. Perianal abscess due to Enterobius vermicularis. Report of a case Dis. Col. & Rect 1984; 27: 677–678.

Mortier E, Zahar JR, Gros I et al. Primary Infection with Human Immunodeficiency Virus that presented as Stevens–Johnson Syndrome. Clin Infect Dis 1994; 19: 798.

Moses S, Bailey RC, Ronald AR. Male circumcision: assessment of health benefits and risks. Sex Transm Infect 1998; 74: 368–373.

Moss JR, Stevenson CJ. Incidence of male genital vitiligo: report of a screening programme. Br J Vener Dis 1981; 57: 145–146.

Moss RL, Shewmake SW. Idiopathic calcinosis of the scrotum. Int J Dermatol 1981; 20: 134–136.

Mouly MR. A propos des suppurations perineo–fessieres chroniques et de leur traitment chirurgical Bulletin de la Societe Fr Dermatologie et Syphiligr 1969; 76: 23.

Moyle G, Barton S, Gazzard BG. Penile ulceration with foscarnet therapy. AIDS. 1993; 7(1): 140–1.

Moyle G, Gazzard BG. Opportunistic infections and tumours. Cytomegalovirus infection. In: AIDS Care Handbook. Gazzard BG ed. Mediscript London; 2002.

Muehlberger T, Homann HH, Kuhnen C et al. Etiology, clinical aspects and therapy of penoscrotal lymphedema. Chirurg 2001; 72(4): 414–418. German.

Muir CS, Nectoux J. Epidemiology of carcinoma of the testis and penis. Nat Cancer Inst Monogr 1979; 53: 157–164.

Mukai H, Eto H, Yamamoto T. Ano–sacral cutaneous amyloidosis. Japan J Dermatol 1986; 96(12): 1247–1251.

Mulcahy JJ, Schileru G, Donmezer MA et al. Lymphangioma of scrotum Urology. 1979; 14(1): 64–65.

Mullhaupt B, Bauerfeind P, Kurrer MO et al. Anal squamous cell carcinoma in a patient with Peutz–Jeghers syndrome. Digest Dis Sci 2001; 46(2): 273–277.

Munro CS, Cox NH. Pyoderma gangrenosum associated with Behçet's syndrome – response to thalidomide. Clin Exp Dermatol 1988; 13: 408–410.

Murali TR, Raja NS. Cavernosal cold abscess: a rare cause of impotence. Br J Urol 1998; 82(6): 929–930.

Murata Y, Kumano K, Tani M. Underpants–pattern erythema: a previously unrecognized cutaneous manifestation of extramammary Paget's disease of the genitalia with advanced metastatic spread. J Am Acad Derm 1999; 40(61): 949–956.

Murphy M, Buckley M, Corr J et al. Fournier's gangrene of scrotum in a patient with AIDS. Genitourin Med. 1991; 67: 339–341.

Murray WJ, Fletcher MS, Yates–Bell AJ et al. Plasma cell balinitis of Zoon. Br J Urol 1986; 58(6): 689–691.

Murthy KVN. Primary cutaneous carcinoma of the scrotum. J Occup Med 1993; 35(9): 889–889.

Mutailik S. Fixed drug eruption caused by erythromycin. Int J Dermatol 1991; 30(10): 751.

Myers DA, Strandjord SE, Marcus RB Jr et al. Histiocytosis presenting as a primary penile lesion J Urol. 1981; 126: 268–269.

Myhr GE, Myrvold HE, Nilsen G et al. Perianal fistulas: Use of MRI imaging for diagnosis. Radiology. 1994; 191(2): 545–549.

Myslovaty B, Kyzer S, Koren R et al. Kaposi sarcoma limited to the glans penis. Plast Reconst Surg 1993; 92: 764.

N

Nagore E, Sanchez–Motilla JM, Febrer MI et al. Median raphe cysts of the penis: a report of five cases. Pediatr Dermatol. May 1998; 15(3): 191–193.

Naib ZM In: The Hurman Herpesviruses, Nahmias AJ et al, eds. New York: Elsevier; 1981.

Nakamura M, Sakurai T, Yoshida K et al. Sclerosing lipogranuloma of the penis: chemical analysis of lipid from the lesional tissue. J Urol 1985; 133: 1046–1048.

Nakamura S, Imai T, Nakayama K. Calcinosis of the scrotum. J Dermatol 1985; 12: 369–371.

Nakamura S, Kanamori S, Nakayama K et al. Verrucitorm xanthoma of the scrotum. J Dermatol 1989; 16: 397–401.

Narayana AS, Olney LE, Loening SA et al. Carcinoma of the penis. Cancer 1982; 49: 2185–2191.

Narouz N, Allan PS, Wade AH. Penile granuloma annulare. Sex Trans Infect 1999; 75(3): 186–187.

Nasca MR, Innocenzi D, Micali G. Penile cancer among patients with genital lichen sclerosus. J Am Acad Dermatol 1999; 41(6): 911–914.

Nazzari G, Drago F, Malatto M et al. Epidermoid anal canal carcinoma metastic to the skin. A clinical mimic of prostate adenocarcinoma metastases. J Dermatol Surg Oncol 1994; 20: 765–766.

Neff JH. Congenital canals and cysts of the genito–perineal raphe. 1936; 31: 308–315.

Nehra A, Hall SJ, Basile G et al. Systemic sclerosis and impotence: A clinicopathological correlation. J Urol 1995; 153: 1140–1146.

Neill ME, Swash M. Chronic perianal pain: an unsolved problem. J Roy Soc Med 1982; 75: 96–101.

Neill SM, Tatnall FM, Cox NH. Guidelines for the management of lichen sclerosus. Br J Dermatol 2002; 147: 640–649.

Neinstein LS, Goldenring J. Pink pearly papules: An epidemiologic study. J Pediatr 1984; 105: 594–595.

Nelson GS. 'Hanging groin' and hernia, complications of onchocerciasis. Trans Roy Soc Trop Med Hyg 1958; 52: 272–275.

Nelson JH. III, Winter CC. Priapism: evolution of management in 48 patients in a 22–year series. J Urol 1977; 117: 455–458.

Nelson R, Gregory JC. Gonococcal infections of penile prostheses. Urology 1988; 31: 391–394.

Neri I, Bardazzi F, Marzaduri S et al. Perianal streptococcal dermatitis in adults. Br J Dermatol 1996; 135: 796–798.

Neri I, Bardazzi F, Raone B et al. Ectopic pearly penile papules: a paediatric case. Genitourin Med 1997; 73(2): 136.

Nesbit RM, Hodgson NB. Thromboangutis obliterans of the spermatic cord. Trans Amer Ass of Genito–Urinary Surg 1959; 51: 92–94.

Neuhofer J, Fritsch P. Treatment of localized scleroderma and lichen sclerosus with etretinate. Acta Derm Venereol 1984; 64(2): 171–174.

Neumann HAM, Faber WR. Pyodermite vegetante of Hallopeau. Immunofluorescence studies performed in an early disease stage. Arch Dermatol 1980; 116(10): 1169–1171.

Newman PL, Fletcher CDM. Smooth muscle tumours of the external genitalia: clinicopatological analysis of a series. Histopathology 1991; 18(6): 523–529.

Newson R. Appropriate controls are essential in assessing the relationship between circumcision and penile dermatoses. Reply. Arch Dermatol 2001; 137(4): 503–504.

Ng CS. Carcinoma erysipeloides from prostate cancer presenting as cellulitis. Cutis 2000; 65(4): 215–216.

Nickel JC, Morales A. Necrotizing fasciitis of the male genitalia (Fournier's gangrene). Can Med Ass J 1983; 129: 445–448.

Nico MM, Cymbalista NC, Hurtado YC et al. Perianal cytomegalovirus ulcer in an HIV infected patient: case report and review of literature. J Dermatol 2000; 27(2): 99–105.

Niederauer HH, Weindorf N, Schultz–Ehrenburg U. Ein fall von condyloma acuminatum giganteum. Der Hautarzt 44(12). 1993; 795–799.

Nishigori C, Taniguchi S, Hayakawa M et al. Penis tuberculides: papulonecrotic tuberculides on the glans penis. Dermatologica 1986; 172: 93–97.

Nishimura M, Matsuda T, Muto M et al. Balanitis of Zoon. Int J Dermtol 1990; 29: 421–423.

Nitidandhaprabhas P. Artificial penile nodules: case reports from Thailand. Br J Urol 1975; 47: 463.

Nnoruka EN, Agu CE. Successful treatment of scabies with oral ivermectin in Nigeria. Trop Dis 2001; 31(1): 15–18.

Noble WC, Somerville DA. In: Microbiology of Human Skin vol 2: Major Problems in Dermatology, Rook AJ, ed. London: Saunders, 1974.

Noel JC, de Dobbeleer G. Development of human papillomavirus–associated Buschke–Lowenstein penile carcinoma during cyclosporine therapy for generalized pustular psoriasis. J Am Acad Dermatol 1994; 31(2 Pt. 1): 299–300.

Noel JC, Vandenbossche M, Peny MO et al. Verrucous carcinoma of the penis: importance of human papillomavirus typing for diagnosis and therapeutic decision. Eur Urol 1992; 22: 83–85.

Nomland R. Nevoxanthoendothelioma: A benign xanthomatous disease of infants and children. J Invest Dermatol 1954; 22: 207.

Noone TC, Clark RL. Primary isolated urethral amyloidosis. Abdom Imaging. Jul 1997; 22(4): 448–449.

Noordeen SK, Pannikar VK. Leprosy. In: Manson's Tropical Diseases. 20th edition Cook GC. Saunders, London. 1997; 1016–1044.

Nouri M, Koutani A, Tazi K et al. Fractures of the penis: apropos of 56 cases. Prog Urol 1998; 8(4): 542–547. French.

Novick NL. Angiokeratoma vulvae. J Am Acad Dermatol 1985; 12: 561–563.

Novick NL, Gribetz ME. Annular constriction of the glans penis. J Am Acad Dermatol 1986; 15: 351.

Nunez M, Miralles ES, Hilara Y et al. Concurrent cytomegalovirus, M tuberculosis and M avium–intracellulare cutaneous infection in an HIV patient. J Dermatol 1997; 24(6): 401–404.

Nuovo GJ, Becker J, Margiotta M, et al. Histological distribution of polymerase chain reaction–amplified human papillomavirus 6 and 11 in penile lesions. Am J Surg Pathol 1992; 16(3): 269–275.

NybergLM, Bias WB, Hochberg MC. Identification of an inherited form of Peyronie's disease with autosomal dominant inheritance and association with Dupuytren's contracture and histocompatability B7 cross–reacting antigens. J Urol 1982; 128: 48–51.

O

Oates JK. Pearly penile papules. Genitourin Med 1997; 73(2): 137–138.

Oates JK, Greenhouse PR. Retention of urine in anogenital herpetic infection. Lancet 1978; i: 691–692.

Obalek S, Jablowska S, Beaudenon S et al. Bowenoid papulosis of the male and female genitalia: Risk of cervical neoplasia. J Am Acad Dermatol 1986; 14: 433–444.

O'Brien TS, Luzzi GA. Improving visualization of intrameatal warts: use of the otoscope. Br J Urol 1995; 75(6): 793.

O'Brien WM, O'Connor KP, Lynch JH. Priapism: current concepts. Ann Emerg Med 1989; 18(9): 980–983.

Occella C, Bleidl D, Rampini P et al. Argon laser treatment of cutaneous multiple angiokeratomas. Dermatol Surg 1995; 21(2): 170–172.

Ochonisky S, Wechsler J, Marinho E et al. Eccrine syringofibroadenomatosis (Mascaro) with mucous involvement. Arch Dermatol 1994; 130(7): 933–934.

Odds FC. Genital candidiasis. Clin Exper Dermatol 1982; 7: 345–354.

Oertel YC, Johnson FB. Sclerosing lipogranuloma of male genitalia. Arch Pathol Lab Med 1977; 101: 321–326.

O'Farrell N, Egger M. Circumcision in men and the prevention of HIV infection: a 'meta–analysis' revisited. Int J STD AIDS 2000; 11: 137–142.

Ogawa A, Watanabe. Genitourinary neurofibromatosis in a child presenting with an enlarged penis and scrotum. J Urol 1986; 135: 755–757.

Oh C, Lee C, Jacobson JH II. Necrotizing fasciitis of the perineum. Surgery 1982; 91: 49–51.

Ohnishi T, Kano R, Nakamura Y et al. Genital Bowen disease associated with an unusual human papillomavirus type 57b. Arch Dermatol 1999; 135(7): 858–859.

Ohtake N, Maeda S, Kanzaki T et al. Leiomyoma of the Scrotum. Dermatology 1997; 194: 299–301.

Oldbring J, Mikulowski P. Malignant melanoma of the penis and male urethra. Report of nine cases and review of the literature. Cancer 1987; 59: 581–587.

Oliet FJ, Estes SA. Perianal comedones associated with chronic topical fluorinated steroid use. J Am Acad Dermatol 1982; 7: 405–407.

Olsen EA, Kelly FF, Vollmer RT et al. Comparitive study of systemic interferon alfa–nl and isotretinoin in the treatment of resistant condylomata acuminata. J Am Acad Dermatol 1989; 20(6): 1023–1030.

O'Neil CA, Hansen RC. Pearly penile papules on the shaft. Arch Dermatol 1995; 131(4): 491–492.

Onel JD, Ridgeway GL, eds. Current topics in infection–genital infections by Chlamydia trachomatis. London: Arnold; 1982.

Oranje AP, Brouwer J, Vuzevski VD. Condyloma–like penis carcinoma. Dermatologica 1976; 152: 47–54.

Orchard GE, Jones EW, Jones RR. Verruciform xanthoma: an immunocytochemical study. Br J Biomed Sci 1994; 51(1): 28–34.

Orhan I, Onur R, Ardicoglu A et al. Behcet's disease and spontaneous Haematocele: an unusual complication. Br J Urol International 1999; 84(6): 739–740.

Oriel JD. Natural history of genital warts. Br J Vener Dis 1971; 47: 1–13.

Orihuela E, Tyring SK, Pow–Sang M et al. Development of human papillomavirus type 16 asssociated squamous cell carcinoma of the scrotum in a patient with Darier's disease treated with systemic isotreinoin. J Urol 1995; 153(6): 1940–1943.

Orkin M, Maibach HI. Scabies therapy– Semin Dermatol. 1993; 12(1): 22–25.

Orkin M, Maibach HI. Current views of scabies and pediculosis pubis. Cutis 1994; 33: 85–97.

Orme RL, Nordlund JJ, Barich L et al. The MAGIC syndrome (mouth and genital ulcers with inflamed cartilage). Arch Dermatol 1990; 126: 940–944.

Ortiz Cabria R, Adriazola Semino M, Blanco Parra MA et al. Skin lesions of the penis. Prostatic adenocarcinoma metastasis Report of a case. Actas Urol Esp 1999; 23(2): 153–155. Spanish.

Ortiz de Saracho J, Castrodeza Sanz R, Guzman Davila G. Penile metastasis and pulmonary carcinoma. Arch Bronconeumol 1998; 34(4): 226–227. Spanish.

Ortiza H, Marti J, Jauneta E et al. Lord's procedure: a critical study of its basic principle. Br J Surg 1978; 65: 281–284.

Ortonne JP, Perrot H, Thivolet J. Granulome gluteal infantile (GGI): etude ultrastructurale. Annales de Dermatologie et de Venereologie 1980; 107: 631–634.

Osborne GE, Chinn RJ, Francis ND et al. Magnetic resonance imaging in the investigation of penile lymphangioma circumscriptum. Br J Dermatol 2000; 143: 467–468.

Osborne GE, Francis ND, Bunker CB. Synchronous onset of penile lichen sclerosus and vitiligo. Br J Dermatol 2000; 143: 218–219.

Oshin DR, Bowles WT. Congenital cysts and canals of the scrotal and perineal raphe. J Urol 1962; 88(3): 406–408.

Øster J. Further fate of the foreskin. Incidence of preputial adhesions, phimosis, and smegma among Danish schoolboys. Arch Dis Child 1968; 43: 200–203.

P

Padma–Nathan H, Goldstein I, Krane RJ. Treatment of prolonged of priapistic erections following intracavernosal papaverine therapy. Sem Urol 1986; 4: 236.

Paget J. On disease of the mammary areola preceding carcinoma of the mammary gland. St Barts Hosp Rep 1874; 10: 87–89.

Palder SB, Shandling B, Bilik R et al. Perianal complications of pediatric Crohn's disease, J Pediatr Surg 1991; 26(5): 513–515.

Palefsky JM. Human papillomarvirus–associated anogenital neoplasia and other solid tumours in human immunodeficiency virus infected individuals. Curr Opin Oncol 1991; 3(5): 881–885.

Palmer AE, Amolsch AL, Shaffer LW. Histoplasmosis with mucocutaneous manifestations. Report of a case. Arch Derm Syphil 1942; 45: 912–916.

Bibliography

Pande SK, Mewara PC. Fournier's gangrene: a report of 5 cases. Br J Surg 1976; 63: 479–481.

Pandey SS, Chandra S, Guha PK et al. Dermatophyte infection of the penis. Association with a particular undergarment. Int J Dermatol 1981; 20: 112–114.

Pantuck AJ, Kraus SL, Barone JG. Hair strangulation injury of the penis. Pediatr Emerg Care 1997; 13(6): 423–424.

Paradisi M, Cianchini G, Angelo C et al. Efficacy of topical erythromycin in treatment of perianal streptococcal dermatitis. Pediatr Dermatol 1993; 10(3): 297–298.

Paradisi M, Cianchini G, Angelo C et al. Perianal streptococcal dermatitis: Two familial cases. Cutis 1994a; 54(5): 341–342.

Paradisi M, Cianchini G, Angelo C et al. Perianal streptococcal dermatitis. Minerva Pediatrica 1994b; 46(6): 303–306.

Pardy B, Eastcott HHG. Diabetic scrotal gangrene. Proc Roy Soc Med 1982; 75: 829–830.

Paricio Rubio JF, Revenga AF, Alfaro TJ et al. Squamous cell carcinoma of the penis arising on lichen sclerosus et atrophicus. J Eur Acad Dermatovenereol 1999; 12: 153–156.

Park HG, Moon DC, Kwon KS et al. A case of familial benign chronic pemphigus improved with oral etretinate (Tigason). 718.

Park HS, Lee YS, Chun DK. Squamous cell carcinoma in vitiligo lesion after long-term PUVA therapy. J Eur Acad Dermatol Venereol. 2003; 17(5): 578–80.

Park HJ, Kim YC, Cinn YW, Yoon TY. Granulomatous pyoderma gangrenosum: two unusual cases showing necrotizing granulomatous inflammation. Clin Exp Derm 2000; 25(8): 617–620.

Park KC, Kim KH, Youn SW et al. Heterogeneity of human papillomavirus DNA in a patient with Bowenoid papulosis that progressed to squamous cell carcinoma. Br J Derm 1998; 139(6): 1087–1091.

Park SK, Lee JY, Kim YH et al. Molluscum contagiosum occurring in an epidermal cyst–report of 3 cases. J Dermatol 1992; 19(2): 119–121.

Parkash S, Ramakrishnan K, Ananthakrishnan N et al. Amoebic ulcer of the penis. Postgrad Med J 1982; 58: 375–377.

Parker SW, Stewart AJ, Wren MN et al. Circumcision and sexually transmissible disease. Med J Austral 1983; 2(6): 288–290.

Parks AG, Porter NH, Hardcastle J. The syndrome of descending perineum. Proc Roy Soc Med 1966; 59: 477–482.

von Parra CA. Solitares neurinom der glans penis. Dermatologica 1968; 137: 150–155.

Parry EL, Foshee WS, Hall W et al. Diaper dermatophytosis. Am J Dis Child 1982; 136: 273–274.

Parsad D, Saini R. Oral stanozolol in lichen sclerosus et atrophicus. J Am Acad Dermatol 1998; 38(2 Pt 1): 278–279.

Parsons RW. A case of keloid of the penis. Plast Reconstr Surg 1966; 37: 431–432.

Pasieczny TAH. The treatment of balanitis xerotica obliterans with testosterone propionate ointment. Acta Dermato–Venereologica 1977; 57: 275–277.

Patel B, Hashmat A, Reddy V et al. Spindle cell carcinoma of the penis. Urology 1982; 19(1): 93–95.

Patrizi A, Costa AM, Fiorillo L et al. Perianal streptococcal dermatitis associated with guttae psoriasis and/or balanoposthitis: A study of five cases. Pediatr Dermatol 1994; 11(2): 168–171.

Patterson JW, Kas GF, Graham JH et al. Bowenoid papulosis. Cancer 1986; 57: 823–836.

Paul AB, Johnston CAB, Nawroz I. Masson's tumour of the penis. Br J Urol 1994; 74(2): 261–262.

Pautrier LM. In: Les lichénifications. Nouvelle Pratique Dermatologique, vol 7 Darier J, ed. Paris: Masson. 1936; 497.

Pegum JS, Wright JT. Epidermolysis bullosa acquisita and Crohn's disease. Proc Roy Soc Med 1973; 66: 234–235.

Pehoushek J, Smith KJ. Imiquimod and 5% fluorouracil therapy for anal and perianal squamous cell carcinoma in situ in an HIV–1 positive man. Arch Dermatol 2001; 137:14–.

Peleg D, Steiner A. The Gomco circumcision: common problems and solutions. Am Fam Phys 1998; 58(4): 891–898.

Pelisse M. Lichen sclerosus. Ann Dermatol Venereol 1987; 114(3): 411–419. French.

Pellice i Vilalta C, Casalots i Casado J, Cosme i Jiménez MA. Zoon's balanoposthitis. A preliminary note Arch Esp Urol. Jan 1999; 52(1): 69–72. Spanish.

Peltola H. Images in clinical medicine. Bacterial perianal dermatitis. N Engl Med J 2000; 342(25): 1877.

Penfield W, Rasmussen T. The cerebral cortex of man. Macmillan, New York; 1950.

Penneys NS, ed. Skin Manifestations of AIDS London: Martin Dunitz; 1990.

Perceau G, Derancourt C, Clavel C, et al. Lichen sclerosus is frequently present in penile squamous cell carcinomas but is not always associated with oncogenic human papillomavirus. Br J Dermatol. 2003; 148(5): 934–8.

Perez VG, Eres Saez FJ, Ramada Benlloch FJ et al. Association of giant condyloma acuminatum of the penis with intraurethral simple condylomata. Apropos of a case. Arch Espan Urol 1991; 44(9): 1103–1105.

Perkins W, Lamont, MacKie RM. Cutaneous malignancy in males treated with photochemotherapy. Lancet 1990; 336(8725): 1248.

Perriard J, Saurat JH, Harms M. An overlap of Cowden's disease and Bannayan–Riley–Ruvalcaba syndrome in the same family. J Am Acad Dermatol 2000; 42(2 Pt 2): 348–350.

Persky L, deKernion J. Carcinoma of the penis. Cancer J Clinic 1986; 36(5): 258–273.

Peters MS, Perry HO. Bowenoid papules of the penis. J Urol 1981; 126: 482–484.

Petersen CS, Zachariae C. Acute balanoposthitis caused by infestation with Cordylobia anthropophaga. Acta Derm Venereol 1999; 79(2): 170.

Petrelli NJ, Cebollero JA, Rodriguez–Bigas M et al. Photodynamic therapy in the management of neoplasms of the perianal skin. Arch Dermatol 1992; 127(12): 1436–1438.

Petros JG, Rimm EB, Robillard RJ. Clinical presentation of chronic anal fissures. Am Surg 1993; 59: 666–668.

Peutherer JF, Smith JW, Robertson DHH. Necrotizing balanitis due to generalized primary infection with herpes simplex virus type 2. Br J Vener Dis 1979; 55: 48–51.

Philip I, Nicholas JL. Congenital giant prepucial sac: case reports. J Pediatr Surg 1999; 34(3): 507–508.

Philippson L. Ueber das sarcoma idiopathicum cutis Kaposi. Ein beitrag zur sarcomlehre. Arch Pathol Anat 1902; 167: 58–81.

Phillips SS, Baird DB, Joshi VV et al. Crohn's disease of the prepuce in a 12–year–old boy: a case report and review of the literature. Pediatr Pathol Lab Med May 1997; 17(3): 497–502.

Picconi MA, Eijan AM, Distefano AL et al. Human papillomavirus (HPV) DNA in penile carcinomas in Argentina: analysis of primary tumors and lymph nodes. J Med Virol 2000; 61(1): 65–69.

Pickering MC, Haskard DO. Behçet's syndrome. J Roy Coll Phys Lond 2000; 34: 169–177.

Pielop J, Rosen T. Penile dermatophytosis. J Am Acad Derm 2001; 44(5): 864–867.

Piepkorn M, Kumasaka B, Krieger et al. Development of human papillomavirus–associated Buschke–Lowenstein penile carcinoma during cyclosporine therapy for generalised pustular psoriasis. J Am Acad Dermatol 1993; 29(2 Pt. 2): 321–325.

Piette W. In: Dermatology. Bolognia J, Jorizzo JL, Rapini RP. Mosbypages. 2003; 367–375.

Pillai KG, Singh G, Sharma BM. Trichorhyton rubrum. Infection of the penis. Dermatologica 1975; 100: 252–254.

Pinol Aguade J. XlVe congres de l'association des dermatologistes et syphiligraphers de langue francaise, Geneve, 1973 II Vascularites.Geneva: Medecine et Hygiene. 1974; 112.

Pinto AP, Lin Mc, Sheets EE et al. Allelic imbalance in lichen sclerosis, hyperplasia and intraepithelial neoplasia of the vulva. Gynecol Oncol 2000; 77: 171–176.

Piot P, Duncan M, van Dyck E et al. Ulcerative balanoposthitis associated with non syphilitic spirochaetal infection. Genitourin Med 1986; 62, 11–16.

Pirone E, Infantin A, Masin A et al. Can proctological procedures resolve perianal pruritus and mycosis? Int J Colorect Dis 1992; 7(1): 18–20.

Poblet E, Alfaro L, Fernander–Segoviano P et al. Human papillomavirus associated penile squamous cell carcinoma in HIV positive patients. Am J Surg Pathol 1999; 23: 1119–1123.

Pohlman RB. Photo quiz. A lesion that should raise suspicion. Am Fam Physician 2000; 62(9): 2095–2096.

Pointon RCS. Carcinoma of the penis. External beam therapy. Proc Roy Soc Med 1975; 68: 779–781.

Polakova K. Atypically localised scrofuloderma. Bratislavske Lekarske Listy 1993; 94(10): 536–538.

Poland RL. The question of routine neonatal circumcision. N Engl J Med 1990; 18(332): 1312–1315.

Ponce de Leon J, Algaba F, Salvador J. Cutaneous horn of the glans penis. Br J Urol 1994; 74(2): 257–258.

Pond HS. Priapism as the presenting complaint of myelogenous leukemia. South Med J 1969; 62: 465–467.

Ponsky LE, Ross JH, Knipper N et al. Penile adhesions after neonatal circumcision. J Urol 2000; 164(2): 495–496.

Porras–Luque JI, Valks R, Casal EC et al. Generalized exanthem with palmoplantar involvement and genital ulcerations. Acute primary HIV infection. Arch Dermatol 1998; 134(10): 1279, 1282.

Porter WM, Grabczynska S, Francis N et al. The perils and pitfalls of penile injections. Br J Dermatol 1999; 141(4): 736–738.

Porter W, Bunker CB. Treatment of pearly penile papules with cryotherapy. Br J Dermatol 2000; 142: 847–848.

Porter WM, Dinneen M, Hawkins DA et al. Disease spectrum in penile intaepithelial neoplasia. Br J Dermatol 2000; 143 (Suppl 57): 49–50.

Porter WM, Dinneen M, Bunker C. Chronic penile lymphoedema. Arch Dermatol 2001; 137: 1108–1110.

Porter WM, Bewley A, Dinneen M et al. Nodular lichen simplex of the scrotum treated by surgical excision. Br J Dermatol 2001; 144: 915–916.

Porter WM, Dinneen M, Hawkins DA et al. Erosive penile lichen planus responding to circumcision. JEADV 2001; 15: 266–268.

Porter WM, Du P. Menage H, Philip G et al. Porokeratosis of the penis. Br J Dermatol 2001; 144: 643–644.

Porter WM, Bunker CB. The dysfunctional foreskin. Int J STD AIDS. 2001; 12(4): 216–20.

Porter WM, Francis N, Hawkins D et al. Penile intraepithelial neoplasia: clinical spectrum and treatment of 35 cases. Br J Dermatol 2002; in press.

Post B, Janner M. Lichen sclerosus et atrophicus penis. Z Hautkr 1975; 50(16): 675–681. German.

Potts P. Cancer Scroti. Chirurgical Works 1779; 3: 225–229.

Pouget F, Chemaly P, Wechsler J et al. Hyperkeratose epidermolytique genitale masculine. Annales de Dermatologie et de Venereologie 1993; 120: 850–851.

Pounder DJ. Ritual mutilation. Subincision of the penis among Australian Aborigines. Am J Forensic Med Pathol. 1983; 4(3): 227–9.

Powell FC, Venencie PY, Winkelmann RK. Metastatic prostate carcinoma manifesting as penile nodules. Arch Dermatol. 1984; 120: 1604–1606.

Powell J, Robson A, Cranston D et al. High incidence of lichen sclerosus in patients with squamous cell carcinoma of the penis. Br J Dermatol 2001; 145: 85–89.

Powell II, Wojnarowska F. Lichen sclerosus. Lancet 1999; 353(9166): 1777–1783.

Pow–Sang MR, Orihuela E. Leiomyosarcoma of the penis. J Urol 1994; 151(6): 1643–1645.

Preminger B, Gerard PS, Lutwick L et al. Histoplasmosis of the penis. J Urol 1993; 149: 848–850.

Pretorius ES, Siegelman ES, Ramchandani P et al. Imaging of the penis. Radiographics 2001; 21:S283–98, discussion S. 298–9.

Pripwie SR, Krippen S, Dass et al. Bowen carcinoma in renal transplant recipient. Urology 1979; 13: 290–299.

Pride HB, Miller OF, Tyler WB. Penile squamous cell carcinoma arising from balanitis xerotica obliterans. J Am Acad Dermatol 1993; 29: 469–473.

Priesley JB. Physical signs of sexual abuse in children. J Roy Coll Phys 1997; 31: 580–581.

Prose NS. Mucocutaneous disease in pediatric human immunodeficiency virus infection. Pediatr Clin North Am. 1991; 38(4): 977–90.

Prošvic P, Moravek P, Stefan H et al. Uncommon finding of penile carcinoma: case record. Rozhl Chir 1997; 76: 454–7. Czech.

Provet JA, Rakham J, Mennen J et al. Primary amyloidosis of urethra. Urology 1989; 34: 106–108.

Pueblitz S, Mora–Tiscareno A, Meneses–Garcia AA et al. Epithelioid sarcoma of penis. Urology 1986; 28(3): 246–249.

Puissant A, Pringuet R, Noory JY et al. Condylome acumine geant (syndrome de Buschke–Lowenstein). Action de la bleomycine. Bulletin de la Societe Francaise Dermatologie et Syphiligraphie 1975; 79: 9–12.

Putkonen T, Wangel GA. Renal hyperparathyroidism with metastatic calcification of the skin. Dermatologica 1959; 118: 127–144.

Puy–Montburn T, Denis J, Ganansia R et al. Anorectal lesions in human immunodeficiency virus–infected patients. Int J Colorect Dis 1992; 7(1): 26–30.

Q

Qazi NA, Morlese JF, Walsh JC et al. Severe cutaneous ulceration secondary to cytomegalovirus inclusion disease during successful immune reconstitution with HAART Aids Read. 2002; 12: 452–457.

Quante M, Patel NK, Hill S et al. Epithelioid hemangioendothelioma presenting in the skin: a clinicopathologic study of eight cases. Am J Dermatopathol 1998; 20(6): 541–546.

Queyrat M. Erythroplasie du gland. Bulletin de la Societie de Dermatologie et de Syphiligraphie 1911; 22(1): 378–382.

Quiles DR, Mas IB, Martinez AZ et al. Gonocaccal infection of the penile median raphe. Int J Dermatol 1987; 26(4): 242–243.

Quintela R, Delmas V, Cannistra C et al. Plastic surgery of the penis after circumcision. Prog Urol 2000; 10(3): 476–478. French.

R

Raaschou–Nielsen W, Revmann F. Familial benign chronic pemphigus Acta Dernato– Venerelogica (Stockh) 1959; 39: 280–291.

Rabinowitz R, Lewin EB. Gangrene of the genitalia in children with pseudomonas sepsis. J Urol 1980; 124: 431–432.

Radaelli F, Volpe AD, Colombi M et al. Acute gangrene of the scrotum and penis in four hematologic patients. Cancer 1987; 60: 1462–1464.

Rademaker M, Forsyth A. Allergic reactions to rubber condoms. Genitourin Med 1989; 65: 194–195.

Ramam M, Khaitan BK, Singh MK et al. Frictional sweat dermatitis. Contact Dermatitis 1998: 4938.

Ramlogan D, Coulsom IH, McGeorge A. Cicatricial pemphigoid: a diagnostic problem for the urologist. J Roy Coll Surg Edin 2000; 45(1): 62–3.

Ramm Z, Findler G, Spiegelman R et al. Intermittent priapism in spinal canal stenosis. Spine 1987; 12: 377–378.

Randazzo RF, Hulette CM, Gottlieb MS et al. Cytomegaloviral epididymitis in a patient with the acquired immune deficiency syndrome. J Urol 1986; 136: 1095–1097.

Ranki A, Lassus J, Niemi K. Relation of p53 tumor suppressor protein expression to human papilloavirus (HPV) DNA and to cellular atypia in male genital warts and in premalignant lesions. Acta Derm Venereol (Stockh) 1995; 75: 180–186.

Rankin GB. National cooperative Crohn's disease study. Gastroenterol 1979; 77: 814.

Rao RN, Spurlock BO, Witherington R. Angiolymphoid hyperplasia with eosinophilia: Report of a case with penile lesions. Cancer 1981; 47: 944–949.

Rashid AMH, Menai Williams R, Parry D et al. Actinomycosis associated with pilonidal sinus of the penis. J Urol 1992; 148: 405–406.

Ravindran M. Cauda equina compression presenting as spontaneous priapism. J Neurol Neurosurg Psychiatry. 1979; 42(3): 280–2.

Ray B, Whitmore WF Jr. Experience with carcinoma of the scrotum. J Urol 1977; 117: 741–745.

Ray TL, Levine JB, Weiss W et al. Epidermolysis bullosa acquisita and inflammatory bowel disease. J Am Acad Dermatol 1982; 6: 242–252.

Read SI, Abell E. Pseudoepitheliomatous, keratotic, and micaceous balanitis. Arch Dermatol 1981; 117: 435–437.

Recondo G, Sella A, Ro JY et al. Perianal ulcer in disseminated histoplasmosis. South Med J 1991; 84(7): 931–932.

Reddy CRRM, Devendranath V, Pratap S. Carcinoma of the penis: role of phimosis. Urology 1984; 24(1): 85–88.

Redondo P, Idoate M, Espana A et al. Pruritus ani in an elderly man. Extramammary Paget's disease. Archiv Dermatol 1995; 131(8): 952–953.

Rehder PA, Eliezer ET, Lane AT. Perianal cellulitis. Arch Dermatol 1988; 124: 702–704.

Reinberg Y, Chelimsky G, Gonzalez R. Urethral atresia and the prune belly syndrome. Br J Urol 1993; 72(1): 112–114.

Reiter H. Ueber eine bisher unerkannte. Dtsch Med Woschensch 1916; 42: 1535–1536.

Remond B, Dompmartin A, de Pontville M et al. Malakoplakie cutanee chez un transplante cardiaque, Annales de Dermatologie et de Venereologie. 1993; 120(11): 805–808.

Revuz J, Clerici T. Penile melanosis. J Am Acad Dermatol 1989; 20(4): 567–570.

Reynolds VH, Madden J, Franlin ID et al. Preservation of anal function after total excision of the anal mucosa for Bowen's disease. Ann Surg 1984; 199: 563–568.

Rhodes AR, Harrist TJ, Momtaz TK. The PUVA–induced pigmented macule: a lentiginous proliferation of large, sometimes cytologically atypical, melanocytes. J Am Acad Dermatol 1983; 9(1): 47–58.

Rhodes AR, Silverman RA, Harrist TJ et al. Mucocutaneous lentigines, cardiomucocutaneous myxomas, and multiple blue nevi: The "LAMB" syndrome. J Am Acad Dermatol 1984; 10: 72–82.

Richens J. National guideline for the management of donovanosis (granuloma inguinale). Clinical Effectiveness Group (Association of Genitourinary Medicine and the Medical Society for the Study of Venereal Diseases. Sexually Transmitted Infections should be added to the Fp & LP 1999. 1999; 75(Suppl 1): 38–39.

Rickwood AM. Medical indications for circumcision. Br J Urol Int 1999; 83(Suppl. 1): 45–51.

Rickwood AM, Walker J. Is phimosis overdiagnosed in boys and are too many circumcisions performed in consequence? Ann R Coll Surg Engl 1989; 71(5): 275–277.

Rickwood AM, Hemalatha V, Batcup G et al. Phimosis in boys. Br J Urol 1980; 52(2): 147–150.

Riddell L, Edwards A, Sherrard J. Clinical features of lichen sclerosus in men attending a department of genitourinary medicine. Sex Trans Infect 76(4. 2000; 311–313.

Ridley CM. Lichen sclerosus et atrophicus. Br Med J 1987; 295: 1295–1296.

Ridley CM. Lichen sclerosus et atrophicus. Arch Dermatol 1987; 123: 457–460.

Ridley CM. Perianal streptococcal dermatitis: Diagnostic considerations. Pediatr Dermatol 1991; 8(1): 91.

Ridley CM. Lichen sclerosus. Dermatol Clin 1992; 10(2): 309–318.

Ridley CM. Genital lichen sclerosus (lichen sclerosus et atrophicus) in childhood and adolescence. J Roy Soc Med 1993; 86(2): 69–75.

Ridley CM, Neill SM. Circumcision. Br Med J 1993; 306(6877): 583–584.

Riedl CR, Plas E, Engelhardt P et al. Iontophoresis for treatment of Peyronie's disease. J Urol 2000; 163(1): 95–99.

Ring J et al. LAV/HTLV. III infection and atopy; serum IgE and specific IgE antibodies to environmental allergens. Acta Derm Venereol (Stockh) 1986; 66: 530–532.

Risse L, Négrier P, Dang PM et al. Treatment of verrucous carcinoma with recombinant alfa–interferon. Dermatology 1995; 190(2): 142–144.

Roberts JA. Does circumcision prevent urinary tract infection. J Urol 1986; 135: 991–992.

Robertson DHH, McMillan A, Young H. Homosexual transmission of amoebiasis. J Roy Soc Med 1982; 75: 564.

Robey EL, Schellhammer PF. Four cases of metastases to the penis and a review of the literature. J Urol 1984; 132: 992–994.

Robinson SS, Tasker S. Angiomas of the scrotum (angiokeratoma, Fordyce). Arch Dermatol Syphilol 1946; 54: 667–674.

Rock B, Shah KV, Farmer EV. A morphologic, pathologic, and virologic study of anogenital warts in men. Arch Dermatol 1992; 128: 495–500.

Rogozinski TT, Janniger CK. Bowenoid papulosis. Am Fam Phys 1988; 38: 161–164.

Rogus BJ. Squamous cell carcinoma in a young circumcised man. J Urol 1987; 138: 861–862.

Rohde H. Routine anal cleansing, so–called hemorrhoids, and perianal dermatitis: cause and effect? Dis Col Rect 2000; 43(4): 561–563.

Romeu J, Roig J, Bada JL, et al. Adult human toxocariasis acquired by eating raw snails. J Infect Dis. 1991; 164(2): 438.

Romero LI, Pincus SH. In situ localization of Interleukin–6 in normal skin and atrophic cutaneous disease. Int Arch Allergy Immunol 1992; 99(1): 44–49.

Ronan SG, Bolano J, Manaligod JR. Verruciform xanthoma of the penis. Urology 1984; 23(6): 600–603.

Roos TC, Alam M, Roos S et al. Pharmacotherapy of ectoparasitic infections. Drugs 2001; 61(8): 1067–1088.

Rosen T, Brown TJ. Genital ulcers. Evaluation and treatment. Dermatol Clin 1998; 16(4): 673–685.

Rosen T, Krawczynska AM, McBride ME et al. Naftifine treatment of trichomycosis pubis. Int J Dermatol 1991; 30(9): 667–669.

Rosenbaum EH, Thompson HE, Glassberg AB. Priapism and multiple myeloma. Urology 1978; 12(2): 201–202.

Rosenbaum SN. Circumcision–syphilis. J Cutan Genito–Urin Dis 1899; 7: 317.

Rosenberg PH, Shuck JM, Tempest BD et al. Diagnosis and therapy of necrotizing soft tissue infections of the perineum. Ann Surg 1978; 187: 430–434.

Rosin RD. Paget's disease of the anus. J Roy Soc Med 1991; 84: 112–113.

Rossi R, Urbano F, Tortoli E et al. Primary tuberculosis of the penis. JEADV 1999; 12: 174–176.

Roszkiewicz A, Roszkiewicz J, Lange M et al. Kaposi's sarcoma following long–term immunosuppressive therapy: clinical, histologic, and ultrastructural study. Cutis. Mar;61(3):137–141; quiz. 1998; 152.

Roth AD, Berney CR, Rohner S et al. Intra–arterial chemotherapy in locally advanced or recurrent carcinomas of the penis and anal canal an active treatment modality with curative potential. Br J Cancer. 2000; 83(12): 1637–1642.

Rousselot M, Privat Y, Bonerandi JJ. Granulome eosinophile du visage. Bulletin de la Societe Francaise Dermatologie et Syphiligrahpie 1975; 82: 44–45.

Rowell NR, Goodfield MJD. The 'Connective Tissue Diseases', Textbook of Dermatology. Rook/Wilkinson/Ebling. Champion RH, ed. 1998.

Rubin MA, Kleter, B, Zhou M et al. Detection and typing oh human papillomavirus DNA in penile carcinoma. Evidence for multiple independent pathways of penile carcinogenesis. Am J Pathol 2001; 159; 1211–1217.

Rubinstein I, Baum GL, Hiss Y. Sarcoidosis of the penis: report of a case. J Urol 1986; 135: 1016–1017.

Rubio FA, Robayna G, Herranz P et al. Necrotizing vasculitis of the glans penis. Br J Dermatol 1999; 140(4): 756–757.

Russell AI, Lawson WA, Haskard DO. Potential new therapeutic options in Behçet's syndrome. BioDrugs 2001; 15(1): 25–35.

Rustin MHA, Gilkes JJH, Robinson TWE. Pyoderma gangrenosum associated with Behçet's disease: treatment with thalidomide. J Am Acad Dermatol 1990; 23(5): 941–944.

Ruszczak Z, Stadler R, Schwartz RA. Case report. Kaposi's sarcoma limited to penis treated with cobalt–60 radiotherapy. J Med 1996; 27: 211–220.

Ruth EB. The os priapi: A study in bone development. Anat Rec 1934; 60: 231–249.

Rutkow IM. A remarkable injury of the perinaeum, scrotum, and penis. Arch Surg 1997; 132(11): 1242.

Ryan AK, Bartlett K, Clayton P et al. Smith–Lemli–Opitz syndrome: a variable clinical and biochemical phenotype. J Med Genetics 1998; 35(7): 558–565.

S

Sachs W, Sachs PM. Erythroplasia of Queyrat. Arch Dermatol Syphilol 1948; 58: 184–190.

Sadikoglu B, Kuran I, Özcan H et al. Cutaneous lymphatic malformation of the penis and scrotum. J Urol 1999; 162(4): 1445–1446.

Saenz De San Pedro Morera B, Enriquez JQ, Lopez JF. Fixed drug eruptions due to betalactams and other chemically unrelated antibiotics. Contact Dermatitis 1999; 40(4): 220–221.

Sagar SM, Retsas S. Metastasis of the penis from malignant melanoma: Case report and review of the literature. Clin Oncol 1992; 4(2): 130–131.

Sagerman PM, Kadish AS, Niedt GW. Condyloma accuminatum with superficial spirochetosis simulating condyloma latum. Am J Dermatopathol 1993; 15(2): 176–179.

Sagi A, Rosenberg L, Rosenberg L et al. Squamous cell carcinoma arising in a pilonidal sinus: A case report and review of the literature. J Dermatol Surg Oncol 1984; 10: 210–212.

Salvatore P, Pokia I, Vocatura A. The presence of HPV types 6/11, 16/18, 31/33/51 in Bowenoid papulosis demonstrated by DNA in situ hybridization. Int J STD AIDS 2000; 11(12): 823–824.

Samenius B. Primary syphilis of anorectal region. Proc Roy Soc Med 1966; 49: 629–631.

Sami N, Ahmed AR. Penile pemphigus. Arch Dermatol 2001; 137(6): 756–758.

Samsoen M, Deschler JM, Servelle M et al. Le lymphoedeme penoscrotal two observations. Annales de Dermatologie et de Venereologie 1981; 108: 541–546.

Sanchez MH, Sanchez SR, del Cerro Heredero M et al. Pyoderma gangrenosum of penile skin. Int J Dermatol 1997; 36(8): 638–639.

Sanchez–Perez J, Cordoba S, Cortizas CF et al. Allergic contact balanitis due to tetracaine (amethocaine) hydrochloride. Contact Dermatitis 1998; 39(5): 268.

Sand PK, Bowen LW, Blischke SO et al. Evaluation of male consorts of women with genital human papilloma virus infection. Obstetr Gynecol 1986; 68: 679–681.

Sand Petersen C, Menne T. Anogenital warts in consecutive male heterosexual patients referred to a CO_2–laser clinic in Copenhagen. Acta Dermato–Venereologie 1992; 73(6): 465–466.

Sand Petersen C, Bjerring P, Larsen J et al. Systemic interferon alpha–2b increases the cure rate in laser treated patients with multiple persistent genital warts: a placebo–controlled study. Genitourin Med 1991; 67(2): 99–102.

Sanders TJ, Venable DD, Sanusi ID. Primary malignant melanoma of the urethra in a black man: a case report. J Urol 1986; 135: 1012–1014.

Sanusi ID, Fielding RE, McClure D. Petroleum jelly lipogranuloma of the penis treated with excision and native skin coverage. Urology 2000; 56(2): 331.

Sanusi ID, Gonzalez E, Venable DD. Pyoderma gangrenosum of penile and scrotal skin. J Urol 1982; 127: 547–549.

Sapan N. Food induced pruritus ani. A variation of allergic target organ? Eur J Pediatr 1993; 152(8): 701–702.

Sarihan H. Idiopathic scrotal necrosis. Br J Urol 1994; 74(2): 259.

Sarkany J. A method of studying the microtopography of the skin. Br J Dermatol 1962; 74: 254–59.

Sarma DP, Weilbaecher TG. Scrotal calcinosis; calcification of epidermal cysts. J Surg Oncol 1984; 27: 76–79.

Sasson I, Haley N, Hoffmann D et al. Cigarette smoking and neoplasia of the uterine cervix: smoke constituents in cervical mucus. N Engl J Med 1985; 312: 315–316.

Sathaye UV, Goswami AK, Sharma SK. Skin Bridge–a complication of pediatric circumcision. Br J Urol 1990; 66(2): 214.

Sawada Y, Kanekasu K, Toribatake Y et al. Spinal metastasis of sweat gland carcinoma. Spine 1991; 16(11): 1344–1346.

Sawh RN, Borkowski J, Broaddus R. Metastatic renal cell carcinoma presenting as a hemorrhoid. Arch Pathol Lab Med 2002; 126(7): 856–858.

Schapiro L, Platt N, Torres–Rodriguez VM. Idiopathic calcinosis of the scrotum. Arch Dermatol 1970; 102: 199.

Schempp C, Bocklage H, Lange R et al. Further evidence for Borrelia burgdorferi infection in morphea and lichen sclerosus et atrophicus confirmed by DNA amplification. J Invest Dermatol 1993; 100: 717–720.

Schiavino D, Sasso F, Nucera E et al. Immunologic findings in Peyronie's disease: a controlled study. Urology 1997; 50(5): 764–768.

Schlappner OLA, Rosenblum GA, Rowden G et al. Concomitant erythrasma and dermatophytosis of the groin. Br J Dermatol 1979; 100: 147–151.

Schmidt ME, Yalisove BL, Parenti DM et al. Rapidly progressive penile ulcer: An unusual manifestation of Karposi's sarcoma. J Am Acad Dermatol 1992; 27(2 Pt.1): 267–268.

Schmitt EC, Pigatto PD, Boneschi V et al. Erosiver lichen planus der glans penis. Der Hautarzt 1993; 44(1): 43–45.

Schneider A, Kirchmayr R, De Villers E–M et al. Subclinical human papilloma virus infection in male partners of female carriers. J Urol 1988; 140: 1431–1434.

Schnitzler L, Halligon J, Schubert B et al. Quatre cas de 'tuberculose cutanée'. Role possible des mycobacteries atypiques. Bulletin de la Societe Francaise Dermatologie Syphiligraphie 1972; 79: 571–577.

Schnitzler L, Sayag J, Sayag J et al. Épithélioma spino–cellulaire aigu de la verge et lichen scléro–atrophique. Annales de Dermatologie et de Venereologie 1987; 114: 979–981.

Schoen EJ. The status of circumcision of newborns. N Engl J Med 1990; 322(18): 1308–1312.

Schoen EJ, Anderson G, Bohon C et al. (AAP. Task Force on Circumcision) Report of the Task Force on Circumcision. Pediatrics 1989; 84: 388.

Schoen EJ, Oehrli M, Colby CJ et al. The highly protective effect of newborn circumcision against invasive penile cancer. Pediatrics 2000; 105(3): E 36.

Schoeneich G, Perabo FG, Muller SC. Squamous cell carcinoma of the penis. Andrologia 1999; 31(suppl 1): 17–20.

Schrek R, Lenowitz H. Etiological factors in carcinoma of the penis. Cancer Res 1947; 7: 180–187.

Schubach A, Cuzzi–Maya T, Goncalves–Costa SC et al. Leishmaniasis of glans penis. J Eur Acad Dermatol Venereol 1998; 10(3): 226–228.

Schultheiss D, Truss MC, Stief CG et al. Uncircumcision: a historical review of preputial restoration. Plast Reconstr Surg 1998; 101(7): 1990–1998.

Bibliography

Schultz ES, Diepgen TL, von den Driesch P et al. Systemic corticosteriods are important in the treatment of Fournier's gangrene: a case report. J Dermatol 1995; 133: 633–635.

Schurmann D, Bergmann F, Temmesfeld–Wollbruck B et al. Topical cidofovir is effective in treating extensive penile condylomata acuminata. AIDS 2000; 14(8): 1075–1076.

Schwartz RA. Buschke–Loewenstein tumor. Verrucous carcinoma of the penis. J Am Acad Dermatol 1993; 23(4 Pt.1): 723–727.

Schwartz RA, Janniger CK. Bowenoid papulosis. J Am Acad Dermatol 1991; 24(2 Pt.1): 261–263.

Schwartz RA, Nychay SG, Lyons MD et al. Buschke–Lowenstein tumour. Verrucous carcinoma of the anogenitalia. Cutis 1991; 47: 263.

Schwartz RA, Cohen JB, Watson RA et al. Penile Kaposi's sarcoma preceded by chronic penile lymphoedema. Br J Dermatol 2000; 142: 153–156.

Schweigel JF, Shim SS. A comparison of the treatment of gas gangrene with and without hyperbaric oxygen. Surg Gynaecol Obstetr 1973; 136: 969–970.

Scolaro MJ, Gunnill LB, Pope LE, et al. The antiviral drug docosanol as a treatment for Kaposi's sarcoma lesions in HIV type 1-infected patients: a pilot clinical study. AIDS Res Hum Retroviruses. 2001; 17(1): 35–43.

Scott GR. European guidelines for the management of scabies. Int J STD AIDS 2001; 12(Suppl. 3): 58–61.

Seemayer TA, Dionne PG, Tabah EJ. Epithelioid sarcoma. Can J Surg 1974; 17: 37–42.

Seftel AD, Sadick NS, Waldbaum RS. Kaposi's sarcoma of the penis in a patient with the acquired immune deficiency syndrome. J Urol 1986; 136: 673–675.

Sehgal VH, Gangwani OP. Genital fixed drug eruptions. Genitourin Med 1986; 62: 56–58.

Seidman B, Schiff H, Bruckner H et al. Mycosis fungiodes causing urethral obstruction. Urology 1982; 20(2): 170–171.

Selli C, Scott CA, De A et al. Squamous cell carcinoma arising at the base of the penis in a burn scar(1). Urology 1999; 54(5): 923.

Senoh K, Miyazaki T, Kikuchi I et al. Angiomatous lesions of the glans penis. Urology 1981; 17(2): 194–196.

Serota AI, Weil M, Williams RA. Anal doacogenic carcinoma. Arch Surg 1981; 116: 456–459.

Serrano Ortega S, Sanchez Hurtado G, Dulanto Campos MC et al. Avulsion complete de piel de pene. Actas Dermo–Sifilographicas 1980; 71: 381–382.

Seseke F, Kugler A, Hermanns M et al. Langerhans–cell histiocytosis of the penis. Urologe A 1999; 38(1): 42–5. German.

Severo LC, Kauer CL, Oliveira F et al. Paracoccidioidomycosis of the male genital tract. Report of eleven cases and a review of Brazilian literature. Revista do Instituto de Medicina Tropical de Sao Paulo 2000; 42(1): 37–40.

Shafer WG. Verruciform xanthoma. Oral Surg 31. 1971; 784–789.

Shah SS, Varea EG, Farsaii A et al. Giant epidermoid cyst of the penis. Urology 1979; 14(4): 389–391.

Shankar KR, Rickwood AM. The incidence of phimosis in boys. Br J Urol Int 1999; 84(1): 101–102.

Shapiro L, Platt N, Torres–Rodriguez VM. Idiopathic calcinosis of the scrotum. Arch Dermatol 1970; 102: 199–204.

Shapiro PE. "Cello scrotum" questioned. J Am Dermatol 1991; 24(4): 665.

Shelley WB, Arthur RP. The neurohistology and neurophysiology of the itch sensation in man. Arch Dermatol 1957; 76: 296–323.

Shelley WB, Crissey JT, Bowen JT. In: Classics in Dermatology, Shelley W B Crissey J T eds. Springfield, Ill., Charles C Thomas; 1953.

Shelley WB, Shelley ED. Scrotal dermatitis caused by 5–fluororacil (Efudex). J Am Acad Dermatol 1988; 19(5 Pt.2): 929–931.

Shelley WB, Shelley ED. Beçhet's syndrome. In: Advanced Dermatologic Diagnosis. Saunders, Philadelphia; 1992; 316–329.

Shelley WB, Shelley ED. Genital lesions–penis. In: Advanced Dermatologic Diagnosis. Saunders, Philadelphia; 1992; 609.

Shelley WB, Shelley ED, Grunenwald MA et al. Long–term antibiotic therapy for balanitis xerotica obliterans. J Am Acad Dermatol 1999; 40(1): 69–72.

Shenot P, Rivas DA, Kalman DD et al. Latex allergy manifested in urological surgery and care of adult spinal cord injured patients. Arch Phys Med Rehabil 1994; 75(11): 1263–1265.

Shenoy MU, Rance CH. Surgical correction of congenital megaprepuce. Pediatr Surg Int 1999; 15(8): 593–594.

Shenoy MU, Srinivasan J, Sully L et al. Buried penis: surgical correction using liposuction and realignment of skin. Br J Urol Int 2000; 86(4): 527–530.

Sherertz EF. Symptomatic dermographism as a cause of genital pruritus. J Am Acad Dermatol 1994; 31(6): 1040–1041.

Shindo Y, Mikoshiba H, Mochizuku M. Two cases of verruciform xanthoma of the scrotum. Japan J Clin Dermatol 1981; 35: 365–369.

Shukla VK, Hughes LE. A case of squamous cell carcinoma complicating hidradenitis suppurativa. Euro J Surg Oncol 1995; 21(1): 106–109.

Shum DT, Guenther L. Intracellular elastin in cutaneous giant cell reaction. J Am Acad Deramtol 1987; 16(3 Pt.1): 617–618.

Siami GA, Siami FS. Intensive tandem cryofiltration apheresis and hemodialysis to treat a patient with severe calciphylaxis, cryoglobulinemia, and end–stage renal disease. ASAIO J 1999; 45(3): 229–233.

Siboulet A, Catalant F, Deubel M. Balanites et 'mycoplasma.' Bulletin de la Societe Francaise Dermatology et Syphilology 1975; 82: 419–422.

Sieber PR, Duggan FE. Sarcoidosis and testicular tumors. Urology 1988; 31(2): 140–141.

Siegal GP, Gaffey TA. Solitary leiomyomas arising from the tunica dartos scroti. J Urol 1976; 116: 69–71.

Sills M, Schwartz A, Weg JG et al. Conjugal histoplasmosis. A consequence of progressive dissemination in the index case after steroid therapy. Ann Intern Med 1973; 79: 221–224.

Silver RI, Docimo SG. Hair coil strangulation of the penis. Urology 1997; 49(5): 773.

Simeon CP, Fonollosa V, Vilardell M et al. Impotence and Peyronie's disease in systemic sclerosis. Clin Exper Rheumatol 1994; 12(4): 464.

Simmons PD, Langlet F, Thin RNT. Cryotherapy versus electrocautery in the treatment of genital warts. Br J Vener Dis 1981; 57: 273–274.

Simon F, Namssenmo A, Klotz F. Ulcerations cutanees perianales en zone tropicale. Proposition d'arbre decisionnel diagnostique et therapeutique. Medecine Tropicale 1993; 53(2): 159–166.

Simonart T, Noël JC, De Dobbeleer G et al. Carcinoma of the glans penis arising 20 years after lichen sclerosus. Dermatology 1998; 196(3): 337–338.

Simonart T, Dargent JL, Hermans P et al. Penile intraepithelial neoplasia overlying Kaposi's sarcoma lesions: role of viral synergy? Am J Dermatopathol 1999; 21(5): 494–497.

Skierlo P, Heise H. Testosteronpropionat–Salbeein Therapieversuch beim Lichen sclerosus et atrophicus. [Testosterone propionate ointment—a therapeutic trial in lichen sclerosus et atrophicus.] Hautarzt 1987; 38: 295–297.

Skiles MS, Covert GK, Fletcher HS. Gas producing clostridial and nonclostridial infections. Surg Gynaecol Obstetr 1978; 147: 65–67.

Slaney G, Muller S, Clay J et al. Crohn's disease involving the penis. Gut 1986; 27: 329–333.

Slater G, Greenstein A, Aufses A. Anal carcinoma in patients with Crohn's disease. Ann Surg 1984; 199: 348–350.

Slauf P, Antos F, Novak J et al. Perianal pyoderma. Rozhledy V Chirurgii 1993; 72(7): 331–333.

Sloan PJM, Goepel J. Lichen sclerosus et atrophicus and perianal carcinoma. Clin Exper Dermatol 1981; 6: 399–402.

Smith BH. Subclinical Peyronie's disease. Am J Clin Pathol 1969; 52: 385–390.

Smith GL, Bunker CB, Dineen MD. Fournier's gangrene. Br J Urol 1998; 81; 347–355.

Smith HR, Mark MM. Basal cell carcinoma of the penis. Br J Dermatol 1999; 140(2): 361–362.

Smith JN, Winship DH. Complications and extraintestinal problems in inflammatory bowel disease. Med Clin N Am 1980; 64: 1161–1171.

Smith KJ, Skelton HG Ad, James WD et al. Concurrent epidermal involvement of cytomegalovirus and herpes simplex virus in two HIV–infected patients. Military Medical Consortium for Applied Retroviral Research (MMCARR). J Am Acad Dermatol 1991; 25: 500–506.

Smith LE, Henrichs D, McCullah RD. Prospective studies on the etiology and treatment of Pruritis Ani. Dis Col. & Rect 1982; 25: 358–363.

Smith PG, Kinlen LJ, White GC et al. Mortality of wives of men dying with cancer of the penis. Br J Cancer 1980; 41: 422–428.

Smith RA, Ross JS, Branfoot AC et al. Panniculitis with pseudomonas septicaemia in AIDS JEADV. 1995; 4: 166–169.

Smith SR. Skin changes in short bowel syndrome. Ann Dermatol Venereol 1977; 113: 657–659.

Snoeck R, Van Laethem Y, De Clercq E et al. Treatment of a bowenoid papulosis of the penis with local applications of cidofovir in a patient with acquired immunodeficiency syndrome. Arch Intern Med 2001; 161: 2382–2384.

Snow SN, Desouky S, Lo JS et al. Failure to detect human papillomavirus DNA in extramammary Paget's disease. Cancer. 1992; 69(1): 249–251.

Snoy FJ, Wagner SA, Woodside JR et al. Management of penile incarceration. Urology 1984; 24(1): 18–20.

Sobera JO, Elewski BE. Fungal diseases. In: Bolognia JL, Jorizzo JL, Rapini RP, eds. Dermatology. London: Mosby; 2003: 1171–98.

Sobrado CW, Mester M, Nadalin W et al. Radiation–induced total regression of a highly recurrent giant perianal condyloma: report of case. Dis Col Rect 2000; 43(2): 257–260.

Sodal G, Ly B, Borchgrevink HH. Thrombosis of the inferior vena cava, disseminated intravascular coagulation and gangrene of the penis. Acta Med Scand 1978; 203: 535–538.

Sola Casas MA, de Delas JS, Bellon PR et al. Syringomas localized to the penis. Clin Exper Dermatol 1993; 18(4): 384–385.

Soler C, Allibert P, Chardonnet Y et al. Detection of human papillomavirus types 6, 11, 16 and 18 in mucosal and cutaneous lesions by the multiplex polymerase chain reaction. J Virol Methods 1991; 35: 143–157.

Soler C, Chardonnet Y, Allibert P et al. Detection of multiple types of human papillomavirus in a giant condyloma from a grafted patient. Analysis by immunohistochemistry, in situ hybridisation, Southern blot and polymerase reaction. Virus Res 1992; 23(3): 193–208.

Somers WJ, Lowe FC. Localized gangrene of the scrotum and penis: A complication of herion injection into the femoral vessels. J Urol 1986; 136: 111–113.

Sønderbo K, Nyfors A. Skin lesions in sadomasochism. Dermatologica 1986; 172: 196–200.

Song DH, Lee KH, Kang WH. Idiopathic calcinosis of the scrotum: histopathologic observations of fifty–one nodules. J Am Acad Dermaol 1988; 19: 1095–1101.

Sonnex C, Dockerty WG. Pearly penile papules: a common cause of concern. Int J STD AIDS 1999; 10(11): 726–727.

Sonnex C, Scholefield JH, Kocjan G et al. Anal human papillomavirus infection in heterosexuals with genital warts: prevalence and relation with sexual behaviour. Br Med J 1991; 303(6812): 1243.

Sonnex C, Scholefield JH, Kocjan G et al. Anal human papillomavirus infections a comparative study of cytology, colposcopy and DNA hybridisation as methods of detection. Genitourin Med 1991; 67: 21–25.

Sonnex TS, Dawber RPR, Ryan TJ et al. Zoon's (plasma–cell) balanitis: treatment by circumcision. Br J Dermatol 1982; 106(5): 585–588.

Soria J–C, Fizazi K, Piron D et al. Squamous cell carcinoma of the penis: multivariate analysis of prognostic factors and natural history in a monocentric study with a conservative policy. Ann Oncol 1997; 8: 1089–1098.

Soria J–C, Théodore C, Gerbaulet A. Carcinome épidermoïde de la verge (Squamous cell carcinoma of the penis). Bull Cancer 1998; 85(9): 773–784.

Southcyrand P, Wong E, MacDonald DM. Zoon's balanitis (balanitis circumscripta plasmacellularis). Br J Dermatol 1981; 105(2): 195–199.

South LM, O'Sullivan JP, Gazet JC. Giant condylomata of Buschke and Lowenstein. Clin Oncol 1977; 3: 107–115.

Sowmini CN, Vijayalakshmi K, Chellamuthiah C et al. Infections of the median raphe of the penis: report of three cases. Br J Vener Dis 1972; 49: 469–474.

Spirnak JP, Resnick Ml, Hampel N et al. Fournier's gangrene: Report of 20 cases. J Urol 1984; 132: 289–291.

Srigley JR, Ayala AG, Ordonez NG et al. Epithelioid hemangioma of the penis. A rare and distinctive vascular lesion. Arch Pathol Lab Med 1985; 109: 51–54.

Srinivas V, Morse MJ, Herr HW et al. Penile cancer: Relation of extent of nodal metastasis and survival. J Urol 1987; 137: 880.

van de Staak WJBM. Non–venereal sclerosing lymphangitis of the penis following herpes progenitalis. Br J Dermatol 1977; 96: 679–680.

Stables GI, Stringer MR, Ash DV. The treatment of erythroplasia of Queyrat by topical aminolaevulinic acid photodynamic therapy. Br J Dermatol 1995; 133(supp.45): 30.

Stables GI, Stringer MR, Robinson DJ et al. Erythroplasia of Queyrat treated by topical aminolaevulinic acid photodynamic therapy. Br J Dermatol 1999; 140(3): 514–517.

Stack RJ, Bickley LK, Coppel IG. Miliary tuberculosis presenting as skin lesions in a patient with acquired immunodeficiency syndrome. J Am Acad Dermatol 1990; 23(5 Pt.2): 1031–1035.

Staley TE, Nieh PT, Ciesielski TE et al. Metastatic basal cell carcinoma of the scrotum. J Urol 1983; 130: 792–794.

Stallmann D, Schmoeckel C. Morbos Hailey–Hailey mit Dissemination und Eczema herpeticatum unter Etretinattherapie. Hautarzat 1988; 39(7): 454–456.

Stamm WE, Handsfield HH, Rompalo AM et al. The asssociation between genital ulcer disease and aquisition of HIV infection in homosexual men. J Am Med Ass 1988; 260(10): 1429–1433.

Stankler L. Striae of the penis. Br J Dermatol 1982; 107(3): 371–372.

Staubitz WJ, Lent MH, Oberkincher OJ. Carcinoma of the penis. Cancer 1955; 8: 371–378.

Stearns MW, Urmacher C, Sternberg SS et al. Cancer of the anal canal. Curr Prob Cancer. 1980; 4: 1–44.

Steele RJ, Eremin O, Krajewski AS, et al. Primary lymphoma of the anal canal presenting as perianal suppuration. Br Med J (Clin Res Ed). 1985; 291(6491): 311.

Stehbens WE, Ludatscher RM. Fine structure of senile angiomas of human skin. Angiology 1968; 19: 581–592.

Steinberg JL, Cibley LJ, Rice PA. Genital warts: diagnosis, treatment, and counselling for the patient. Curr Clin Topics Infect Dis 1993; 13: 99–122.

Steinhardt J, McRoberts JW. Total distal penile necrosis caused by condom catheter. J Am Med Ass 1980; 244: 1238.

Stellon AJ, Wakeling M. Hidradenitis suppurativa associated with use of oral contraceptives. Br Med J 1989; 298: 28–29.

Stern RS, Bagheri S, Nichols K; PUVA Follow Up Study. The persistent risk of genital tumors among men treated with psoralen plus ultraviolet A (PUVA) for psoriasis. J Am Acad Dermatol. 2002; 47(1): 33–9.

Stern RS. Genital tumours among men with psoriasis exposed to psoralens and ultraviolet A radiation (PUVA) and ultraviolet B radiation. N Engl J Med 1990; 322(16): 1093–1097.

Stern RS, Thibodeau LA, Kleinerman RA et al. Risk of cutaneous carcinoma in patients treated with oral methoxalen

265

photochemotherapy for psoriasis. N Engl J Med 1979; 300(15): 809–813.

Stern RS, Laird N, Melski J et al. Cutaneous squamous–cell carcinoma in patients treated with PUVA. N Engl J Med 1984; 310(18): 1156–1161.

Strescobich D, Donadio R, Aguilar OG et al. Fistulas anales de etiologia poco frecuente. Prensa Med Argent 1969; 56: 622–623.

Stewart RC, Beason ES, Hayes CW. Granulomas of the penis from self–injection with oils. Plast Reconst Surg 1979; 64: 108–111.

Stillwell TJ, Zincke H, Gaffey TA et al. Malignant melanoma of the penis. 1988; 140(1): 72–75.

Stirling DI. Thalidomide and its impact in dermatology. Semin Cutan Med Surg 1998; 17: 231–242.

Stirn A. Body piercing: medical consequences and psychological motivations. Lancet. 2003; 361(9364): 1205–15.

Strand A, Andersson S, Zehbe I et al. HPV prevalence in anal warts tested with the MY09/MY11 SHARP Signal system. Acta Dermato–Venereologica 1999; 79(3): 226–229.

Strauss SE, Takiff HE, Seidlin M et al. Suppression of frequently recurring genital herpes. N Engl J Med 1984; 310: 1545–1550.

Strickler HD, Schiffman MH, Shah KV et al. A survey of human papillomavirus 16 antibodies in patients with epithelial cancers. Eur J Cancer Prev 1998; 7(4): 305–313.

Sturm HM. Bowen's disease and 5–fluorouracil. J Am Acad Dermatol 1979; 1: 513–522.

Sturm JT, Christenson CE, Vecker JH et al. Squamous cell carcinoma of the anus arising in a giant condyloma acuminatum. Dis Col Rect 1975; 18: 147–151.

Subramaniam TK. Bone in the penis. J Indian MA 1952; 21: 137.

Sugathan P. Bulleetus. International Journal of Dermatology 1987; 26(1): 51.

Sulzberger ME, Satenstein DL. Erythroplasia of Queyrat. Arch Dermatol 1933; 28: 798–806.

Sumithra S, Jayaraman M, Yesudian P. Desmoplastic trichoepithelioma and multiple epidermal cysts. Int J Dermatol 1993; 32(10): 747–748.

Summerton DJ, McNally J, Denny AJ et al. Congenital megaprepuce: an emerging condition– how to recognize and treat it. Br J Urol Int 2000; 86(4): 519–522.

Sundaravej K, Suchato C. Tancho's nodules. Australas Radiol. 1974; 18(4): 453–4.

Suss R, Al–Ayoubi M, Ruzicka T. Cyclosporine therapy in Behçet's disease. J Am Acad Dermatol 1993; 29(1): 101–102.

Sussman SJ, Schiller RP, Shashikumar VL. Fournier's syndrome. Report of three cases and a review of the literature. Am J Dis Child 1978; 132: 1189–1191.

Sutton RL. A clinical and histopathological study of angiokeratoma of the scrotum. J Am Med Ass 1911; 57: 189–192.

Swinehart JM, Golitz LE. Scrotal calcinosis. Arch Dermatol 1982; 118: 985–988.

Swinyer LJ. Connubial contact dermatitis from perfumes. Contact Derm 1980; 6: 226.

Syed TA, Lundin S. Topical treatment of penile condylomata acuminata with podophyllotoxin 0.3% solution, 0.3% cream and 0.15% cream. Dermatology 1993; 187(1): 30–33.

Szylit JA, Grossman ME, Luyando Y et al. Becker's nevus and an accessory scrotum. J Am Acad of Dermatol 1986; 14(5 Pt.2): 905–907.

T

Tait WF, Sykes PA. Unusual presentation of anorectal carcinoma. Br Med J 1982; 285: 1742.

Takayama H, Pak K, Tomoyoshi T. Electron microscopic study of mineral deposits in idiopathic calcinosis of the scrotum. J Urol 1982; 127: 915–918.

Tanabe H, Kishigawa T, Sayama S et al. A case of giant extramammary Paget's disease of the genital area with squamous cell carcinoma. Dermatology 2001; 202(3): 249–251.

Tanaka M, Nameki H, Saito Y. Generalized familial benign chronic pemphigus. Skin Res 1992; 34(supp.12): 236–237.

Tanaka Y, Sasaki Y, Kobayashi T et al. Granular cell tumor of the corpus cavernosum of the penis. J Urol 1991; 146(6): 1596–1597.

Taniguchi S, Inoue A, Hamada T. Angiokeratoma of Fordyce: a cause of scrotal bleeding. Br J Urol 1994; 73(5): 589–590.

Tanii T, Hamada T, Asai Y et al. Mondor's phlebitis of the penis: a study with factor VIII related antigen. Acta Dermato–Venereologica 1984; 64: 337–340.

Tannebaum MH, Becker SW. Papillae of the corona at the glans penis. J Urol 1965; 93: 391–395.

Taplin D, Meinking TL, Chen JA et al. Comparison of crotamiton 10% cream (Eurax) and permethrin 5% cream (Elimite) for the treatment of scabies in children. Pediatr Dermatol 1990; 7(1): 67–73.

Tappeiner J, Pfleger L. Granuloma gluteale infantum. Hautarzt 1971; 22: 383–388.

Tappero JW, Conant MA, Wolfe SF, et al. Kaposi's sarcoma. Epidemiology, pathogenesis, histology, clinical spectrum, staging criteria and therapy. J Am Acad Dermatol. 1993; 28(3): 371–95.

Tarry WF, Duckett JW, Snyder HMC. Urological complications of sickle cell diease in a pediatric population. J Urol 1987; 138: 592.

Tash JA, Eid JF. Urethrocutaneous fistula due to a retained ring of condom. Urology 2000; 56(3): 508.

Tavadia S, Mortimer E, Munro CS. Genetic epidemiology of Darier's disease: a population study in the west of Scotland. Br J Dermatol 2002; 146(1): 107–109.

Taylor DR Jr, South DA. Bowenoid papulosis: a review. Cutis 1981; 27: 92–98.

Taylor JS, Pradiswan P. Latex allergy: review of 44 cases including outcome and frequent association with allergic hand eczema. Arch Dermatol 1996; 132: 265–271.

Taylor JS, Cassettari J, Wagner W et al. Contact urticaria and anaphylaxis to latex. J Am Acad Dermatol 1989; 21(4 Pt.2): 874–877.

Taylor TV, Engler P, Pullan BR et al. Ablation of neoplasia by direct current. Br J Cancer 1994; 70(2): 342–345.

Taylor–Robinson D, McCormack WM. The genital mycoplasmas II. N Engl J Med 1980; 302: 1063 1067.

Teichman JM, Lilly JD, Schmidt JD. Rectourethral fistula caused by Kaposi's sarcoma. J Urol 1991; 145: 144–145.

Tessler AN, Applebaum SM. The Buschke–Lowenstein tumor. Urology 1982; 20(1): 36–39.

Testori A, Mazzarol G, Viale G et al. Medical decision making for melanoma of the glans penis. J Exp Clin Cancer Res 1999; 18(2): 219–221.

Thami GP, Jaswal R, Kanwar AJ. Fibrous hamartoma of infancy in the scrotum. Pediatr Dermatol 1998; 15(4): 326.

Theuvenet WI, Nolthewus–Puylaert T, Juvaha ZLG et al. Massive deformation of the scrotal wall by idiopathic calcinosis of scrotum. Plast Reconstruct Surg 1984; 74: 539–543.

Thianprasit M, Schuetzenberger R. Prioderm lotion in the treatment of scabies. Southeast Asian J Trop Med Public Health 1984; 15(1): 119–121.

Thomas AJ Jr, Timmons JW, Perlwitter AD. Progressive penile amputation. Tourniquet injury secondary to hair. Urology 1977; 9: 42–44.

Thomas JA, Matanhelia SS, Rees RWM. Recurrent adult idiopathic penile oedema: a new clinical entity? Hospital Update 1993; 667–8.

Thomson JPS, Grace RH. The treatment of perianal and anal condylomata acuminata: a new operative technique. J Roy Soc Med 1978; 71: 180–185.

Thomson KF, Highet AS. Penile ulceration in fatal malignant atrophic papulosis (Degos' disease). Br J Dermatol 2000; 143(6): 1320–1322.

Thune P, Andersson T, Skjorten F. AIDS manifesting as anogenital herpes zoster eruption: demonstration of virus–like particles in lymphocytes. Acta Dermato–Venereologie 1983; 63: 540–543.

Tietjen DN, Malek RS. Laser therapy of squamous cell dysplasia and carcinoma of the penis. Urology 1998; 52(4): 559–565.

Tiwari SM, Hemal AK. Penile Horn. Urologia Internationalis 1992; 49(2): 123–124.

Tolia BM, Castro VL, Mouded IM et al. Bowen's disease of the shaft of the penis. Successful treatment with 5–fluorouracil. Urology 1976; 7: 617–619.

Tomasini C, Aloi F, Pippione M et al. Dermoid cyst of the penis. Dermatology 1997; 194: 188–190.

Tomaszewski JE, Korat OC, LiVolsi VA et al. Paget's disease of the urethral meatus following transitional cell carcinoma of the bladder. J Urol 1986; 135: 368–370.

Tomera KM, Gaffey TA, Goldstein IS et al. Leiomyoma of the scrotum. Urology 1981; 18(4): 388–389.

Tomioka S, Fuse H, Wakisaka M et al. Sclerosing lipogranuloma in the scrotum. Japan J Clin Urol 1987; 41: 911.

Toome BK, Bowers KE, Scott GA. Diagnosis of cutaneous cytomegalovirus infection: a review and report of a case. J Am Dermatol 1991; 24: 857–863.

Toonstra J, van Wichen DF. Immunohistochemical characteristics of plasma cells in Zoon's balanoposthitis and (pre)malignant skin lesions. Dermatologica 1986; 172: 77–81.

Toribio J, Muno MG, Perez–Oliva N et al. Papulosis bowenoide genital. Actas Dermo–Sifilographicas 1981; 72: 545–550.

Trap R, Wiebe B. Granuloma annulare localized to the shaft of the penis. Scand J Urol Nephrol 1993; 27(4): 549–551.

Tremaine RDL, Miller RAW. Lichen sclerosus et atrophicus. Int J Dermatol 1989; 28(1): 10–16.

Tripp BM, Chu F, Halwani F, et al. Necrotizing vasculitis of the penis in systemic lupus erythematosus. J Urol. 1995; 154(2 Pt 1): 528–9.

Tsai TF, Su IJ, Lu YC et al. Cutaneous angiocentric T–cell lymphoma associated with Epstein–Barr virus. J Am Acad Dermatol 1992; 26(1): 31–38.

Tschen JA, McGavran MH, Kettler AH. Pagetoid dyskeratosis: A selective keratinocytic response. J Am Acad Dermatol 1988; 19: 891–894.

Tsujii T, Iwai T, Inoue Y et al. Cutaneous hemangioma of the penis successfully treated with sclerotherapy and ligation. Int J Urol 1998; 5(4): 396–397.

Tsur H, Urson S, Schewach–Millet M. Lymphangioma circumscriptum of the glans penis. Cutis 1981; 28: 642–643.

Tsurusaki T, Maruta N, Iwasaki S et al. Idiopathic bilateral panniculitis of the spermatic cord in an elderly male patient. J Urol 2000; 164: 1657–1658.

Tsutsumi Y, Kawai K, Hori S et al. Ultrastructural visualisation of human papillomavirus DNA in verrucous and precancerous squamous lesions. Acta Pathologica Japonica 1991; 41(10): 757–762.

Tulpule A, Groopman J, Saville MW, et al. Multicenter trial of low-dose paclitaxel in patients with advanced AIDS-related Kaposi sarcoma. Cancer. 2002; 95(1): 147–54.

Tulpule A, Joshi B, DeGuzman N, et al. Interleukin-4 in the treatment of AIDS-related Kaposi's sarcoma. Ann Oncol. 1997; 8(1): 79–83.

Turjanmaa K, Alenius H, Makinen–Kiljunen S et al. Natural rubber latex allergy. Allergy 1996; 51: 593–602.

Turk CO, Schacht M, Ross L. Diagnosis and management of testicular sarcoidosis. J Urol 1986; 135: 380–381.

Turner AG. Pagetoid lesions associated with carcinoma of the bladder. J Urol 1980; 123: 124–126.

Tyring SK, Arany II, Stanley MA et al. Mechanism of action of imiquimod 5% cream in the treatment of anogenital warts. Prim Care Update Ob Gyns 1998; 5: 151–152.

U

Udall DA, Drake DJ, Rosenberg RS. Acute scrotal swelling: a physical sign of primary peritonitis. J Urol 1981; 125: 750–751.

Uemura S, Hutson JM, Woodward AA et al. Balanitis xerotica obliterans with urethral stricture after hypospadias repair. Pediatr Surg Int 2000; 16(1–2): 144–145.

Urabe A, Tsuneyoshi M, Enjoji M. Epithelioid hemangioma versus Kimura's disease. A Comparative clinicopathologic study. Am J Surg Pathol 1987; 11(10): 758–766.

Urahashi J, Hara H, Yamaguchi Z et al. Pigmented median raphe cysts of the penis. Acta Dermato–Venereologica 2000; 80(4): 297–298.

Usha V, Gopalakrishnan Nair TV. A comparative study of oral ivermectin and topical permethrin cream in the treatment of scabies. J Am Acad Dermatol 2001; 45(4): 637–638.

Uwyyed K, Korman SH, Bar–Oz B et al. Scrotal abscess with bacteremia caused by salmonella group D after ritual circumcision. Pediatr Infect Dis J 1990; 9(1): 65–66.

Uygur MC, Gulerkaya B, Altug U et al. 13 years' experience of penile fracture. Scand J Urol Nephrol 1997; 31(3): 265–266.

V

Valadez RA, Waters WB. Leiomyosarcoma of the penis. Urology 1986; 27(3): 265–267.

Val–Bernal JF, Azcarretazabal T, Garijo MF. Pilonidal sinus of the penis. A report of two cases, one of them associated with actinomycosis. J Cutan Pathol 1999; 26(3): 155–158.

Val–Bernal JF, Garijo MF. Pagetoid dyskeratosis of the prepuce. An incidental histologic finding resembling extramammary Paget's disease. J Cutan Pathol 2000; 27(8): 387–391.

Val–Bernal JF, Hernandez–Nieto E. Benign mucinous metaplasia of the penis. A lesion resembling extramammary Paget's disease. J Cutan Pathol 2000; 27(2): 76–79.

Valsecchi R, Cainelli T. Nonpigmenting fixed drug reaction to piroxicam. J Am Acad Dermatol 1989; 21(6): 1300.

van der Meer JB, de Jong MCJM. Recent aspects of pathogenesis and therapy of fulminant elapsing necrosis. Neth J Med. 1992; 40: 244–253.

van der Meer JB, van der Wal T, Bos WH et al. Fournier's gangrene: the human counterpart of the local Shwartzman phenomenon? Arch Dermatol 1990; 126: 1376–1377.

Van Ginkel CJ, Rundervoort GJ. Increasing incidence of contact allergy to the new preservative. 1,2–dibromo–2,4–dicyanobutane (methyldibromoglutaronitril. Br J Dermatol 1995; 132: 918–920.

Van Gulik TM, Jansen JW, Taat CW. Kimura's disease in the spermatic cord, an unusual site of a rare tumor. Neth J Surg 1986; 38(3): 93–95.

Van Howe RS. Variability in penile appearance and penile findings: a prospective study. Br J Urol 1997; 80(5): 776–782.

Van Howe RS. Does circumcision influence sexually transmitted diseases? A literature review. Br J Urol International 1999; 83(Suppl. 1): 52–62.

Van Howe RS, Svoboda JS, Dwyer JG et al. Involuntary circumcision: the legal issues. Br J Urol Int 1999; 83(Suppl. 1): 63–73.

van de Scheur MR, van der Waal RI, van der Waal I, et al. Ano-genital granulomatosis: the counterpart of oro-facial granulomatosis. J Eur Acad Dermatol Venereol. 2003; 17(2): 184–9.

van de Scheur MR, van der Waal RI, Volker-Dieben HJ, et al. Orofacial granulomatosis in a patient with Crohn's disease. J Am Acad Dermatol. 2003; 49(5): 952–4.

Vanheuverzwyn R, Delannoy A, Michaux JL, et al. Anal lesions in hematologic diseases. Dis Col Rectum. 1980; 23: 310–312.

Vapnek JM, Quivey JM, Carroll PR. Aquired immunodeficiency syndrome–related Kaposi's sarcoma of the male genitalia: management with radiation therapy. J Urol 1991; 146(2): 333–336.

Vassileva S, Pramatarov K, Popova L. Ultraviolet light induced confluent and reticulated papillomatosis. J Am Acad Dermatol 21 1989; 413–440.

Veien NK, Hattel T, Justesen O et al. Dermatoses in coffee drinkers. Cutis 1987; 40: 421–422.

Bibliography

Vélez A, Moreno JC. Febrile perianal streptococcal dermatitis. Pediatric Dermatology 1999; 16(1): 23–24.

Venkataramaiah NR, Reinaerta HHM, Van Roalte JE et al. Pseudomalignant cutaneous amoebiasis. Trop Doctor 1982; 12: 162–163.

Venn SN, Mundy AR. Urethroplasty for balanitis xerotica obliterans. Br J Urol 1998; 81(5): 735–737.

Verbov J. Pruritis ani and its management – a study and reappraisal Clin Exp Dermatol. 1984; 9: 46–52.

Veress B, Malik MAO. Idiopathic scrotal calcinosis. A report of six cases from the Sudan. East African Med J 1975; 52: 705–710.

Vermooten V. Metaplasia in the penis: the presence of bone, bone marrow and cartilage in the glans. N Engl J Med 1933; 209(8): 368–370.

Vesper JL, Messina J, Glass LF et al. Profound proliferating pearly penile papules. Int J Dermatol 1995; 34(6): 425–426.

Vickers D, Morris K, Coulthard MG et al. Anal signs in haemolytic uraemic syndrome. Lancet 1998; 1: 998.

Vieyra F, Luna–Perez P, Pena JP et al. [Associated clinical features in 41 patients with anal epidermoid carcinoma, studied at a cancer center]. [Article in Spanish.] Rev Gastroenterol Mex 1997; 62(2): 89–93.

Villa LL, Lopes A. Human papillomavirus DNA sequences in penile carcinomas in Brazil. Int J Cancer 1986; 37: 853–855.

de Villez RL, Stevens CS. Bowenoid papules of the genitalia. J Am Acad Dermatol 1980; 3: 149–152.

Voltz JM, Drobacheff C, Derancourt C et al. Papillomavirus–induced anogenital lesions in 121 HIV seropositive men. Clinical, histological, viral study, and evolution. Ann Derm Vener 1999; 126(5): 424–429.

von Happle R. Chirurgische Behandlung des Lichen sclerosus et atrophicus penis. Surgical treatment of penile lichen sclerosus et atrophicus. Dermatol Monatsschr 1973; 159: 975–977.

Voog E, Ricksten A, Olofsson S et al. Demonstration of Epstein–Barr virus DNA and human papillomavirus DNA in acetowhite lesions of the penile skin and the oral mucosa. Int J STD AIDS 1997; 8(12): 772–775.

Vordermark JS, Hudson LD. Behcet disease with genitourinary involvement treated with colchicine. Urology 1984; 23(3): 290–292.

Voron DA, Hatfield HH, Kalkhoff RK. Multiple lentignes syndrome. Am J Med 1976; 60: 447–456.

W

Wade TR, Kopf AW, Ackerman AB. Bowenoid papulosis of the genitalia. Arch Dermatol 1979; 115: 306–308.

Wahba A, Cohen HA. Herpes simplex virus isolation from pyoderma gangrenosum lesions in a patient with chronic lymphatic leukaemia. Dermatologica 1979; 158: 373–378.

Wakelin SH, White IR. Natural rubber latex allergy. Clin Exp Dermatol 1999; 24: 245–248.

Walboomers JMM, Meijer CJLM. Do HPV–negative cervical carcinomas exist? J Pathol 1997; 181: 253–254.

Walker GJA, Johnstone PW. Interventions for treating scabies (Cochrane Review). In: The Cochrane Library, Issue 2, Oxford: Update Software Ltd; 2002.

Walker RR. Chronic papular dermatitis of the scrotum due to Schistosoma mansoni. Arch Dermatol 1979; 115: 869–870.

Wallace HJ. Lichen sclerosus et atrophicus. Trans St John's Hospital Dermatol Soc 1969; 57(1): 9–30.

Wallace HJ. Lichen sclerosus et atrophicus. Trans St John's Hospital Dermatol Soc 1971; 57: 9–30.

Wallace HJ. Anderson–Fabry disease. Br J Dermatol 1973; 88: 1–23.

Walther PJ, Andriani RT, Maggio MI et al. Fournier's gangrene: A complication of penile prosthetic implantation in a renal transplantaion patient. J Urol 1987; 137: 299.

Wan SP, Soderdahl DW, Blight EM. Nonpsychotic genital self–mutilation. Urology 1985; 26(3): 286–287.

Ward CS, Dundas DD, Dow J et al. Scrotal swelling due to perianeurysmal fibrosis. Br J Urol 1988; 61: 536–538.

Warwick DJ, Dickson WA. Keloid of the penis after circumcision. Postgrad Med J 1993; 69(809): 236–237.

Wasadikar PP. Incarceration of the penis by a metallic ring. Postgrad Med J 1997; 73(858): 255.

Washecka RM, Sidhu G, Surya. Leiomyosarcoma of scrotum. Urology 1989; 34(3): 144–146.

Watanabe K, Ogawa A, Komatsu H et al. Malignant fibrous histiocytoma of the sacrotal wall: a case report. J Urol 1988; 140(1): 151–152.

Watanabe T, Murakami T, Okochi H et al. Ulcerative porokeratosis. Dermatology 1998; 196(2): 256–259.

Watt P, Parkinson R, Bogiatzis G et al. Enterobiasis in young Australian adults. Med J Austral 1991; 154(7): 496.

Waugh MA. Herpes zoster of the anogenital area affecting urination and defaecation. Br J Dermatol 1974; 90: 235.

Waugh MA. Balanitis. Dermatol Clin 1998; 16(4): 757–762. xii.

Weaver SM, Keelly AP. Herpes zoster as a cause of neurogenic bladder. Cutis 1982; 29: 611–612.

Weber P, Rabinovitz H, Garland L. Verrucous carcinoma in penile lichen sclerosus et atrophicus. J Dermatol Surg Oncol 1987; 13: 529.

Wei H, Friedman KA, Rudikoff D. Multiple indurated papules on penis and scrotum. J Cutan Med Surg 2000; 4(4): 202–204.

Weigand DA. Lichen sclerosus et atrophicus, multiple dysplastic keratoses, and squamous cell carcinoma of the glans penis. J Dermatol Surg Oncol 1980; 6: 45–50.

Weigand DA. Microscopic features of lichen sclerosus et atrophicus in acrochordons: a clue to the cause of lichen sclerosus et atrophicus? J Am Acad Dermatol 1993; 28(5 Pt 1): 751–754.

Weinberger GI, Wajsman Z, Beckley S et al. Primary sarcoma of penis. Urology 1982; 19(2): 193–194.

Weiss J, Elder D, Hamilton R. Melanoma of the male urethra: surgical approach and pathological analysis. J Urol 1982; 128: 382–385.

Weiss SW, Enzinger FM. Epithelioid hemangioendothelioma. A vascular tumor often mistaken for a carcinoma. Cancer 1982; 50: 970–981.

Wen LM, Estcourt CS, Simpson JM et al. Risk factors for the acquisition of genital warts: are condoms protective? Sex Trans Infect 1999; 75(5): 312–316.

Werdin R, Kupczyk–Joeris D, Schumpelick V. Malignant eccrine poroma. Case report of a rare tumour of the skin. Chirurg 1991; 62(4): 350–352.

Wesselmann U, Burnett AL, Heinberg LJ. The urogenital and rectal pain syndromes. Pain 1997; 73: 269–294.

Wessels H. Genital skin loss: unified reconstructive approach to a heterogeneous entity. World J of Urol 1999; 17(2): 107–114.

Wester RC, Maibach HI, Bucks DA et al. Malathion percutaneous absorption after repeated administration to man. Toxicol Appl Pharmacol 1983; 68(1): 116–119.

Whimster IW. The natural history of endogenous skin malignancy as a basis for experimental research. Trans St John's Hospital Dermatol Soc 1973; 59: 195–224.

White Jr JW, Olsen KD, Banks PM. Plasma cell orificial mucositis. Arch Dermatol 1986; 122: 1321–1324.

White SW, Smith J. Trichomycosis pubis. Arch Dermatol 1979; 115: 444–445.

White C, Sparks RA. Prepucial occlusion and circumcision after genital herpes infection. Int J STD AIDS. 1991; 2: 209–10.

White WB, Barrett S. Penile ulcer in heroin abuse: a case report. Cutis 1981; 29: 62–72.

Whitfield H. Circumcision. Br J Urol Int 1999; 83(Suppl. 1): 1–113.

Whitlock FA, ed. Psychophysiological aspects of skin disease. London: Saunders. 1976; 118–121.

Wieland U, Jurk S, Weissenborn S et al. Erythroplasia of Queyrat: coinfection with cutaneous carcinogenic human papillomavirus type 8 and genital papillomaviruses in a carcinoma in situ. J Invest Dermatol 2000; 115: 396–401.

Wigbels B, Luger T, Metze D. Imiquimod: a new treatment possibility in bowenoid papulosis? Hautarzt 2001; 52(2): 128–131. German.

Wijesinha SS, Atkins BL, Dudley NE et al. Does circumcision alter the periurethral bacterial flora? Pediatr Surg Int 1998; 13(2–3): 146–148.

Wikstrom A, Hedblad MA, Johansson B et al. The acetic acid test in evaluation of subclinical genital papillomavirus infection: a comparative study on penoscopy, histopathology, virology and scanning electron microscopy findings. Genitourin Med 1992; 68(2): 90–99.

Wikstrom A, Von Krogh G, Hedblad M–A et al. Papillomavirus–associated balanoposthitis. Genitourin Med 1994; 70: 175–181.

Wilde H, Canby JP. Penile venereal edema. Arch Dermatol 1973; 108: 263.

Wilkinson DS. Necrolytic migratory erythema with carcinoma of the pancreas. Trans St John's Hospital Dermatol Soc 1973; 59: 244.

Wilkinson DS, ed. The nursing and management of skin diseases, 4th edn. London: Faber; 1977.

Wilkinson JD, Hambly EM, Wilkinson DS. Comparison of patch test results in two adjacent areas in England. Acta Dermato–Venereologica 1980; 60: 245–249.

Wilkström A, Lindbrink P, Johansson B et al. Penile human papillomavirus carriage among men attending Swedish STD clinics. Int J STD AIDS 1991; 2(2): 105–109.

Wille S, Niesel T, Breul J et al. Elephantiasis of the legs with lichen sclerosus et atrophicus of the penis and scrotum. J Urol 1997; 157(6): 2262.

Williams JL, Crawford BH. A method for urethroplasty for urethral strictures. Br J Urol 1968; 40: 712–716.

Williams N, Kapila L. Complications of circumcision. Br J Surg 1993; 80(10): 1231–1236.

Willkens RF, Arnett FC, Bitter T et al. Reiter's syndrome. Arthritis and Rheumatism 1981; 24(6): 844–849.

Willsher MK, Daley KJ, Conway JF et al. Penile horns. J Urol 1984; 132: 1192–1193.

Wilson Jones E, Grice K. Rehculate pigmented anomaly of the flexures: Dowling Degos disease, a new genodermatosis. Arch Dermatol 1976; 114: 1150–1157.

Wilson LS, Lockhart JL, Bergman H et al. Fibrosarcoma of the penis: case report and review of the literature. J Urol 1983; 129: 606–607.

Wiltz OH, Torregrosa M, Wiltz O. Autogenous vaccine: The best therapy for perianal condyloma acuminata. Dis Col Rect 1995; 38(8): 838–841.

Winkelmann RK, Su WP. Pemphigoid vegetans. Arch Dermatol 1979; 115(4): 446–448.

Winkelstein W. Smoking and cancer of the uterine cervix: hypothesis. Am J Epidemiol 1977; 106: 257–259.

Winner HL, Hurley R, eds. Symposium on Candida Infections. Edinburgh: Livingstone; 1966.

Winter CC, Khanna R. Peyronie's disease: results with dermo–jet injection of dexamethasone. J Urol 1975; 114: 898–900.

Wiswell TE, Enzenauer RW, Cornish D et al. Declining frequency of circumcision: implications for the changes in the absolute incidence and male to female sex ratio of urinary tract infections in early infancy. Pediatr 1987; 79(3): 338–342.

Wiswell TE, Geschke DW. Risks from circumcision during the first month of life compared with those for uncircumcised boys. Pediatr 1989; 83(6): 1011–1015.

Wiswell T, Curtis J, Dobek AS et al. Staphylococcus aureus colonization after neonatal circumcision in relation to the device used. J Pediatr 1991; 119(2): 302–304.

Wolbarst AL. Circumcision and penile cancer. Lancet 1932; 1: 150–153.

Wolber RA, Dupuis BA, Wick MR. Expression of C–erb–2 oncoprotein in mammary and extramammary Paget's disease. Am J Clin Pathol 1991; 96: 243–247.

Wolf P, Kerl H. Artificial penile nodules and secondary syphilis. Genitourin Med 1991; 67(3): 247–249.

Wong E, Souteyrand P, MacDonald DM. Zoon's balanitis (balanitis circumscripta plasma cellularis) (abstr). Br J Dermatol 1981; 105(Suppl. 19): 28–29.

Wong TY, Milm Jr MC. Acantholytic dermatosis localized to genitalia and crural areas of male patients: A report of three cases. J Cutan Pathol 1994; 21(1): 27–32.

Woodrow JC, Graham DR, Evans CC. Behcets syndrome in HLA–identical siblings. Br J Rheumatol. 1990; 225–227.

Woodruff JD, Sussman J, Shakfeh S. Vulvitis circumscripta plasma cellularis. J Reprod Med 1989; 34: 369–372.

Worheide J, Bonsmann G, Kolde G et al. Plattenepithyelkarzinom auf dem Boden eines lichen ruber hypertrophicus an der glans penis. Der Hautarzt 1991; 42(2): 112–115.

Wortman PD. Infection with Penicillium marneffei. Int J Derm 1996; 35(6): 393–399.

Wright LF, Bicknell SL. Systemic necrotizing vasculitis presenting as epididymitis. J Urol 1994; 136: 1094.

Wright RA, Judson FN. Penile venereal edema. J Am Med Ass 1979; 241: 157–158.

Wright S, Navsaria H, Leigh IM. Idiopathic scrotal calcinosis is idiopathic. J Am Acad Dermatol 1991; 24(5 Pt.1): 727–730.

Wynne JM. Perineal amoebiasis. Arch Dis Child 1980; 55: 234–236.

Wynne JM, Hobbs CJ. Examination of children who may have been sexually abused. Arch Dis Child 2000; 82(3): 268.

X

Xavier Bosch F, Michele Manos M, Munoz N et al., International Biological Study on Cervical Cancer (IBSCC) Study Group. Prevalence of human papillomavirus in cervical cancer: a worldwide perspective. J Natl Cancer Inst 1995; 87: 796–802.

Xu X, Zhu W, Wu Y. Experience of the treatment of severe electric burns on special parts of the body. Ann N Y Acad Sci 1999; 888: 121–130.

Y

Yagi H, Igawa M, Shiina H et al. A study of growth pattern in giant condyloma acuminatum. Urologia Internationalis 1998; 61(3): 188–91.

Yamamoto S, Maeda H, Mori H, Shindo M, Fujinaga K. Flat wart of the urethra caused by human papillomavirus type 16 Urologica Internationalis. 1993; 51(2): 108–110.

Yanagihara M. Ano–sacral cutaneous amyloidosis. Japan J Dermatol 1981; 91(4): 463–471.

Yanagihara M, Fukishima N, Mori S. Anosacral amyloidosis. 16th Congress on Dermatology. Tokyo: Tokyo University Press. 1982; 922.

Yeager JK, Findlay RF, McAleer IM. Penile verrucous carcinoma. Arch Dermatol 1990; 126: 1208–1210.

Yildirim S, Akoz T, Akan M. A rare complication of circumcision: concealed penis. Plast Reconst Surg 2000; 106(7): 1662–1663.

Yoganathan S, Bohl TG, Mason G. Plasma cell balanitis and vulvitis (of Zoon). J Reprod Med 1994; 39: 939–944.

Yokokawa K, Nakano E, Takaha M. Accessory scrotum: a case report. J Urol 1986; 135: 593–594.

Yoneta A, Yamashita T, Jin HY et al. Development of squamous cell carcinoma by two high–risk human papillomaviruses (HPVs), a novel HPV–67 and HPV–31 from bowenoid papulosis. Br J Dermatol 2000; 143(3): 604–608.

Yoshida M, Kitamura S, Fujininaga T. Intrascrotal sclerosing lipogranuloma. A case report. Acta Urologica Japonica 1987; 33: 137.

Yuhan R, Orsay C, DelPino A et al. Anorectal disease in HIV–infected patients. Dis Colon Rectum 1998; 41: 1367–1370.

Yun K, Joblin L. Presence of human papillomavirus DNA condylomata acuminata in children and adolescents. Pathology 1993; 25(1): 1–3.

Bibliography

Z

Zabbo A, Stein B. Penile intraepithelial neoplasia in patients examined for exposure to human papilloma virus. Urology 1993; 41(1): 24–26.

Zachariae H, Larsen PM, Sogaard H. Recombinant interferon alpha–2A (Roferon–A) in a case of Buschke–Lowenstein giant condyloma. Dermatologica 1988; 177: 175–179.

Zalla JA, Perry HO. An unusual case of syringoma. Arch Dermatol 1971; 103: 215–217.

Zambolin T, Simeone C, Baronchelli C et al. Kaposi's sarcoma of the penis. Br J Urol 1989; 63(6): 645–646.

Zampogna JC, Flowers FP, Roth WI, Hassenein AM. Treatment of primary limited cutaneous extramammary Paget's disease with topical imiquimod monotherapy: two case reports. J Am Acad Dermatol. 2002; 47(4 Suppl): S229–35.

Zapolski–Downar A, Nowak A, Bielecka–Grzela S. Lichen sclerosus et atrophicus in a married couple. Dermatol Monatsschr 1987; 173(3): 141–145. German.

Zawahry ME. Cutaneous amoebiasis. Indian J Dermatol 1966; 11: 77–78.

Zax RH, Kulp–Shorten CL, Callen JP. Leukemia cutis presenting as a scrotal ulcer. J Am Acad Dermatol 1989; 21(2 Pt.2): 410–413.

Zbar AP, Fenger C, Efron J et al. The pathology and molecular biology of anal intraepithelial neoplasia: comparisons with cervical and vulvar intraepithelial carcinoma. Int J Colorectal Dis 2002; 17(4): 203–215.

Zderkiewicz B. Lichen sclerosus et atrophicus hemorrhagicus treated by a new method. Przegl Dermatol 1972; 59(1): 55–59. Polish.

Zeinberg VH, Kays S. Anorectal carcinomas of extramucosal origin. Ann Surg 1957; 145: 344–354.

Zhu W–Y, Leonardi C, Penney NS. Polymerase chain reaction in detection of human papillomavirus DNA and types of condyloma acuminata. Chinese Med J 1993; 106(2): 141–144.

Zimbelman J, Lefkowitz J, Schaeffer C et al. Unusual complications of warfarin therapy: skin necrosis and priapism. J Pediatr 2000; 137(2): 266–268.

Zochow KR, Ostrow RS, Bender M et al. Detection of human papillomavirus DNA in anogenital neoplasias. Nature 1982; 300: 771–773.

Zoon JJ. Verenigingsverslagen. Nederl Tijdschr. Geneesk 1950; 94(2): 1528–1530.

Zoon JJ. Balanoposthite chronique cironscrite benigne a plasmocytes. Dermatologica 1952; 105(1): 1–7.

Zouboulis CC, Keitel W. A historical review of early descriptions of Adamantiades–Behçet's disease. J Invest Dermatol 119. 2002; 201–205.

Zufall R. Lymphangiectasis of the penis. Urology 1982; 19(1): 53–54.

zur Hausen H. Genital papillomavirus infections. Prog Med Virol 1985; 32: 15–21.

Index

Page numbers in **bold** refer to figures; page numbers in *italics* refer to tables.

Index

Page numbers in **bold** refer to figures; page numbers in *italics* refer to tables.

Page numbers in **bold** refer to figures; page numbers in *italics* refer to tables.

Index

Page numbers in **bold** refer to figures; page numbers in *italics* refer to tables.

Page numbers in **bold** refer to figures; page numbers in *italics* refer to tables.

Index

Page numbers in **bold** refer to figures; page numbers in *italics* refer to tables.

Page numbers in **bold** refer to figures; page numbers in *italics* refer to tables.

Index

Page numbers in **bold** refer to figures; page numbers in *italics* refer to tables.

278

Page numbers in **bold** refer to figures; page numbers in *italics* refer to tables.

Index

Page numbers in **bold** refer to figures; page numbers in *italics* refer to tables.

Page numbers in **bold** refer to figures; page numbers in *italics* refer to tables.

Index

Page numbers in **bold** refer to figures; page numbers in *italics* refer to tables.

Page numbers in **bold** refer to figures; page numbers in *italics* refer to tables.

Index

Page numbers in **bold** refer to figures; page numbers in *italics* refer to tables.

Page numbers in **bold** refer to figures; page numbers in *italics* refer to tables.